Livestock Health and Housing

Livestock Health and Housing

Third Edition

DAVID SAINSBURY MA PhD BSc MRCVS

Lecturer in Animal Health, University of Cambridge; Member, Joint FMC and NFU Development Trust; Unit for Study of Intensive Livestock Production

PETER SAINSBURY NDDH Diploma in Dairying (University of Reading)

Baillière Tindall

This book is printed on acid-free paper.

Baillière Tindall 24–28 Oval Road
W.B. Saunders London NW1 7DX, England

The Curtis Center
Independence Square West
Philadelphia, PA 19106–3399, USA

55 Horner Avenue
Toronto, Ontario M8Z 4X6, Canada

Harcourt Brace Jovanovich (Australia) Pty Ltd,
30–52 Smidmore St
Marrickville, NSW 2204, Australia

Harcourt Brace Jovanovich Japan Inc.
Ichibancho Central Building, 22–1 Ichibancho
Chiyoda-ku, Tokyo 102, Japan

First published as *Animal Health and Housing* 1967

Second Edition 1979
Third Edition 1988

A CIP record for this book is available from the British Library

ISBN 0–7020–1161–4

Typeset by Profile Ltd, Salisbury, Wilts
Printed in Great Britain at the Alden Press, Oxford

Contents

Preface to Third Edition

The preface to the first edition stated the aim of *Livestock Health and Housing* is to assist all those who are concerned with the 'housing of farm animals and who are determined they are provided with the best possible environmental conditions'. This aim remains unchanged in this fully revised version of the book. Although the subject has almost no professional barriers as it involves the farmer, animal husbandry specialist, architect, surveyor, engineer and veterinarian, the book is particularly addressed to students in agricultural colleges and veterinary schools.

The subject is dynamic and changing, but whatever the degree of intensification, environmental conditions must be controlled with great care and standards of hygiene and housing raised to the highest levels if good health and productivity are to be achieved. The growth and well-being of all livestock are effected by three principal factors: their genetic constitutions, their nutrition and the climatic environment. In addition, the health status of the animals is of profound importance. Knowledge of the fundamental environmental requirements have improved the understanding of the practical requirements of the housed animal and these advances have been incorporated in the text. But perhaps the most interesting feature of the last few years has been the signs of certain fundamental changes in livestock husbandary. Up to about ten years ago, it had been moving really in only one direction – ever greater intensivism. Now it is very nearly taking a 'U-turn' away from this, searching for less intensive and more agriculturally balanced and natural systems of management.

There are several reasons for this. In many countries of the world there is over-production of animal products and intensive methods tend to be the most expensive in capital investment and the least flexible in adapting themselves to changing circumstances. There have also been a rising number of low-grade infections with intensive systems which can be eliminated by using alternative methods. Pressure from the welfarists has also had its effect in persuading an increasing number of farmers to seek more natural methods of housing with less restriction on the movement of the stock.

There is also a view becoming prevalent that large isolated intensive units having no connection with the surrounding land are something of an anachronism. The fodder and bedding for the stock may have to be imported from far afield and the manure may be wasted or may be a heavy liability. It is far more sensible, argue many farmers and economists, to keep livestock in smaller units in harmony with the land around them, so that a high proportion of the fodder is produced locally and the dung can be economically utilised on the surrounding fields. The smaller units can produce a healthier herd or flock and the more natural methods tend to be preferred by the stockman. Housing and general capital input may be less and the buildings can be of a less specialised nature. It is potentially very useful if a building can be turned over to different types of livestock as market requirements vary.

In many respects what the farmer is looking for is a more relaxed method of keeping his animals and the public wants to be assured that animals are kept in a humane and healthy way. There is also a growing demand for less total reliance on drugs and vaccines to maintain health, turning more to the fundamentals of good hygiene, housing and management. All these factors taken together have had a profound effect on housing and it is hoped they are adequately reflected in the new emphasis in this edition, though indeed these always have been the major criteria of *Livestock Health and Housing*.

In preparing the new edition, we would particularly like to acknowledge the frank appraisal of the text made by colleagues in agricultural colleges. Their valuable comments will go far to ensure that this text is a practical and useful source of guidance to agricultural students.

David Sainsbury
Peter Sainsbury

Preface to First Edition

The aim of this book is to break new ground and present a new and positive approach to the interrelated fields of the environment, health and housing of livestock. There is no other text in this field, but no doubt this is because so many of the innovations in animal husbandry connected with these subjects have been made comparatively recently.

As a veterinarian, my approach is obviously weighted in favour of the welfare of the animals and I have given particular attention to the housing of livestock, and ventilation and thermal insulation of buildings, as good practice in these matters is the basis of satisfactory intensive management. Housing systems are reviewed in some detail to try to place them in perspective, emphasizing their limitations from the livestock and hygienic points of view.

I have been fortunate enough to have the collaboration of my brother who is an agriculturist with special interest in cattle and dairy hygiene. We have given particular consideration to dairy and building hygiene and disinfection, and to the need for pure and wholesome water. Details are also given of the very important part which the state veterinary services have played in the development of a practical and scientific approach to animal husbandary in the United Kingdom. It is hoped that this book will help not only the student of agriculture in his veterinary science or animal hygiene course and the student of veterinary medicine in his animal husbandry and veterinary hygiene courses, but also farmers, advisers and others concerned in a practical manner with this dynamic field.

Acknowledgements

There must be few authors more indebted than ourselves to many individuals and organisations for the generous help given in the preparation of a text book. First, we must express our gratitude to the Farm Electric Centre of the Electricity Council currently under the direction of Dr Dan Mitchell and formerly directed by Mr Peter Wakeford, for a great deal of assistance given over many years. Reference is made to the material they have allowed us to reproduce in the list at the end of this section and within the text.

We have also been permitted to reproduce a number of drawings and other material from various publications of the Ministry of Agriculture, Fisheries and Food and the Scottish Farm Buildings Investigation Unit. Associated with these latter bodies it is a pleasure to acknowledge the great contributions made to the whole field of livestock housing by Mr David Soutar OBE, Mr Jan Cernak, Dr James Bruce, Dr David Charles, Dr Mandy Hill, Mr Arnold Elson, Mr Seaton Baxter and Dr Mike Baxter. Material from the expert and wise pen of Professor John Webster of Bristol University's Veterinary School is quoted in the text and deserves especial thanks in connection with the environmental requirements of ruminants.

Finally we thank Miss Margaret McKeen, who typed the script and corrected many a fault and, from the publishers, we shall always be grateful for the help of Mr Aidan Reynolds and Miss Lynne Baxter.

The full list of acknowledgements:

Professor A J F Webster	Table 3.2
Maywick (Hanningfield) Ltd	Figs 3.7 and 3.8
Farm Buildings Information Centre	Figs 5.13–5.17
Ministry of Agriculture, Fisheries and Food	Figs 5.35, 10.5, 10.6, 10.7–10.10, 10.15–10.17
Turbair Ltd	Fig. 6.4
Antec International Ltd	Figs 6.6–6.8
Ambic Dairy Equipment Ltd	Fig. 7.1
The Council of the Scottish Agricultural Colleges	Figs 7.2–7.10
Milk Marketing Board	Fig. 7.4(b)
Loheat Ltd	Figs 7.5, 7.6
West of Scotland Agricultural College	Figs 10.21, 10.22
Dr Dan Mitchell	Figs 11.5, 11.8
Mr D S Soutar	Figs 13.5, 13.7, 13.15, 14.2–14.4

1

The Animal's Requirements

In recent years livestock units, and the buildings within them, have tended to increase in size and complexity. It is not uncommon nowadays to have many hundreds of cattle in one building and as many as 10,000 pigs or 100,000 or more poultry on one site. The momentum of the change has been so great that it has presented the veterinarian and animal husbandman with problems that have often outstripped his knowledge. The disease pattern too has changed radically. Instead of acute, specific, diagnosable and preventable or treatable diseases which can be controlled using vaccines, sera or antibiotics, there has been a trend towards chronic, insidious and complex groups of diseases caused by organisms which are often normal inhabitants of the animal body but which circumstances allow to become pathogenic. These disease conditions are difficult to diagnose, have a large and confusing number of causal agents, create a massive morbidity and financial loss, and require for their control great expertise in the exercise of husbandry, housing and management skills rather than recourse to the routine use of vaccines or drugs. The challenge they present is one of the most stimulating ever found in the long history of livestock production, not least because the search for new solutions demands the cooperation of agriculturists, architects, engineers and veterinarians. In dealing with health in the modern livestock unit it is essential to ensure that the unit is planned on the right lines from the outset. 'Putting out the fire' after it has started may often be impossible without closing down the unit and redesigning or rebuilding it.

In planning a livestock building or conversion, the physiological and health requirements of the livestock should undoubtedly be given absolute priority together with the basic needs of the stockman. It is only then, after satisfying these biological needs, as we may term them, that the questions of labour economy and such aids as easy or automatic methods of feeding, muck disposal and the handling of the animals should be considered. Therefore, the first chapters in this book are concerned with environmental needs because it is primarily to meet these that the buildings should be planned. This does not mean that there need be a conflict between the various essentials: good design brings all the requirements together harmoniously.

When a livestock building is being designed, consideration must always be given to what will happen if an infectious disease breaks out. In recent years large buildings, or groups of buildings, in restricted areas have been favoured. An outbreak of disease can lead to the closing down of such a unit because the infection passes with great ease to all the other stock. In these circumstances infections can only be arrested by evacuating the whole site of livestock – a tremendously expensive procedure.

LIMITATIONS ON UNIT SIZE

The reader will find in the following pages that the most successful building designs attempt to limit the number of animals kept in close contact; the graph (Fig. 1.1) shows data on this aspect collected by one of the authors at Cambridge.[1] In a survey there was found to be a variation in the finishing weight of broilers varying from 2.1 kg in groups of 20 to 1.4 kg in groups of 30 000 and an almost pro-rata relationship with groups of between 50, 100, 500 and 10 000. These differences occurred with birds from the same genetic background, eating similar food and without any obvious disease. Emmans[2] showed a similar trend, viz. broilers grown in a location size of between a modest 595 m^2 and 738 m^2 gave the best performance. For each doubling of the size beyond this range, weight decreased by 0.09 kg. This decline is almost certainly partly due to the increased disease incidence and with such accurate figures available to the agricultural industry, good use should be made of them in planning new units.

Similar figures have been given for laying birds; that is, above a certain size productivity declines. Yet generally, this knowledge is only heeded by a few farmers and designers and over-large livestock units and buildings are a cause of great problems and enormous economic loss.

It is pertinent to point out, however, that from the point of view of health it is the young, immature animal which is at greater risk from disease and

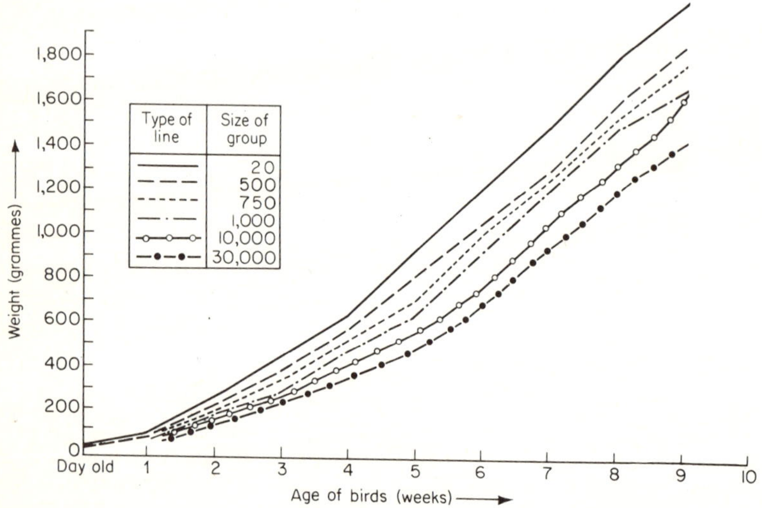

Fig. 1.1 Average weights of various size groups of broilers.

mismanagement. Therefore, while the unit size for the young animal should be limited to a reasonably low level, it can be very much higher for the adult. The main reason for this, apart from the extra vulnerability of the young animal to stress caused by bad management, is the differing immunity to disease among the stock. This is unavoidable on a large unit housing animals of different ages and from different sources of origin (see Fig. 1.2). The adult presents a more stable picture in both respects, being a little more resistant to management changes or errors and very much more uniform in its disease resistance or susceptibility.

The economy of small units

Thus we can say that from the point of view of health, the smaller the better. But what is meant by 'small' may vary enormously, depending on the expertise of the organization and the age of animal and type of species. Britton and Berkeley Hill[3,4] have expressed this in helpfully precise terms: '... as a goal increasing the efficiency of British farming has much to commend it in times when we are looking for ways of counteracting rising food prices and improving our balance of payments. On the other hand, the soulless pursuit of efficiency is often blamed for producing changes in the appearance of the countryside and in the rural population which, when a broad view is taken, offset and maybe even negate any gains from the more productive use of national resources. It is also often assumed that the bigger the farm the more efficient it is, so that if

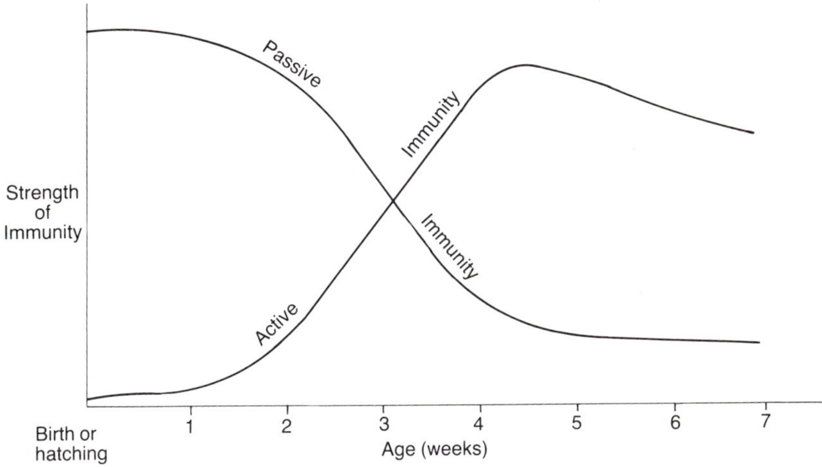

Fig. 1.2 The curves in the diagram represent antibody levels (i.e. immunity) produced by active or passive immunization. Animals or birds derive passive immunity from their dams but it is short-lived. Active immunity comes from vaccines but takes time to develop, or it may be derived from the animal contracting the disease. The latter is usually to be avoided unless it is a very mild infection or a very mild challenge. Note particularly the vulnerability of animals to infection during the first few weeks of life.

farming is to become even more efficient, small and medium-sized farms will be gradually extinguished and we will be left eventually with only superefficient but impersonal mega-agribusinesses. Fortunately this is far from the truth.'

The publications cited show that it is a misconception that efficient production is confined to large farms. Evidence collected strongly suggests that when farm performance is measured by the ratio of the market value of output to the cost of inputs (land, rent, labour and machinery costs, fertilizers, feedingstuffs, etc.) *very* small farms as a group are generally less efficient, but once the three-man unit has been reached, further improvements in performance are small or non-existent. These are only generalizations. Some small farms are as efficient as some larger ones and at all sizes there are instances of high and low efficiency. However there does appear to be a threshold somewhere between the two- and three-man unit below which resources are often less effectively used. This pattern applies to each of the main types of farming, although technological progress has steadily increased the physical size of farms corresponding to this threshold level of labour requirement.

Piecing together the evidence from the economist, the animal husbandman and the veterinarian, the following are suggested as a guide to the maximum number of livestock that should be held on one site:

Dairy cows	200
Beef cattle	1 000
Breeding pigs	500
Fattening pigs	3 000
Sheep	1 000
Commercial laying poultry	70 000
Breeding poultry	12 000
Broiler chickens	200 000

A further question arises as to how far apart sites should be built to ensure a reasonable measure of isolation. This is very difficult to answer, because whereas in the case of mildly contagious conditions a physical separation of a few hundred metres would be quite sufficient, in other cases, such as highly contagious respiratory infections (e.g. Newcastle disease in chickens, or enzootic pneumonia in pigs) there is evidence of air-borne transfer of infection from large conglomerations of at least 30 km.[5] Therefore, in practical terms, the greater the distance the better, especially with large animal populations.

ESSENTIAL CRITERIA FOR GOOD HEALTH

Before discussing the more detailed aspects of the animal's requirements, there are certain fundamentals of intensive husbandry to consider that have a profound effect on the overall design of units and the health of the livestock within them. Apart from the unit size, which has already been discussed, the following points are critical.

Depopulation

So far as possible the practice of periodically depopulating a building or preferably even a whole site should be followed. The benefits of removing the animal hosts to disease-causing agents are well understood and the benefit of being able to clean, disinfect and fumigate a building is also accepted. Nevertheless, in practice, the 'all-in, all-out' policy is more complex than these sentences would indicate. For example, it is particularly important to consider this in the young animal but far less so in the older beast which will have achieved an immunity to many of the local diseases. Much also depends on whether the herd or flock is a 'closed' one with few or no incoming animals, or an 'open' one with a constant renewal of the animal population. If the latter is the case, then the depopulation principle is much more important, as there is little or no opportunity for natural immunity to develop.

Health status

Policy will also be determined by the health status of the animals. At one extreme there is the commercial 'minimal disease' or 'specific pathogen-free' herd which has substantial known freedom from disease. Here depopulation is not such a critical feature as is the maintenance of the complete isolation of the animals from outside infections. Because in most localities this possibility is very serious, it is important to subdivide the unit into smaller groups, so reducing the likelihood of a breakdown and/or enabling isolation and elimination of a sub-group which becomes infected. At the other extreme are those units which receive all their animals from outside and constantly run the risk – usually a near certainty – of introducing animals which are either clinically infected with, or carriers of, disease. Basic design specifications for such units need to be quite different from those for the closed herd. Between the two extremes is the more common arrangement of having a herd or flock which is of a reasonable health status, though certainly not free of some of the most common diseases, and in which only occasionally are new livestock added. In such cases the precautions employed in housing against disease build-up and spread can be relaxed somewhat, but there should still be proper provision for the isolation of incoming and sick animals.

Group size

One of the most important ways of putting the housing on a sound footing is to keep the animals in groups of *minimal* size. At first sight this seems quite an old-fashioned or even a reactionary approach that may counteract all those advantages from automation that large units offer, but this certainly need not be the case. If groups are small it is possible easily to match the animals in them for size, weight and age, and it is well established that it is under these circumstances that fighting and bullying are kept to a minimum – indeed we might prevent it altogether.

Fighting among animals seems to be a highly contagious activity and under conditions of the most intensive management an almost casual accident that draws some blood can escalate into a 'blood-bath'. Pens which keep the animals in small groups will tend to reduce the occurrence of such disasters and with good management, the removal of an animal that has accidentally injured itself or is off-colour and therefore prone to being bullied will stop the trouble before it ever has a chance to erupt.

There is another very important advantage to keeping animals in small groups. It is obviously good practice for a farmer to keep his livestock near the level that has been shown to be the densest possible for optimal productivity. For example, it is known that a broiler chicken will grow to its maximum potential at a stocking rate of about 15 birds/m^2.

If birds are kept in a house to allow this density it is essential that they spread across the house uniformly, so they do in practice occupy and use the whole area. Regrettably this is very rarely the case and especially so when large numbers are housed together without any sub-division at all. The birds crowd in certain parts of the building, which can lead to grossly over-stocked floor areas. This is bad enough in itself but it has further unfortunate side-effects which may be seen also in beef animals and dairy cows, as well as in pigs and sheep. If they crowd excessively in one part of the house, this part may become polluted with dung and exhalations to an abnormal and harmful degree; the humidity becomes high, adequate air movement is impeded and the animals may soon become sick. Sick animals feeling cold tend to huddle together all the more, so the vicious circle is perpetuated and there is seemingly no end to it unless measures are taken to ensure a better distribution of the stock. When this problem arises, it is often impossible to divide up the animals at once. A move in the right direction – that is, encouraging the animals to spread themselves more uniformly over the house – can often be achieved by heating the building by introducing some artificial heat. There are excellent portable gas radiant heaters and oil-fired and electric blower heaters which will fulfil all those requirements if there is no permanent system available.

When animals are kept together in large numbers, the effects of a fright caused by an unusual disturbance can be extremely serious. It is almost impossible to guard against all the extraneous sounds and sights that may adversely affect the stock. The best safeguard, therefore, once all that can be anticipated has been done, is once again to have the animals in small groups so that the effect of a panic movement will be limited and will never escalate to highly dangerous proportions.

BASIC HOUSING TYPES

There are three contrasting types of housing: 'climatic', giving only a cover and protection to the animals; 'controlled environment', which regulates the microclimate as much as is required for the particular stock being housed; and the 'kennel', which is, in a sense, half-way between the first two types and gives two environments in the one building allowing some free and appropriate choice for the animals. The ways of using each of the types, and their suitability for different countries, climatic regions and forms of livestock, vary enormously and must be carefully defined. In our experience some of the greatest errors in livestock housing are made by their incorrect application and it is vital to specify these essential needs and differences. A summary of these may be given as follows:

Climatic housing

The climatic house is most suited to the adult beast which has developed a large measure of adaptability to climatic stress (Fig. 1.3). The house will be cheap because it is basically a cover only, but because the climate cannot be controlled the animals will need a relatively much greater area, especially as there is no powered ventilation: typically, stocking densities will need to be half or less than those in the controlled environment house. A major problem is created by agriculturists when they attempt to apply the highest stocking rates suitable for the controlled environment house to the climatic house, as the building is unable to cope with the demands of the stock. Poor productivity and high disease incidence can result. It is usually the right choice for cattle over about six months, for sheep of all ages, for adult pigs which are bedded, and occasionally for poultry. Climatic housing often requires deep bedding for its success in cooler climatic areas.

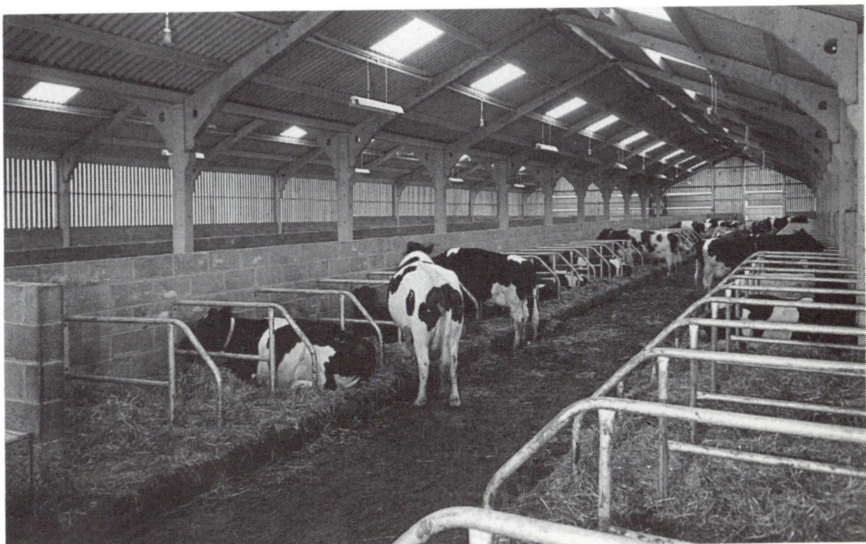

Fig. 1.3 The climatic house.

The controlled environment house

The controlled environment house is quite different. Whilst it can be used for all animals, it is especially appropriate for the young animal, the fattening pig or chicken, animals kept on a bare floor without bedding, and livestock, requiring light control. It is also most economically viable with animals which are fed largely concentrate food rather than substantial quantities of roughage, since the former is too expensive to be utilized as a form of energy (Fig. 1.4). The housing is expensive, sometimes extremely so in areas of climatic stress and where cooling devices are required. For this reason it is usually necessary to stock the buildings as densely as possible to make them economically viable, and this can place a great toll on health control. Management to cope with their special requirements needs to be highly sophisticated and unless these criteria can be observed this is frequently the wrong type of housing to choose. The rewards can be great but the dangers are greater.

Kennel accommodation

This is an increasingly popular system of accommodation which is half-way between the climatic and controlled environment housing, and attempts to combine the virtues of both at low cost, often successfully (Fig. 1.5). The essence of the system is that it keeps the animals in pens or groups which are sufficiently small to allow them to be closely confined, at least while resting, without too great a danger from respiratory or other disease. The close confinement makes it possible to keep the groups warm and draught-free generally by utilizing their

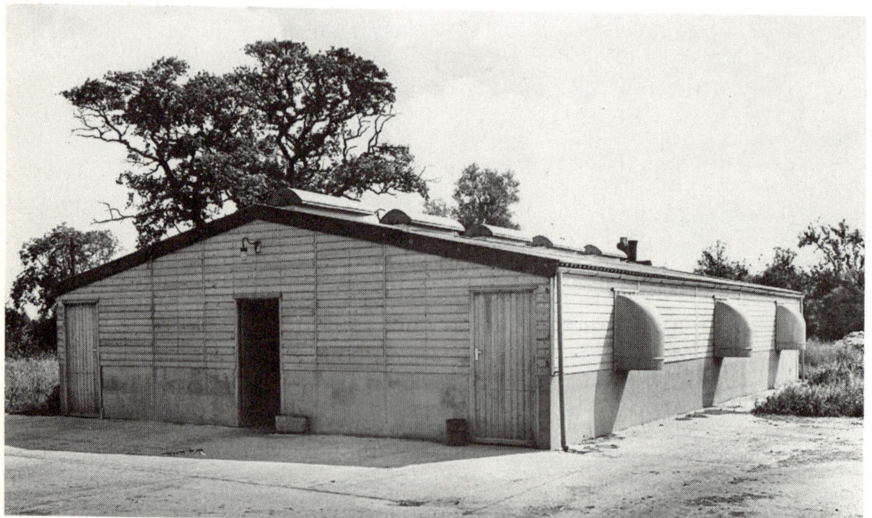

Fig. 1.4 The controlled environment house.

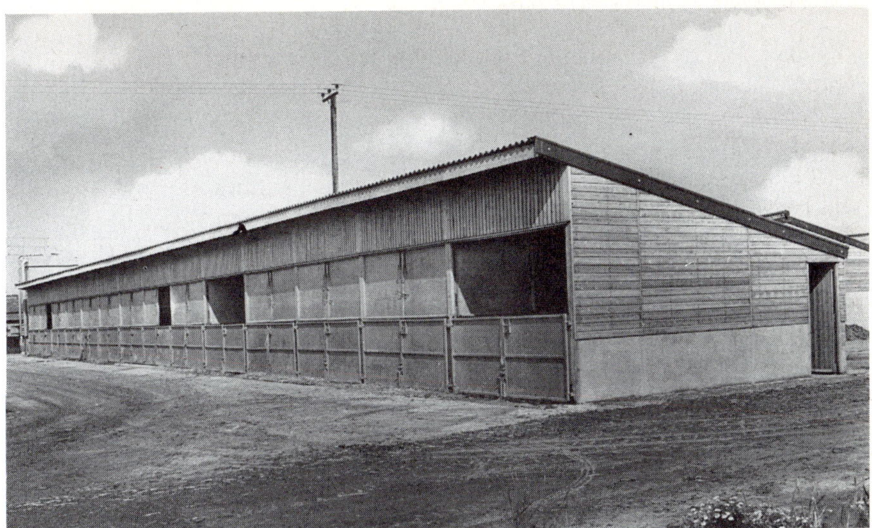

Fig. 1.5 The kennel house.

own body heat and by good insulation of the kennel and a limited cubic air space. This part of the accommodation is roughly a controlled environment house; the rest is the climatic house and can be justified as this is an area where the animals will be moving about freely and will not normally be inactive or lying down. It is likely to contain the dung and often the feeding and watering arrangements too and so must be very well ventilated, usually non-mechanically. In harsh climatic areas it is covered; in milder regions this is unnecessary and the 'yard' can, with benefit to health and productivity, be left uncovered. (See Fig. 1.6.)

It is instructive to look in some detail at the logic of the 'kennel' system.

The cost of the housing can be as low as any, especially with uncovered yarding, and such buildings are also the easiest type for the farmer himself to erect.

Good health is promoted by separating the animals into small groups. The separation of the kennels one from another should be as absolute as possible, as this will limit the build-up and spread of respiratory disease. It will also greatly promote the health of the animals if the muck is not in the warmer or closely confined resting area, a virtue which is easiest to fulfil with the naturally clean pig but is certainly achievable in part with other livestock. It is often possible as well by good design to keep the dunging areas separate so that the muck from different pens is not mixed until after it is out of reach of the animals.

The cheapness of the housing is largely due to the fact that we are controlling the environment only where it is absolutely necessary. It is a definite benefit if the dung can be in an area where the air is moving more freely and the temperature and the humidity possibly much lower – at least in temperate climates. Controlled environment housing is becoming more and more expensive

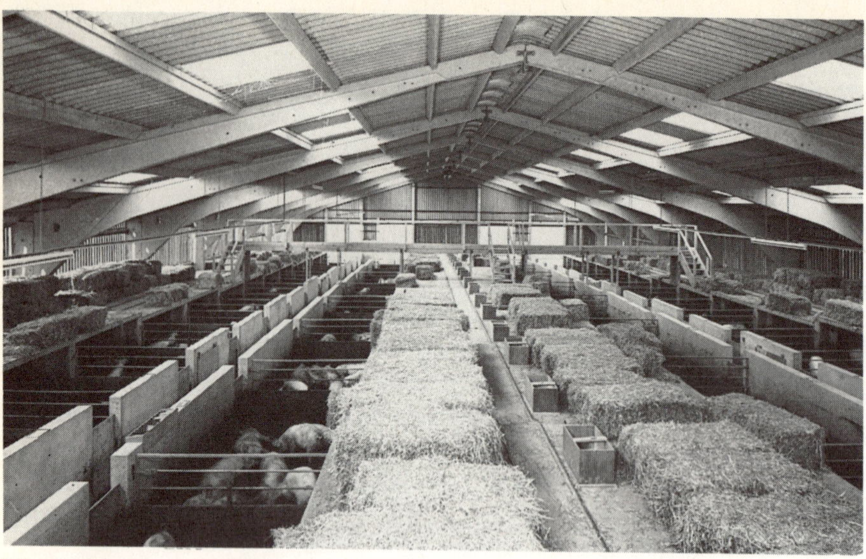

Fig. 1.6 Warmth in kennel housing is readily obtained by using bales of straw on the roof as a temporary measure. The straw can later be used as bedding.

and there is no possible justification for this control to embrace the excreta from the animals, which is not only a considerable expense but also is likely to intensify the disease risk.

THE DISEASE COMPLEX

There are two major groups of diseases that concern us in animal housing design – respiratory and enteric. The problem of disease is also much greater during the rearing stages than in adulthood, as explained earlier in this chapter.

The respiratory complex is probably the worse. Most animals are infected by groups of respiratory viruses, bacteria, mycoplasma and parasites, so that it is almost impossible to look for complete or even any protection by vaccines or hyperimmune antisera. In any case a healthy animal which does not require a vaccine is virtually certain to be more profitable than a vaccinated or challenged one. The design of the accommodation therefore plays a major part in enabling the stock to be reared free from the risks of major outbreaks of respiratory disease.

The second group is the enteric one which is taken to cover all those diseases which are spread primarily by close contact between animals and between animals and their excreta. The isolation principle, which is important with respiratory diseases, helps equally with enteric disorders, but additional measures are needed in the latter to decrease the risk further. Direct contact between animals should be reduced to a minimum, and systems of dung disposal are critical to remove the enormous risk of animals having close contact with dung.

Many modern designs err gravely and fundamentally in neglecting this and consequently there has been an upsurge in non-specific and complex enteric ailments. A number of the newest housing systems increase risks by:

1 Having too close a confinement of the animals.
2 Placing too many animals in one common air space.
3 Reducing both cubic and floor space.
4 Failing to remove muck from the close proximity of the animals.
5 Transferring muck through pens, aiding the transfer of disease.
6 Failing to separate age groups.
7 Neglecting clean feeding and water arrangements.
8 Having poor, or sometimes no drainage.
9 Neglecting the comfort of the stock.

SITING OF THE BUILDING

The siting of livestock buildings is an important factor to consider, whether they are intensively controlled environment houses or those built on more open lines – either climatic or kennel types. The general location of the farm and the climatic region in which it is situated affect several structural details. For example, more ventilation is needed in the south of the U.K. than in the north, and insulation and ventilation *control* must be of a higher standard in the east than in the west. Many farmers will confirm that it is rash to copy buildings from different areas or situations without attention to these details.

Animal accommodation is best built in an open, well-drained site, with a southerly aspect. A moderate slope will not only help drainage but also facilitate the construction of loading bays for the animals' food and dung.

On particularly exposed sites attention should be given to the use of existing trees as windbreaks, or to the planting of quick-growing trees if none is present. Special care must be taken with ventilation both on exposed sites, where special baffling devices will be needed to reduce air flow, and on sheltered sites, where mechanical ventilation is often necessary (see Chapter 5). Dutch barns, implement sheds and stores situated on the north side of the livestock housing give useful protection on exposed sites.

The positioning of the various buildings will depend to a great extent on the need to reduce movement to a minimum and to allow for mechanical handling of food and litter between and within the buildings. A large variety of reliable forms of mechanical handling are available together with bulk storage of food. Every care has to be taken, however, to ensure that attention to mechanization of movement does not result in the livestock buildings being so close together that the risk of disease transfer is greatly increased, or good free ventilation is impaired. A sound rule-of-thumb with naturally ventilated houses is to allow a distance between buildings at least equal to the width of each building.

REFERENCES

1 Sainsbury, D. W. B. (1966) Controlled environment poultry housing. *Proc. 13th World Poultry Congress, Kiev, USSR*. pp. 474–9.
2 Emmans, C. G. (1969) Factors associated with body weights in broiler flocks. *Poultry Rev. VIII*, 63–9.
3 Britton, D. K. and Hill, B. (1975) *Size and Efficiency in Farming*. Farnborough: Saxon House Studies.
4 Britton, D. K. and Hill, B. (1975) Farming, why being big isn't always the best. *The Times*, 17 July.
5 Smith, C. V. (1963) *Agricultural Memo. LX*, Bracknell, UK: Meteorological Office.

2

Construction of Livestock Buildings

Livestock buildings are such highly specialized structures that relatively few designs are adaptable for other purposes. This represents a departure from the generally held view of two or three decades ago that animals could be satisfactorily housed in unspecialized accommodation. Attempts to compromise in this way almost invariably mean that the animals suffer, although there are exceptions, particularly in those buildings where the environment needs a minimum of control – for example, in climatic buildings such as sow and cow yards, and kennel forms of accommodation in general.

APPEARANCE

There are housing types available to satisfy almost every demand of the various farming systems found in the U.K. Although in some respects this helps the farmer, it can paradoxically be a drawback in that inappropriate housing can so easily be chosen. Many designs which are functionally satisfactory are spoiled by poor appearance, general untidiness of the surrounds and inadequate maintenance (Figs. 2.1 and 2.2). Much can be done to blend new buildings into the landscape and to harmonize the new with the old. The choice of materials in prefabricated buildings is to a certain extent fixed but most manufacturers give careful attention to the coordination of the various components.

There are three basic rules to consider in planning a farm enterprise:

1. Contrast the colour and texture between walls and roof with firm eaves, shadow line; generally reduce the dominance of the roof area.
2. Integrate all projections, such as fan chambers, with the main building or make them act as a foil.
3. Make sure that services, electrical supply, fences, concrete perimeters, slurry tanks, and so on are kept neat.

Overriding all design problems is the need for attention to detail and the removal of junk. A pleasing appearance gives beneficial bonuses even to the point of improving productivity and health, because attractive, cleanly finished

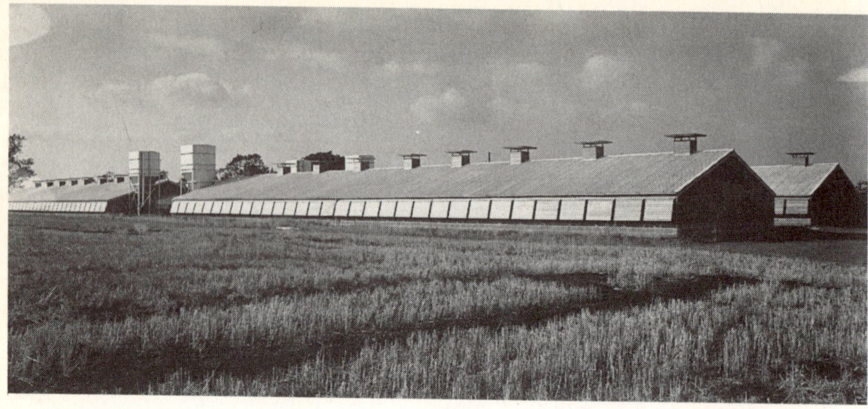

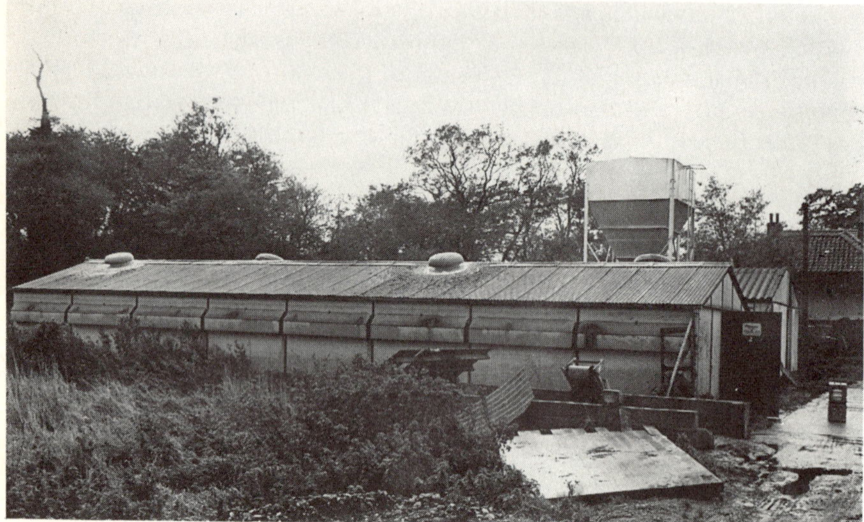

Fig. 2.2 Untidy farm buildings.

and tidy housing and surrounds gives the stockman a genuine pride in his job and helps him maintain hygiene to the highest possible standard.

THERMAL INSULATION

The cornerstone in the construction of a controlled environment house is a high standard of thermal insulation of all the surfaces round the animal: the floor, walls, roof, windows and doors. A good starting point when fully considering the subject is to determine where most of the heat is lost from an animal building so that thermal insulation can be applied in the most cost-efficient and appropriate manner.

Taking as an example a totally covered, uninsulated pig house, the loss of heat from each part is shown in Fig. 2.3, including the heat loss by ventilation, which is shown as a percentage of the total heat loss. Note that it is the roof which loses most heat; indeed this loss, together with that through ventilation, accounts for 80 per cent of the total, However, this does not include heat loss by *conduction* from the animal to any surface with which it has contact, which is considered separately later.

Figure 2.4 shows the vast improvement which results if good insulation principles are applied. This figure shows the heat loss through the surfaces in a well-insulated and an uninsulated animal house per 45 kg pig, contrasted with the heat production of a pig of this weight. The difference between inside and outside temperatures has been taken as 6°C. To gain an idea of the amount of heat involved, seven animals of this weight generate a similar amount of heat to that emitted by a 1 kw electric fire. The heat production is therefore a useful quantity but entirely inadequate to allow any waste by poor insulation or uncontrolled ventilation.

Figure 2.4 also shows that, disregarding the loss of heat by ventilation, a difference of nearly 30°C between inside and outside temperatures is attainable in a well-insulated house making use only of the animals' own heat. Allowing for the ventilation loss, a difference of about 15°C is possible provided that the construction and ventilation are both on sound lines. Without insulation, however, the difference, after allowing for ventilation, is only some 8°C.

Good thermal insulation not only serves to retain the heat in winter but also keeps the building cool in summer. It helps to prevent condensation and damp, keeps heating costs down, and enables the farmer to maintain uniform and near constant conditions in the house. The effects on the stock are economically important – by helping to maintain an optimum environment, food costs are kept to a minimum and growth and good health are promoted. It also assists in helping to buffer the indoor environment against sudden fluctuations outside.

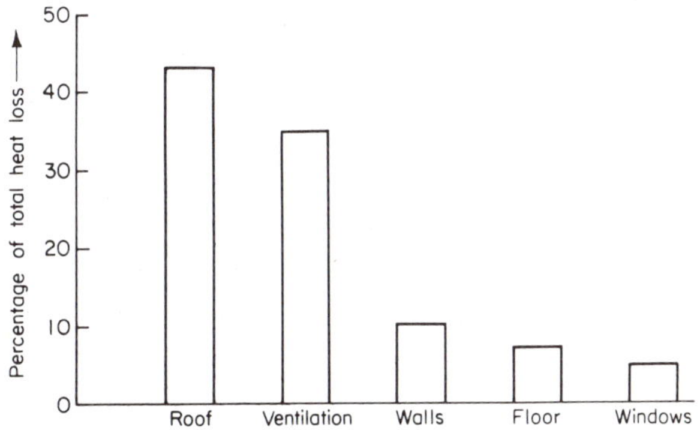

Fig. 2.3 Heat losses from parts of an uninsulated pig house.

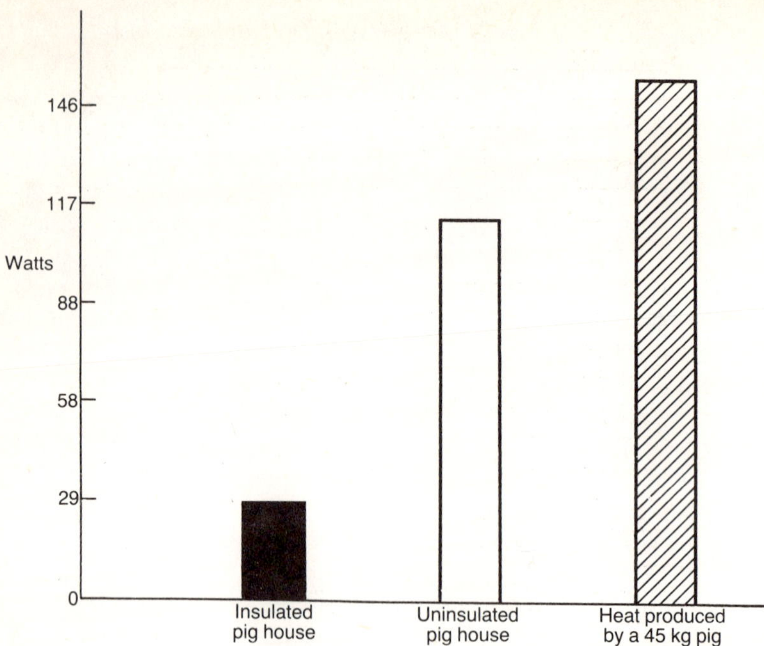

Fig. 2.4 Heat losses through the surfaces of typical insulated and uninsulated pig houses with a difference of 6°C between inside and outside temperatures, contrasted with the heat production of a 45 kg animal.

ASSESSING INSULATION VALUES

Every building material has a thermal conductivity, or K value, which is the measure of a material's ability to conduct heat. It is the amount of heat in watts which passes through 1 m^2 of the material when a temperature difference of 1°C is maintained between opposite surfaces of 1 m thickness. Materials can thus be graded according to their insulating qualities and the figures go some way to answering the question, Which are the best insulators? K values are given in Fig. 2.5. It can be seen that over twice the thickness of straw is needed to give the same insulating value as a given thickness of glass or mineral wool; both can be most useful thermal insulators used in the right circumstances.

However, the K values are of limited use, for surfaces of livestock buildings are generally composite structures. For example, an insulated roof might consist of an outer cladding of corrugated asbestos sheets and an inner lining of mineral wool and fibreboard as well as an air space. What is required is a knowledge of the rate of heat loss (or heat gain during very hot summer weather) throughout the whole structure rather than of the individual materials which compose it. The value which this gives us, and which takes us much further than the K value alone, is known as the U value. The U value is defined as the amount of heat in watts that is transmitted through 1 m^2 of the construction from the air

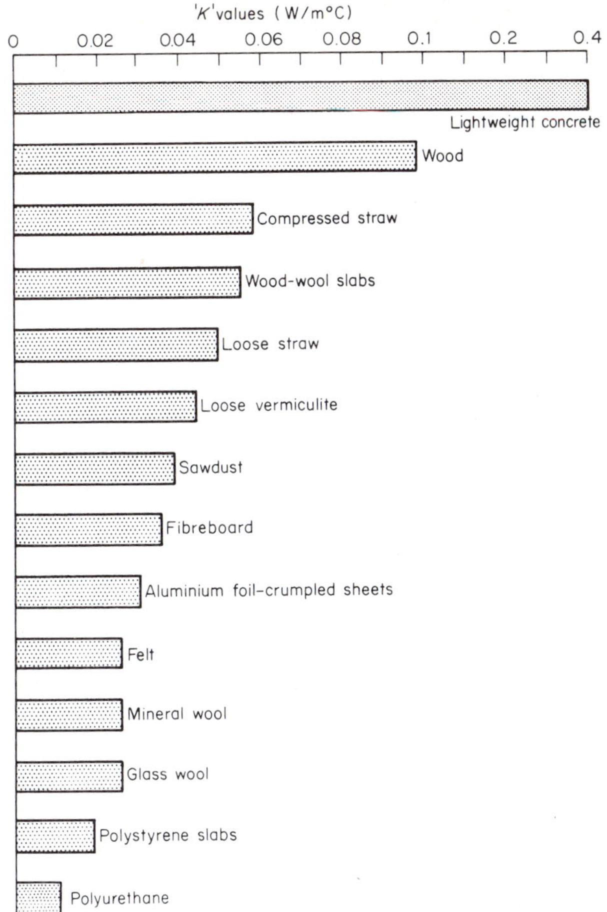

Fig. 2.5 K values of a series of materials used for thermal insulation. The size of blocks is proportional to heat losses through them, so that the materials at the bottom are the best insulators.

inside to the air outside when there is a 1°C difference in temperature between inside and outside. It is possible to build up the U value of a complete wall or roof structure if one has the K values of the individual materials, but this is normally unnecessary as U values for complete structures are available from the manufacturers. As with K values, the lower the U value the better the insulating qualities. Figure 2.6 shows the representative values. The striking reduction in heat loss obtained by insulation is clearly seen, the solid blocks being poor insulators and the cross-hatched blocks reasonable or good ones.

From experience in the housing field we are able to suggest general standards for the U values of a structure. In most controlled environment houses it is good economy to have a U value in the roof of 0.40 or less. The cost of a high

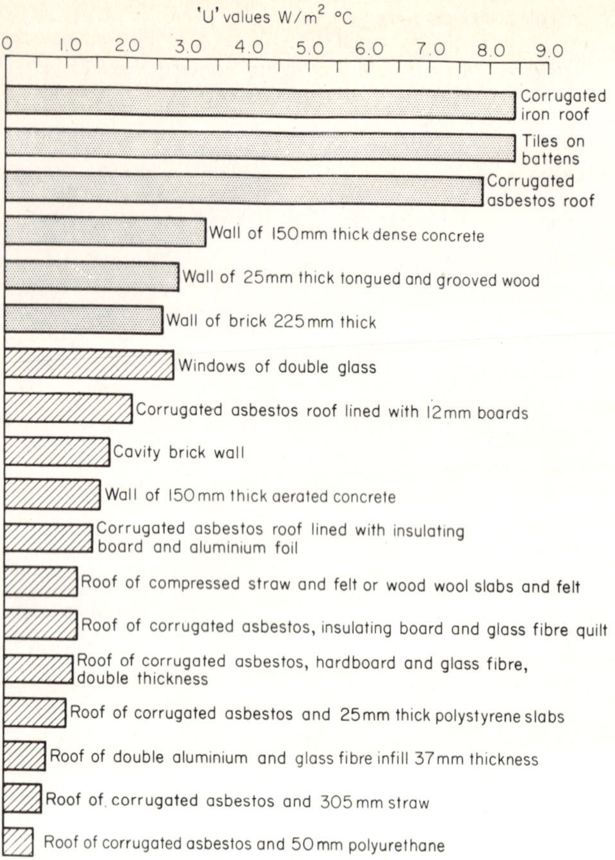

Fig. 2.6 U values of bad (solid blocks) and satisfactory or good (cross-hatched blocks) roof and wall constructions.

standard of insulation is very moderate. For example, mineral wool insulation costs approximately 100 p/m² for each 25 mm thickness and even superb insulation of up to 75–100 mm thickness will not add more than about £2.50/m² to the cost. For the walls a figure of between 1.0 and 1.5 is acceptable; with the floor, however, you should aim to be as near 0.40 as possible.

It is important to eliminate condensation. Table 2.1 shows which U value is able to do this for given differences of temperature between inside and outside.

INSULATING THE ROOF

A good example of the correct construction of an insulated surface is afforded by considering a typically built roof (Fig. 2.7). Whether the outer cladding is already present in an existing building or is to be placed in a new house, it is

Table 2.1. *U value required to overcome condensation*

Relative humidity (%)	Maximum temperature difference (internal–external) 15	20	25	30	35
60	4.6	3.0	2.6	2.3	1.9
65	3.6	2.8	2.3	1.9	1.6
70	3.0	2.4	1.9	1.5	1.4
75	2.6	1.9	1.5	1.3	1.1
80	2.0	1.5	1.2	1.0	0.9
85	1.5	1.1	0.9	0.7	0.8
90	1.1	0.8	0.6	0.5	0.4

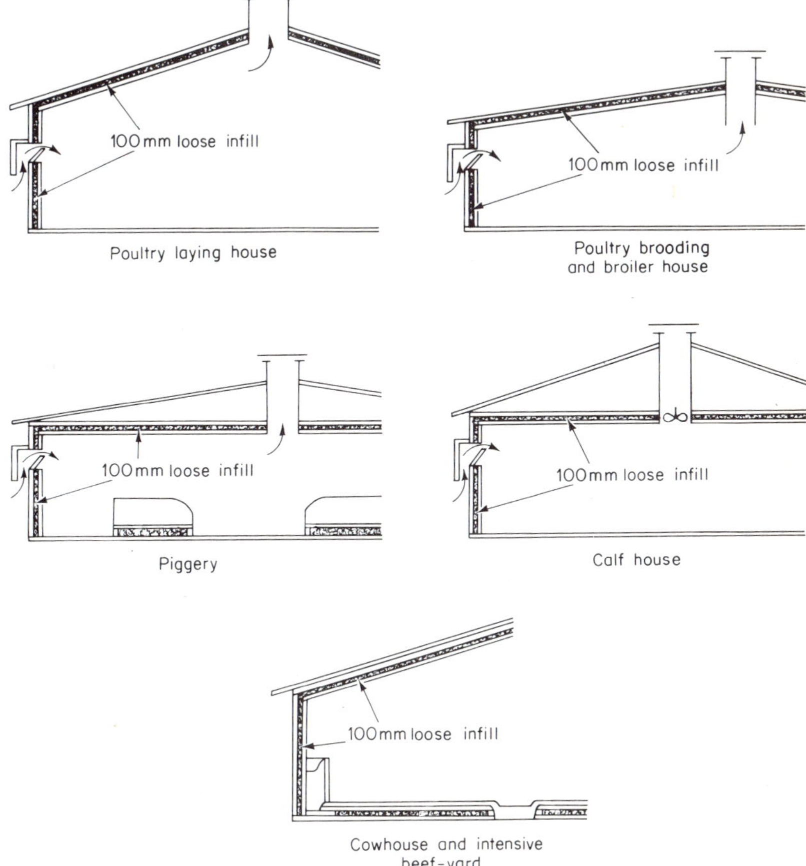

Fig. 2.7 A variety of methods of applying thermal insulation to livestock buildings.

generally of corrugated asbestos or metal. These materials are poor insulators and unsatisfactory when used alone. Below them, therefore, should be placed an insulation lining. This may follow the line of the roof if the pitch is shallow and the walls not too high. However, if the roof is steep and/or the walls are high, it is better to construct a flat 'false' insulated ceiling at a height of around 2 m. A very popular type of insulating material is mineral or glass wool with minimum thickness of 50 mm, although it is preferable to use 75 mm or even 100 mm. In heated buildings, such as poultry and pig houses for young stock, it is now becoming a popular and wise procedure to use a 150 mm glass wool mat. The 'wool' insulation has to be suspended and a variety of materials can be used – for example, aluminium, fibreboard, plywood and flat fibre-cement sheets. Manufacturers use all these materials successfully but the do-it-yourself builder almost always uses a water-repellent plywood, oil-tempered hardboard or fibre-cement sheet.

Vapour seal

To stop moisture within the house permeating the insulation it is essential to place a vapour seal on the warm side or underside of the insulation. Usually the sheets that suspend the insulation are permeable to water vapour, so the vapour seal is placed immediately on top of the sheets (Fig. 2.8). This may consist of polythene sheets, or bitumenized material such as sisalkraft paper. Mineral wool completely sealed in polythene bags and with a built-in overlapping piece is also available. This gives most effective insulation. The insulation material, whether mineral wool or glass wool, must never be compressed, as its insulating qualities depend upon the air spaces between the fibres remaining open.

Working from inside to outside then, the roof will consist of the following layers: first, the inner lining board, then the vapour seal, and finally the insulating material.

Alternative interior linings are as follows:

Fibreboards

As a roof lining a good quality oil-tempered hardboard or an insulation fibreboard can be sucessful if applied in the manner recommended and if

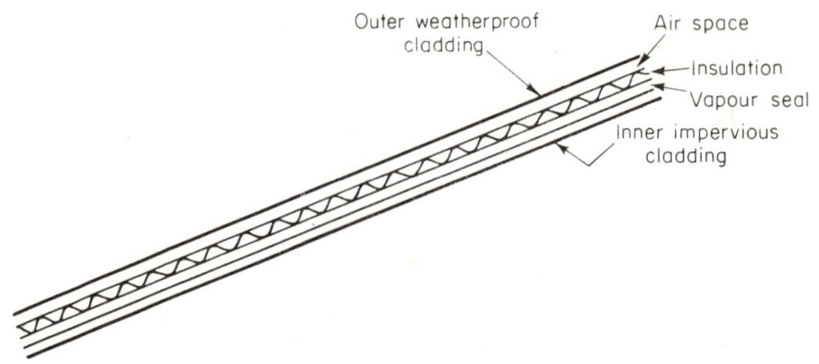

Fig. 2.8 Details of insulated roof construction. The insulation material must never be compressed or its value will be partially lost.

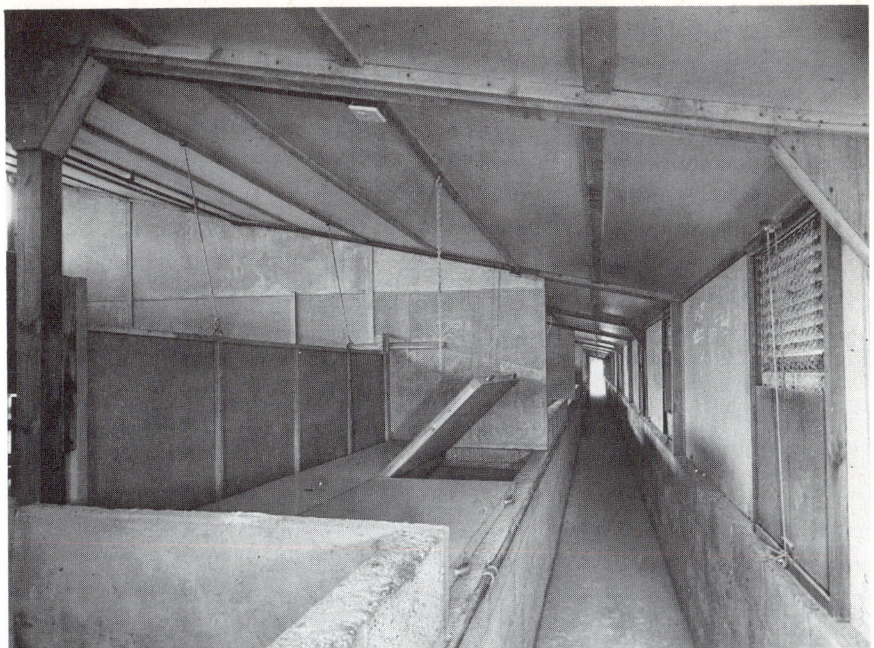

Fig. 2.9 Inner linings to a piggery using suitable fibreboards for roof, walls and kennel tops.

management ensures that the building is kept well ventilated (Fig. 2.9). If an insulation board is likely to be subjected to very damp conditions, it will not prove satisfactory and is best avoided. Oil-tempered hardboard can also form an effective wall lining above the height of the livestock and is able to withstand any amount of dampness without harm.

Asbestos-based boards

The resistance of asbestos-based boards (asbestos insulation boards, partition boards, flexible sheets) to corrosion and moisture makes them a popular choice for internal roof or wall linings; some particularly hard and thick forms of these materials can even be placed in contact with livestock, and are used alone for pen divisions and gates up to 12.5 mm thick. Because of the risk to health of asbestos-based products these are now being replaced by 'fibre cement', asbestos-free products.

Aluminium

As a support for an insulation lining, aluminium is a lightweight lining which only needs a good vapour seal at the joints to make it an acceptable material for this purpose. As a foil, bonded to kraft paper, it is also an acceptable roof lining. Both these constructions for roofs require specialist manufacture and when well built provide a very hygienic surface which is hard-wearing.

Lightweight expanded plastic boards and sprays

The disadvantages of the earliest forms of expanded polystyrene which were very fragile and easily damaged or destroyed by vermin appear to have been largely overcome in the development of the now very hard extruded forms, such as Styrofoam, and these are now widely used as roof linings. They are light enough to make their installation cheap and simple, yet still hard enough to give a clean and hygienic surface.

Another more recently developed expanded plastic – polyurethane – can be used in three ways: it may be pumped into a cavity, forming an insulation material of extremely light weight, rather like candy floss in texture (Fig. 2.10); it may also be sprayed on the underside of the outer cladding, such as asbestos, to form a hard inner insulation lining; and finally, it is made in sheets like polystyrene and may be faced with plastic or aluminium foil. The latter (e.g. Purlboard FP) gives a fine, vapour-proof, light, hygienic surface with good fire-resisting qualities and complying with the spread of flame rating as laid down under BS476, Part 7: 1971 (Fig. 2.11).

Even more recently polyurethane, which has a better insulation value than polystyrene, has been effectively bonded to external cladding materials such as oil-tempered hardboard, resin-bonded plywood, and plastic-coated steel and aluminium sheets. This technique produces in one structure a hard-wearing, well-insulated material that can form the entire roof and walls of animal houses provided that the joints are permanently sealed. The inside surface is normally plastic-coated but where the walls are in contact with the animals, they may be protected with external cladding materials sufficiently strong to withstand the pressure of teeth and feet; for example, 9 mm fully compressed asbestos sheeting is ideal.

Plywood

'Exterior grade' phenolic resin-bonded plywoods can be used successfully as an interior or exterior lining but for external use such boards need good weathering protection. This can take the form of a liquid bitumen preparation applied by brush after construction.

Composition plastic boards

Recently new fibre plastic boards made of compressed plastic waste and paper have proved to be most effective as a lining for animal buildings at animal level and for the construction of livestock building gates and solid divisions, and even for flooring. It is not readily attacked by pigs and other animals and does

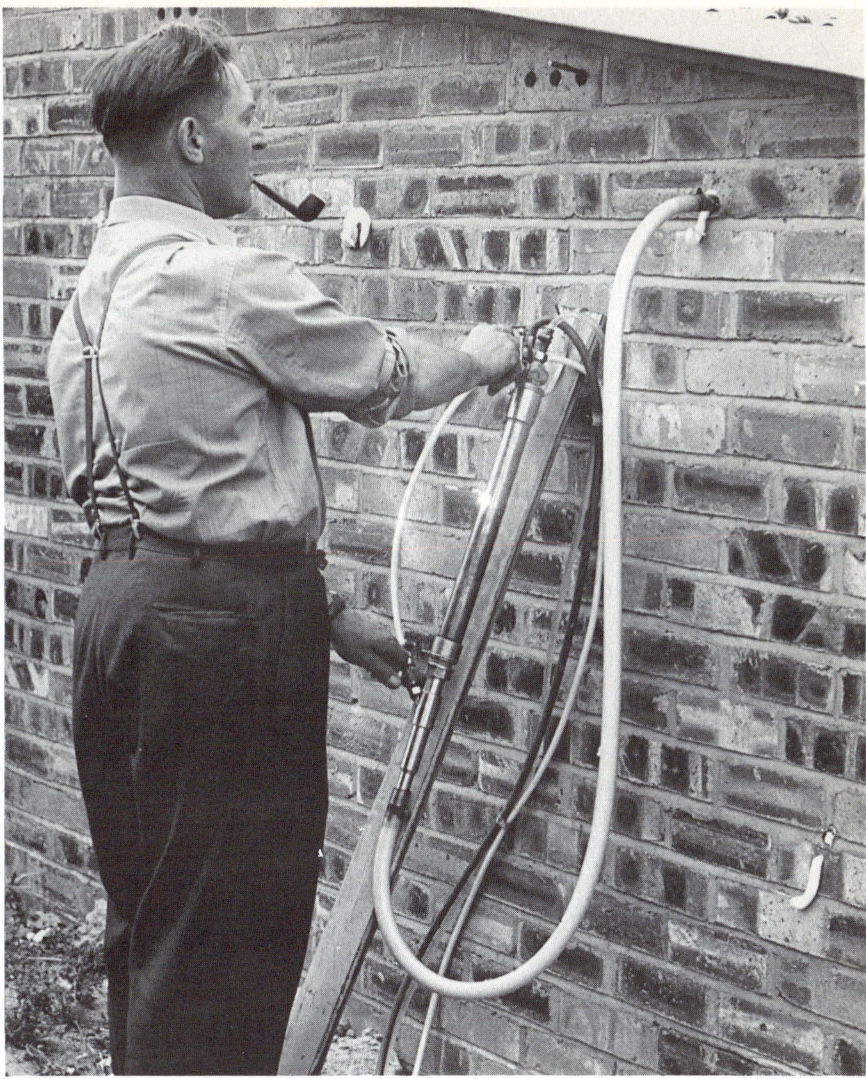

Fig. 2.10 A foamed plastic (Thermalon) being injected under pressure to provide a complete cavity fill.

not corrode, but the manufacturers' instructions on fixing must be carefully followed to avoid 'bowing' under weight, e.g. at the rear of sow stalls.

TRADITIONAL METHODS

Where the more traditional methods of cavity brick or concrete block are used for the walls, many serious errors are still made. First, it should be stressed that

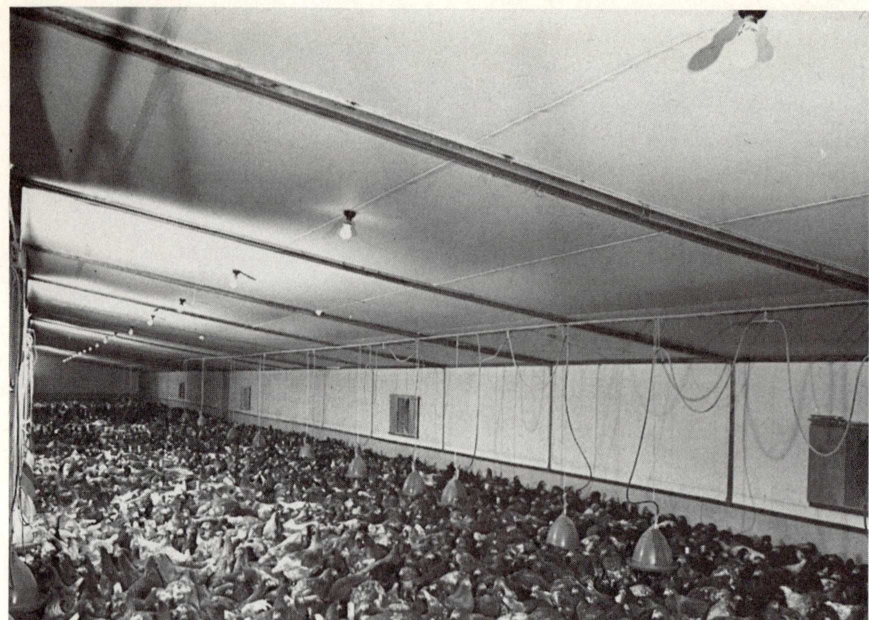

Fig. 2.11 Insulating a poultry house using wall and roof insulation of polyurethane sheets of 'Purlboard FP' with smooth and hygienic finish.

the degree of insulation is not very good with these methods. Cavity brickwork is also very expensive and is used less and less for the insulated animal house. Insulated forms of concrete blocks are frequently used and laid by unskilled labour, but if they are to retain their usefulness, it is vital to protect the outside from the rain either by rendering or by treating with a cheap, liquid-sealing compound. Ordinary hollow blocks in dense concrete are not insulators and can only be recommended where they are used in conjunction with an inner leaf of lightweight insulation blocks, A wall construction of two layers of blocks, the outer being of dense concrete, the inner of insulation-type with an air space between, is a very good construction.

INSULATING THE FLOOR

Floors are of special importance, as stock is frequently in close contact with them and there is usually a need to conserve bedding to the utmost or avoid it altogether. The use of an insulation layer is therefore strongly advised in a building where the animals have direct contact with the floor (Fig. 2.12). Further, in all cases where a concrete floor is installed but the use of thick layer of litter makes insulation unnecessary, a damp-proof course should be built to prevent rising damp. Well made floors therefore consist of the following layers (from bottom to top): hardcore, concrete, damp proof course, insulation layer, cement

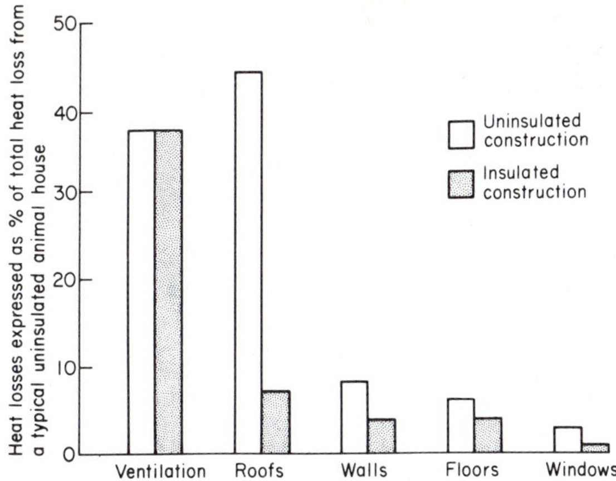

Fig. 2.12 Where heat is lost from insulated and uninsulated animal houses.

screed. The damp proof course can be of polythene, kraft paper, roofing felt or a bituminous liquid. Insulating layers can consist of wood-wool slabs, egg trays, hollow tiles, domed concrete blocks or expanded plastics. The top screed should be as thin as possible – for pig pens, for example, it is usual to make do with a 37 mm thickness – but care must be taken that the screed is thick enough and well made to avoid all risk of collapse. Much damage is done to animals by rough concrete surfaces; the finish must be smooth enough to prevent this, yet not so smooth that the animals slip. A wooden-float finish is best. (Further details of floor finishes are given in those sections of the book dealing with individual species.)

REFLECTIVE INSULATION

The methods of insulation so far described rely on the dead air space within the material reducing the conduction of heat. There is, however, another very useful and often cheap way of reducing heat loss: reflective insulation. A bright shiny surface, such as aluminium, will reflect a relatively high percentage of the heat that is radiated towards it. Thus it is extremely useful to line the inside of a house with aluminium foil as this will conserve the radiation emanating from the livestock heaters or infra-red lamps, or even other parts of the building itself. Reflective insulation is particularly useful as a lining to the inside of piglets' creeps, 'kennels' for fattening pigs, poultry brooding compartments or small calf pens. Reflective insulation on the outside of a building, for example, using an aluminium roof covering and white-painted walls, will materially assist in lowering the inside temperature on hot summer days by reflecting some of the sun's heat.

INSULATING THE WINDOWS

The controlled environment house is often made without windows. Some may deprecate the practice of rearing stock under completely artificial light, but it does have some real advantages. It is possible to control more easily the activity of the stock so that problems such as fighting, cannibalism and sheer over-excitability are mitigated. In addition, from the point of view of insulation, it has the great advantage that a serious source of heat loss and condensation is eliminated. Where, however, windows are used in such buildings, it is essential to use a double thickness of glass with an air space between. This is an inexpensive method which greatly reduces the heat loss (Fig. 2.13). With pigs, the windows should be in or over the dung passage as they tend to go towards the light to dung.

CUBIC AIR SPACE

In connection with thermal insulation, it is worth stressing the merits of reducing the air space in a controlled environment house to reasonable proportions. Buildings will tend to be unnecessarily large and roofs in particular too steeply

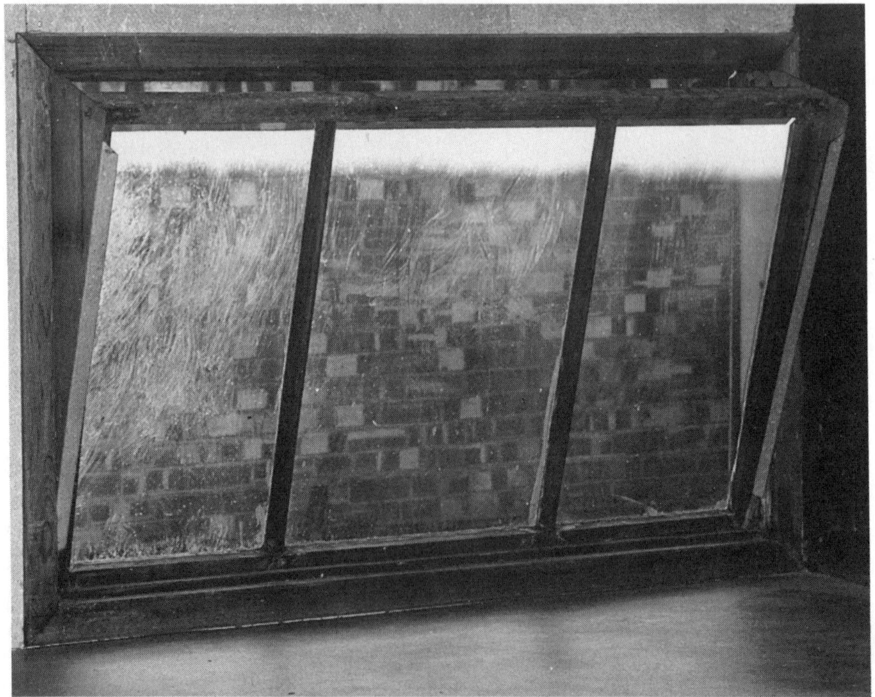

Fig. 2.13 Double-glazed window ideal for controlled environment housing.

pitched. By reducing the cubic area, heat conservation is improved and building costs can be reduced.

It is also important to have efficient drainage around the building. A number of cases occur where the floor becomes permanently wet throughout the winter owing to inefficient drainage. A wet floor is certain to be cold and any litter on it will absorb a great deal of moisture and stock may be chilled.

MATERIALS FOR WALLS

The main materials used in the construction of the walls of farm buildings are:

1. Brickwork
2. Concrete blockwork
3. Concrete walls, either pre-cast or cast *in situ*
4. Timber
5. Metal – galvanized or otherwise protected
6. Plywood
7. Hardboard
8. Asbestos
9. Rendered proprietary insulation materials such as wood-wool and polystyrene or epoxyresin 'glossy white finish' building boards
10. A variety of hard plastic materials

The choice of material will depend on a number of factors – including personal preference – but there are three principal considerations. First, the degree of strength required. Where the larger farm animals are in direct contact with the structure, it must be robust and materials such as brick, blocks or rendered construction may be best, at least for the lower part of the walls. Above animal height, or where the pressure on the material may be slight as in a poultry house, lighter, more fragile materials may be used, such as hardboard, plywood and fibre-cement boards (Fig. 2.14).

The second major consideration is the degree of thermal insulation that is required. From the observations in the next chapter on the climatic needs of stock, it will be seen that mature animals other than poultry may not need an insulated wall. Uninsulated construction is the usual practice in cow and sheep sheds and yards and bull and boar and some sow accommodation. On the other hand, insulated walls are generally chosen for calf houses, most pig accommodation and poultry houses. Common farming practice and the need for heat conservation nowadays demand a high degree of insulation, and prefabricated construction provides this most efficiently (Fig. 2.15). It also costs less than traditional materials and methods.

The third overall need is to consider the construction in relation to hygiene. There is a great risk in all stock buildings of a build-up of disease-causing organisms unless all the materials can be easily and effectively disinfected. This points to the need for smooth and impervious surfaces with a minimum of places

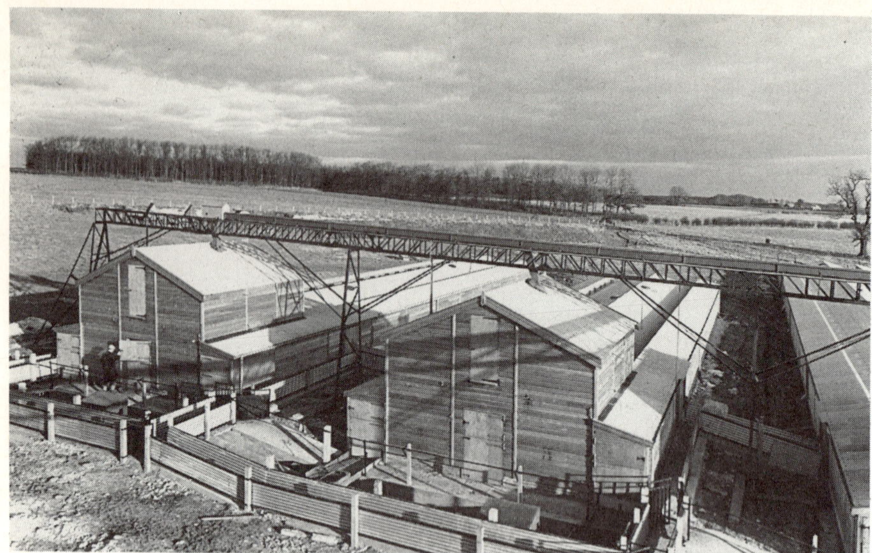

Fig. 2.14 Part of a large pig complex of prefabricated construction with overhead feed conveyors.

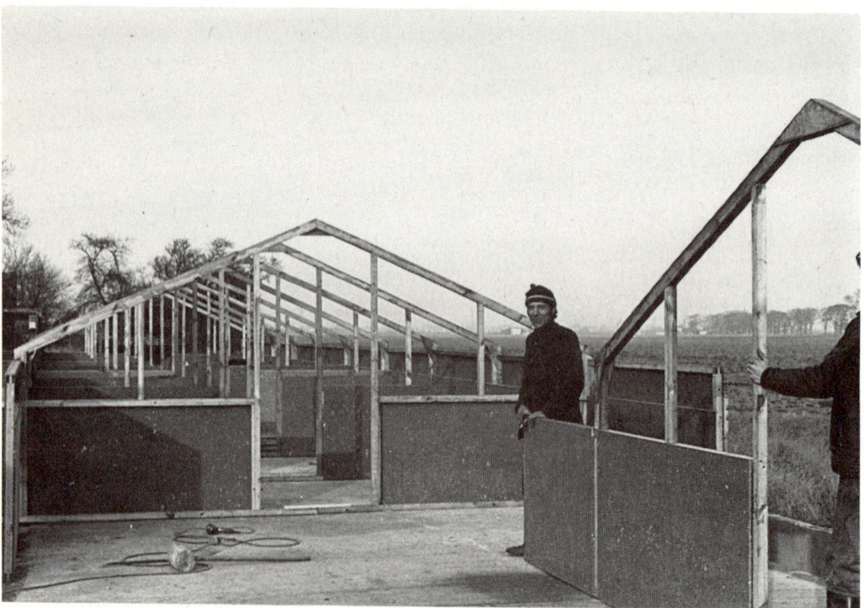

Fig. 2.15 Prefabricated wall sections being erected for weaner pig housing.

where dirt can accumulate. A good cement-rendered surface is clearly satisfactory, although in recent years the more efficient application of prefabricated claddings has provided a cheaper and acceptable alternative.

MATERIALS FOR FLOORS

Floors need to meet certain essential requirements. They must be:

1 Durable
2 Non-slip where there is no bedding
3 Impervious to water or urine
4 Easily cleaned
5 Resistant to chemicals, urine and certain foods, such as whey and skim milk
6 Resistant to rising damp
7 Thermally insulated where in contact with livestock.

Concrete is the material which has everywhere been found the most suitable, although certain bituminous and composition floorings have been used for cow standings to improve the insulation and provide a warmer surface for the cows to stand on. Generally however insulation is best placed as a layer under the top impervious surface. Wood flooring also has its place for certain types of poultry, for pig houses and for calves. Wood floors should be dismountable for cleaning and disinfection. (Floor insulation is dealt with in detail on p. 24; slatted flooring systems are covered under the species in the relevant chapters.)

Floor surfaces

For floors which have to withstand heavy wear, particularly in stables and cowsheds, a granolithic finish is recommended. This is a finely graded concrete with granite chippings as aggregate, the coarse aggregate forming the wear-resistant surface. Cement hardeners producing a non-dusting surface will also improve wear by sealing the pores and making the floor impervious. Materials for this purpose include silicates of soda, and zinc and magnesium silicofluorides, as well as proprietary hardeners. Before it is treated the floor should be not less than two weeks old, and clean and dry. 4.5 litres of commercial silicate of soda added to 1.8 litres of water covers up to 90 m^2. The solution is brushed well into the floor and is washed off with water the day after application. Two or three applications are needed. The finish given to the floor should be non-slip and therefore lightly roughened on the surface apart from the gutters which are best trowelled up. A suitable non-slip surface can be made with a wood float or by 'bouncing' with a broom or light tamping. The best result is usually given by sprinkling carborundum on the finished floor at the rate of 1 kg/m^2.

It frequently happens that the existing floor is so smooth and slippery that the stock cannot gain a proper foothold, and so fall and injure themselves; this makes them timid and frightened to use it. There are various remedies which can be applied to re-texture slippery floor surfaces; most of these are best left to specialist firms:

1 Surface scabbling. A machine chips away the surface of the concrete and leaves an abrasive finish.
2 Surface grooving. A variety of machines will cut grooves in worn concrete to

provide a surface on which cows can get a good grip without causing sore feet.

3 Resin mortars applied to the surface of the concrete and allowed to cure.
4 Acid etching. This uses strong chemicals which can be dangerous to use.

All of this work is best left to specialists and the cost of remedial work should be compared with the cost of relaying the floor.

Cracked and damaged concrete floors may also present a hazard to operators and stock, cause foot problems to livestock, and in the case of milking premises may not conform to statutory requirements. Most badly cracked or worn concrete floors are best completely relaid. There may, however, be small areas where repairs can be made. The essential point is to provide a good 'key' between the existing and the new concrete. This requires really clean surfaces and a proprietary bonding agent incorporated into the cement grout used as a filler. Sufficient curing time is important.

ROOF MATERIALS AND TYPES

The two principal types of roof are: (1) the gable roof and (2) the mono-pitch or lean-to roof. There are several materials available for roofing farm buildings including tiles, slates, cedar shingles, thatch, galvanized and protected steel, and aluminium and fibre-cement tiles and sheets. The most popular are corrugated fibre-cement, steel and aluminium sheets; these have many advantages, the chief being cheapness, fire-resistance, easy fixing and a reasonably long life. Both are tolerably light materials and thus do not require heavy roof structures. Trusses can be constructed with equal success in steel, timber or reinforced concrete, and a convenient spacing is 3 m centres in the cowshed, which is about the width of three cows, and 3–4.5 m in other buildings. The roof must be designed so that it can be easily cleaned.

Low-cost, temporary accommodation for some classes of stock may be provided by plastic-covered framed structures. These structures must be sited carefully to avoid wind damage. To ensure their stability, secure anchorage and a free-draining soil are essential. Because of the temporary nature of the structure the cost of a concrete floor will rarely be justified, but a dry floor is still essential for stock comfort. At one time it was believed that the plastic-covered framed structure would have a considerable future in agriculture and recent experience has shown that there is a definite place for this type of building in the housing of sheep and poultry. Nevertheless such buildings are very vulnerable to damage by wind, livestock and general handling procedures. There may also be environmental problems with condensation, ventilation and overheating in the summer. One of the advantages of cheap structures such as this is the ability it gives the farmer to allow generous space which reduces the risk of disease and vices and also assists generally in management. Buildings such as these may be used only for a year or two before they are taken down and moved to another site, thus removing the risk of a build-up of infectious organisms on animal-sick land.

3

General Environmental Effects

Farm livestock are homeotherms, that is, they must keep their body temperature within a moderately narrow range to work efficiently. To do this they maintain a thermal balance between the heat they produce or gain from the environment and the heat they lose to it. The various routes for heat production and loss are shown in Fig. 3.1. This applies primarily to cattle, but is suited with only a little modification to other farm livestock. It can be seen that heat escapes from the body by a number of routes. A small amount is lost with the faeces and urine but the main losses are by radiation, convection, conduction and evaporation.

Radiation heat loss occurs because a warm body emits heat when it is at a temperature higher than that of its surrounding surfaces. The loss is also affected by the area of the body's surface and its so-called emissivity – that is, its inherent ability to emit heat by this route (see p. 34). Other factors are the position and behaviour of the animal: for example, heat loss will be greatly reduced when groups of animals are close together. Hot surfaces are to be avoided in summer as they prevent the animal from radiating and thus dissipating surplus heat, while in winter cold surfaces will aggravate heat loss in a cool environment and greatly increase the risk of chilling, expecially in the young animal.

Convection loss is governed by the surface area of the animal, its temperature and that of the surrounding air, and the movement of air over the surface, hence the danger of draughts in cold weather as a source of heat dissipation, in contrast to the need for high air movement in warm weather, which can help to relieve the stress of high temperatures.

Conduction loss is due to physical contact of the animal with a surface, and is dependent on the temperature of the surface, its area and its thermal conductivity. It is most important to reduce heat loss by conduction either by providing animals with bedding or by insulating surfaces.

Evaporative heat loss enables an animal to withstand high temperatures even when the loss by radiation, conduction and convection is insignificant or absent. Evaporation of water from the skin plays a minor role in farm animals, which for the most part are sparsely equipped with sweat glands, compared with that from the respiratory surfaces. Evaporation from the skin is dependent, so far as external factors are concerned, on the temperature, humidity and movement of the air; from the lungs it depends on the humidity of the inspired and expired air.

Temperature regulation in farm animals is achieved in various ways. In hot weather heat is lost through a higher breathing rate which increases the evaporation of moisture from the lungs by transudation of moisture through the skin and by an increased intake of water. Livestock also keep cool by avoiding direct sunlight, eating less food and reducing movement to a minimum. They are also helped by postural changes: for example, the chicken in hot weather holds its wings out from its body so that the air can circulate over the poorly ventilated underside. Other animals, especially the pig, wallow to keep cool by evaporation. In very cold weather farm livestock increase their heat production by eating more. They also increase their insulation against cold by depositing larger amounts of fat under the skin, and by growing longer and coarser hair. Heat production is further increased by shivering, and heat is conserved by huddling to reduce the surface area of heat loss.

THE EFFECT OF HUMIDITY

From the aspect of the physiology of the animal, the air humidity has a number of very important influences, for the amount of water vapour in the air controls

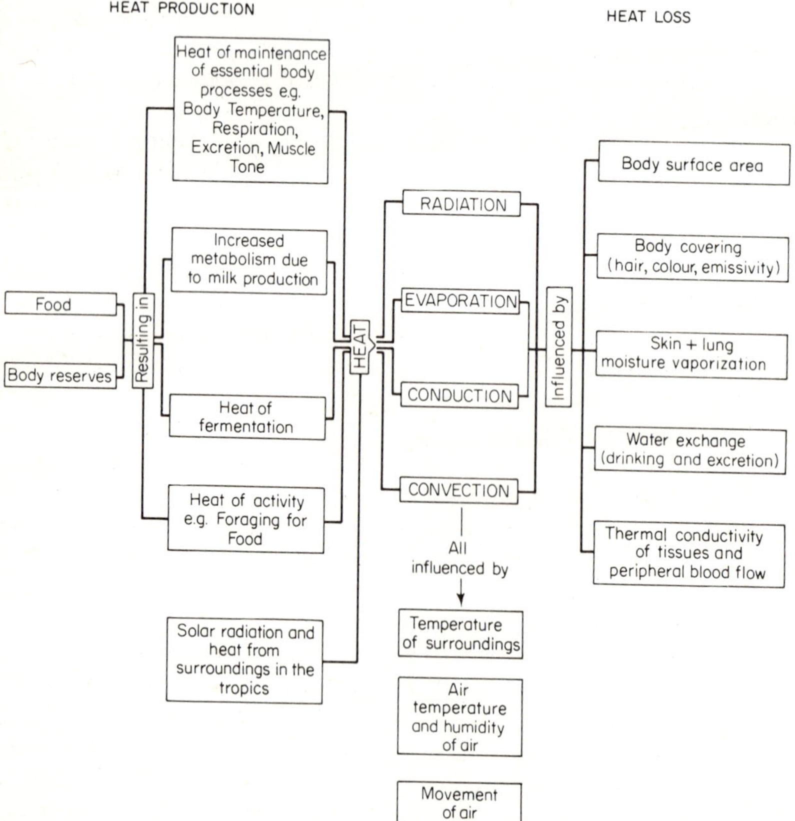

Fig. 3.1 Heat production and heat loss.

the rate of evaporation of moisture from the external surfaces of the animal, especially from the lungs and respiratory tract.

In order to appreciate the role of the air humidity it is necessary to understand certain physical features of water vapour. Water, like other liquids, will tend to saturate the surrounding space with its vapour. In a completely enclosed space the amount of water vapour in a unit volume in the area above the water depends only on the temperature of the system. The pressure developed is termed the true vapour or saturation pressure. If the temperature rises, saturation pressure will increase. When this pressure equals total atmospheric pressure, the water boils.

In a ventilated building where air currents carry the water vapour away, continuous evaporation can take place but the degree to which this happens depends on the rate of air movement and the percentage of saturation of the ambient air. Obviously, if the air moving in the building is already saturated, no evaporation can take place.

The term *relative humidity* (RH) refers to the amount of moisture actually in the air compared to the amount it could contain at the same temperature, and expressed as a percentage. Hence, the amount of moisture in the air at, say, 100 per cent RH will vary depending on the air temperature. Since it is the actual amount of water vapour in the air which influences evaporation, the relative humidity cannot be used to calculate evaporative loss unless the temperature is known.

The following example should make the matter clear. Water vapour in air saturated at a freezing temperature of 0°C exerts a vapour pressure of 5 mmHg – a condition not uncommon through many winter months in temperate climates. When this air is inhaled into the lungs, it meets moist mucous membranes at 37°C which have a vapour pressure of 45 mmHg. At this 40 mmHg difference evaporation occurs quickly, saturating the air now warmed to 37°C. Thus air entering at 0°C 100 per cent RH leaves at 37°C and also 100 per cent RH but with a vastly different moisture content. When the air is exhaled, it cools rapidly and the surplus water vapour condenses out. This moisture is not only seen as a visible cloud, but may also condense and run on any cool surface.

Once the relative humidity and the temperature of the air are found, then any of the other properties of the air can be read from psychometric charts, including the vapour pressure, absolute humidity and dewpoint. In practical terms, in temperate climates livestock may thrive perfectly well over a wide range of humidity, extending from at least 30 to 90 per cent RH. If, however, ambient temperatures are below the correct level, high humidities will intensify the cold stress, owing to the extra moisture surrounding the animal and breathed into its lungs. Likewise, at air temperatures above the normal accepted range, a high humidity will progressively reduce the animal's ability to keep cool by evaporation until, if the air is saturated and as warm as the animal, it will lose this ability altogether. Very dry air, below about 30 per cent RH, may dehydrate the mucous membranes of the respiratory tract and make them more vulnerable to invasion by pathogenic organisms, and create discomfort and a dry, scurfy skin. There will also be indirect effects on the viability of pathogenic organisms (see pp. 56 to 58). It must always be our aim in livestock buildings to ventilate them so that the moisture produced by the animal is liberated from the atmosphere. This is the central theme in Chapter 5.

AIR MOVEMENT

At air temperatures above body temperature, air movement tends to reduce heat dissipation by increasing the flow of heat from the environment through the skin into the body of the animal. The air movement in fact reduces the insulation of the surrounding air and may also reduce that of the hair or feathers. At cold temperatures, on the other hand, excessive air movement in the form of a draught may chill an animal which would otherwise be quite comfortable, and much attention is rightly given to this problem. In subsequent sections dealing with individual species a range of acceptable air movements will be given.

THE EFFECT OF THE ANIMAL'S SURFACE

The animal's body surface is a very important part in its thermoregulatory control. Heat travels to the body surface via the bloodstream and, as we have seen, is dissipated by four routes – convection, radiation, conduction and evaporation. The sweating mechanism of most farm animals is weak – anatomically, cattle, sheep and pigs have sweat glands, but they function poorly. Water vapour is passed through the skin by osmosis ('insensible perspiration') i.e. not associated with sweat glands. The exchange of heat through the body is also affected by the colour of the skin, its physical character and its disposition in relation to the environment.

The amount of solar radiation absorbed by the coat is determined to some extent by its colour. A white coat may absorb only 20 per cent of the visible radiation falling on it; a black coat almost 100 per cent. Half the energy in the solar spectrum is the invisible infra-red portion, which can be completely absorbed on the coat.[1]

The colour of the skin is also important in its reaction to sunburn and photosensitization. A white coat with a smooth and glossy texture minimizes the adverse effects of direct sunlight. Shade reduces the great heat load which may fall on animals. The coat also influences convective and evaporative loss from the skin. If it is thick and/or long, it will trap air and moisture and slow down the convection exchange. It also provides a local climate of high humidity and so renders the exchange of heat by vaporization of water from the skin surface more difficult. Brody[2] showed that in European cattle, as the air temperature rises from -15 to $+35$°C, the heat lost by respiratory vaporization rises from 4 to 30 per cent of the total heat lost; between -15 and $+15$°C the vaporization from the skin surface is of about the same order as the respiratory vaporization rate, but between 15 and 27°C the body surface vaporization rate increases fourfold. At 34°C approximately 26 per cent of the heat is dissipated by vaporization from the outer body surface, and about 15 per cent by non-evaporative cooling. Thus the body surface plays a critical and varying role in temperature regulation in animal production, and it is vital that its healthy state be maintained if it is to fulfil these functions efficiently.

ENVIRONMENT ZONES FOR LIVESTOCK

There are a number of technical definitions applied to the climatic environment which require explanation. In giving these we can show more succinctly the main aims in meeting the needs of housed livestock. It will be apparent at the outset that there is no fixed temperature at which animals must be maintained; every animal, and even more so every group of animals, has a range within which they can given optimal performance. The range one aims to keep all animals in is the so-called 'thermocomfort' zone. (Fig. 3.2). Within this range animals are not only capable of giving an optimal performance, but also feel so comfortable that they have no preference for any particular location – neither huddling nor separating to keep warm or cool, respectively – they are, as it were, in complete harmony with their environment. The 'zone' is difficult to define absolutely because its precise nature will depend on many factors: age, weight, feeding rate, past experience (acclimatization) and husbandry system. It

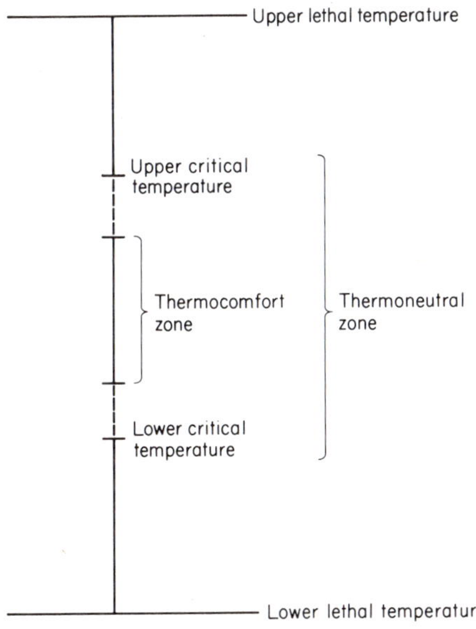

Fig. 3.2 Environment zones for livestock

may be a very narrow zone, as in the day-old chick or piglet, or a very wide zone, as with adult cattle. It is rarely economic to keep animals within the thermocomfort zone at all times, although we should aim for it in our building designs.

On either side of this zone, is the so-called 'thermoneutral' zone. It is vital to try to maintain stock within this at all times if they are housed, and at least most of the time if they are outdoors. It is the zone where there are no metabolic demands on the animals. They maintain homeothermy by quite extensive fluctuations in their behaviour (postural changes, huddling, etc.), by changes in their hair disposition (piloerection in the cold) or blood circulation at the surface, and by perspiration and panting. They can do all these without any measurable metabolic changes, so that productivity can go apace although, because the animal may behave differently in response to them, there may be problems with vices and/or environmental pollution if there is an excessive favouring of certain parts of a pen or building.

If the temperature falls below the lower end of the scale (the lower critical temperature), the animal will need to consume more food to keep warm, so that either the animal produces less if it is on a fixed feeding scale, or eats more to keep warm and still produce at the optimal level. If the animal is principally a roughage consumer, such as adult cattle or sheep, this may matter very little, because the food is relatively cheap, but if it is consuming expensive concentrates, it is a very uneconomic way to keep the animal warm. This is an important reason why non-ruminant livestock, such as pigs and poultry, unlike ruminants are kept in well-insulated housing with controlled ventilation. If the temperature goes above the thermoneutral zone, the animal tries to reduce its heat production, usually by lowering its food consumption and productivity.

If temperatures continue to rise or fall, above or below the upper or lower

Table 3.1. *Ambient temperatures required by housed livestock*

Species	Temperature range (°C)
Adult cattle	Milk production optimum 10–20°, but temperatures from −6 to +25° have little effect on yield
Beef cattle	From −6 to +25° the optimum range
Calves	10–15° at birth, which may fall gradually thereafter; higher temperatures, 15–22°, are used in veal production
Adult pigs on pasture	4–30° a satisfactory range; protection from the sun essential at the higher temperatures
Fattening pigs	At weaning 25°, reducing to 15° at finishing weight of 90–110 kg
Farrowing sows	15–20° for sows; piglets 30° at birth, falling gradually during following weeks to 21° and to 25° at weaning
Laying poultry	20–25° optimum
Broiler chicken	16–25° in house; practical limits 13–30°
Brooders for poultry	35° for day-old chicks; approximately 0.5° drop daily until house temperature optimum reached

critical temperatures, respectively, the animal continues trying to maintain its homeothermy by various metabolic means, but in due course the deep body temperature is altered and it will in extreme conditions eventually collapse and die. Fortunately, in livestock housing we do not often have to face such excessive problems, but even in temperate climates they arise owing to bad design or failure of the environmental control system. The ambient temperatures at which animals succumb are known as the *lethal* temperature, there being one at the top and one at the bottom ends of the scale. Table 3.1 gives a practical guide to the ambient temperatures required by farm livestock.

SPECIES REQUIREMENTS

Cattle

There are certain fundamental differences between ruminant animals and pigs and poultry which makes the approach to environmental control quite different for the two groups of livestock.[3]

Pigs and poultry raised out of doors in temperate and cool climates maintain homeothermy in most circumstances by regulating heat production in order to keep warm. The consequent increase in heat production can usually be achieved with little metabolic distress but at some cost in terms of food energy. Intensive poultry and pig houses have therefore been designed to ensure the best feed conversion efficiency by regulating temperature and ventilation in order to keep the animals in an environment that is warm enough for optimal efficiency of production. It should not be assumed that a cool environment is necessarily uncomfortable for a pig or chicken if it has adequate food.

In most cool, temperate environments, ruminants maintain homeothermy by relating evaporative loss at little metabolic cost in order to keep cool. Morover, ruminants have a very marked ability to alter their thermoneutral zone in response to previous thermal history. There are thus no absolute criteria for the thermal requirements of any class of ruminant livestock, except perhaps the newborn animal; they depend to a very large extent on what the animal has grown accustomed to.

A fundamental difference between the environmental requirements of ruminants and those of pigs and poultry concerns the prevention of disease. Pig and poultry producers can operate closed herds or purchase their stock from pathogen-free units. Vaccines against respiratory and other diseases have been very effective in poultry, and if disease gets into a unit, mass medication is easily administered. However, ruminants such as young calves, for example, arrive on a rearing unit from a variety of sources, which are often unknown and they undoubtedly carry infection onto the premises. No vaccines have been successfully produced against respiratory disease in calves, no doubt because of the complex nature of the disease.

Thermal requirements

Some examples of the lower critical temperatures for ruminants under conditions of varying air movements are shown in Table 3.2. The beasts are standing up, in a dry enclosure, under two types of air movement.

In an unheated building at low air movement the only cattle likely to experience cold sufficient to elevate their heat production are newborn calves, or young calves whose metabolic rate is low by virtue of starvation, sickness or emaciation. Such animals can undoubtedly be stressed by cold in unheated buildings and may require special attention. Increasing air movement to 2 m/s, which is not uncommon in draughty buildings, increases the critical temperature in the newborn calf from +9 to +17°C. This emphasizes the necessity of ensuring that adequate ventilation for calf houses is achieved without allowing excess air movement (or 'draught') to play on the calves.

By one month of age the healthy calf with a good appetite has a critical temperature close to 0°C and is not likely to be stressed by cold when indoors. Well-grown veal calves, by virtue of their very high energy intake and heat production, are particularly tolerant to cold, and by the same criteria, sensitive to heat. The traditional belief that veal calves should be kept in a warm environment because they are not ruminant and are therefore somehow more sensitive to cold is unscientific and untrue.

No other class of cattle is likely to experience a systemic stress of cold when standing in a dry enclosure unless air movement is exceptionally high. For the dairy cow, however, cold stress should not be considered as a systemic but as a local problem. Heat production in the high-yielding cow is again very high and so the critical temperature is low. Milk synthesis, however, depends on blood flow to the mammary glands, which is reduced by local cooling. The production of dairy cows has been shown to fall at temperatures below about 0°C, although it is obvious that direct chilling of the udder depends as much on the thermal properties of the floor as on the air temperature.

Table 3.2 *Lower critical temperature of ruminants housed with very low air movement (0.2 m/s) and in a draught (2 m/s)*

Type of animal	Live wt (kg)	Lower critical temp. (°C) Low air speed	Draught
Calf – newborn	35	+9	+17
1 month old	50	0	+9
Veal	100	−14	−1
Store cattle (maintenance)	250	−32	−20
Beef cow (maintenance)	450	−17	−9
Dairy cow	500	−26	−13
Sheep			
Ewe (maintenance)	50	−11	−4
Ewe (shorn)	50	+17	+20
Newborn lamb	4	+19	+24
Growing lamb	35	−13	−3

From Webster[3]

It is worth stressing that European cattle tend to be tolerant to cold but intolerant to heat. Their 'comfort zone' is between about 0 and 20°C. The critical temperature leading to a decline in milk yield at the higher level is approximately 21–25°C for most European cattle, including Friesians and Jerseys, but as high as 30–32°C with Brown Swiss.[4] In Brahman cattle, however, it may be as high as 38°C before production is affected, so it is clear there are considerable differences between European and tropical cattle. Whereas the tropical breeds, such as the Brahman, withstand high temperatures, European and tropical cross-breeds give an intermediate response and maintain a stable body temperature roughly mid-way between the other two, that is, about 30°C.[4]

The effect of high temperatures may be ameliorated in practice in a number of ways. The provision of shade makes a great difference, as do wallows and artificial showers. For example, great benefit has been found in tropical climates with cattle kept under a so-called desert-cooler consisting of a three-sided shelter open to the north, with an upper roof of aluminium which reflects the heat rays, a ceiling underneath of three layers of old hay, and an evaporative cooler under the roof at the south end of the shelter. In general, shade plus sprinklers are more beneficial to milk production than shade alone. It has been recommended that when temperatures rise above 18°C in the open field, and 22°C in the open barns, some protection should be given.[5] Provision of shadc and sprinklers in summer when average maximum temperatures ranged from 30 to 33.3°C gave up to 2.5 kg more milk per day than shade alone.[6] At high temperatures farm stock also attempt to reduce their heat production by reducing their feed intake. Under hot sunny conditions the temperate breeds in particular spend less time in grazing. In fact, under these conditions most of the grazing will be done at night. There are very marked breed differences, as might be expected, the tropical breeds being least affected.

In loose housing systems with open-fronted barns, protection from solar radiation and maximum provision of air movement represents the limit of environmental improvement. With closed buildings, such as the cowhouse, air conditioning may be used and, in parts of the world where climatic temperatures warrant it, has been found worthwhile.

Cattle floors

With cattle, as with other farm livestock, floor design is critical to thermal comfort, physical comfort, health and security. The animal stands, exercises, moves around, lies down and excretes on the floor so that it must, depending on the needs of the moment, be non-slippery, well-drained and comfortably soft, warm and dry, and also easy to clean mechanically. Of the various materials used, wooden slats, asphalt, rubber mats or damp straw can be said to be neutral types of floor because total sensible heat loss from a calf or an adult dairy cow would not differ significantly, according to whether the animal is standing up or lying down. Concrete, whether wet or dry, has a very high thermal conductivity, which is not improved greatly by underfloor insulation since most of the conductive heat loss from the individual animal is transmitted laterally. A calf lying on concrete is cold when the air temperature falls below 17°C. Straw or other bedding greatly helps in reducing heat loss due to the lowering of conductance heat loss, a generation of warmth within the straw or bedding by fermentation, and a reduction of heat loss by convection. Also, a bedded floor is comfortable and calves therefore lie down for a longer period.

Cows must be on a warm surface but there is also a need, especially for the milking cow, for it to be hygienic. It must also be emphasized that a cow lying on a hard, cold floor is not only more likely to injure her teats each time she changes position, she also changes position more often, presumably because she is uncomfortable. A survey by Murphy[7] has shown that all injuries were much more prevalent on concrete slats, and feet were in much better condition too if there was a good straw bed. However any bedding that is used must be kept thoroughly clean and dry. This means regular attention with renewal of the soiled parts.

Sheep

Sheep have a relatively lower heat production per unit area than cattle because their fleece provides excellent thermo-insulation. The housed adult sheep in full fleece is seldom if ever cold.

Ewes that are housed should be sheared for the following reasons: The ewes take up less space, including trough space, so that about 20 per cent more can be kept per pen; the ewes eat more, they have heavier lambs and pregnancy toxaemia is less likely; it is also easier to spot the off-colour animal; there are fewer problems with lice and keds; and the quality of the shorn fleece is improved.

There are also some disadvantages. Shearing the ewe increases feed costs. It is also most important to use good quality housing if the sheep are not to suffer from cold and draught so that they huddle together, which greatly increases the danger of respiratory disease. Sometimes, too, there is wool loss and rubbing.

One of the main reasons for housing ewes is to ensure individual care at lambing time. Prevention of hypothermia in the newborn lamb is, of course, one consideration, but only a small one. It is common practice, unless the weather is extremely severe, to turn ewes and lambs out of doors as soon as possible to minimize the disease risk especially of enteric disease, even though it is likely that the lambs will be below the lower critical temperature for lambs born in winter or early spring.

To summarize, there is no class of healthy ruminant for which the direct effects of low air temperature *per se* are likely to cause intolerable stress in the temperate and cool zones of the world. Moreover, the effects of air temperature on food conversion efficiency below the critical temperature are likely to affect only the smallest animals and at a time when their daily intake is very small relative to lifetime requirements. Thus there are no sound economic grounds for providing any more environmental control for the healthy ruminant animal than shelter from excessive air movement and precipitation.

PIGS

The young piglet is very poorly endowed with hair or subcutaneous fat and has a thin skin. Losses in piglets are relatively high, generally running at about 10–15 per cent before weaning. Surveys indicate that there is a definite seasonal effect, losses being at their worst from November to March. These losses are reduced by good housing (Fig. 3.3). Moreover many losses are due to chilling and crushing, both factors that can be dealt with by good environmental control and housing. The vast majority of the losses due to poor environmental control occur in the first few days of life: thereafter the effects of poor environment are to cause not so much mortality and disease as a loss in productivity, in respect of both liveweight gain and food conversion efficiency. By adulthood pigs have become reasonably adaptable to a wide range of conditions which are not markedly different from those of other farm livestock.

Piglets

Newborn piglets have a poorly developed heat regulating ability although their homeothermic (i.e. temperature control) mechanisms develop quickly. During the first few hours after birth the body temperature depression under cool housing conditions may be as much as 7°C though the average under satisfactory conditions will be approximately 2°C. The heavier piglet is able to withstand climatic changes and cooling better than the small piglet. It is also much better able to resist crushing. There is significant correlation between the weight of a pig and its ability to withstand cold stress. This underlines the importance of the management of the sow in pregnancy in influencing the viability of the litter. Metabolic rates of pigs at air temperatures of 15, 20, 25 and 30°C showed that the 'critical' temperatures of those pigs fed ad lib exceeded 30°C for pigs weighing 6 kg and under (say, up to 2 weeks) and was 20°C for pigs weighing 10 kg (at say 4 weeks).

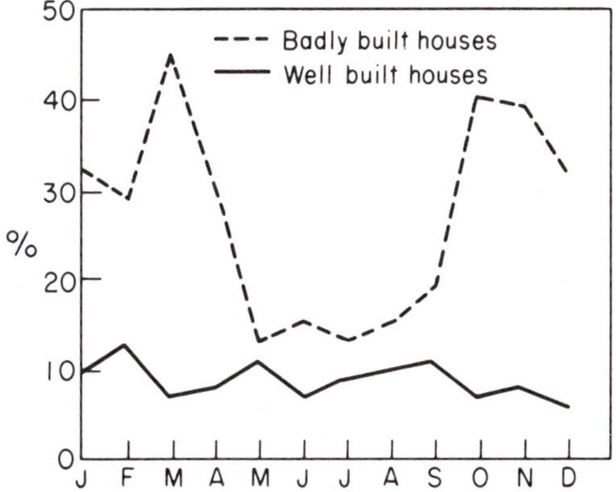

Fig. 3.3 Comparison of piglet losses throughout the year in badly built and well-built houses.

As to the heat loss, evaporative heat loss accounts for only about 10 per cent of total heat loss. The remaining 90 per cent is dependent on the floor. On concrete about 15 per cent is to the floor, 40 per cent by radiation and 35 per cent by convection. On wood only 6 per cent is to the floor; and on polystyrene a mere 2 per cent. Substituting 12 mm of wood for 25 mm of concrete is equivalent to raising the floor temperature by 12°C. Raising the air speed from 0.1 to 0.3 m/s is equivalent to lowering the air temprature by 13°C.[10,11,12]

These findings agree with the observations made by the authors regarding the comfort level of piglets and given in Fig. 3.4, which show that by doubling air velocities the air temperature requirements rise by 12°C. All these facts emphasize the need for straw, shavings or other bedding to be placed over the concrete floor and the necessity for warmth and protection from high air movement. If these exacting provisions are successfully achieved, the piglets are encouraged to lie away from the sow and the danger of crushing is greatly reduced. It has also been shown that the changes in metabolic rate of a *group* of young pigs exposed to falling environmental temperature tend to correspond to those of a *single* pig of the same total weight.

Temperature	Air movement below 0.15 m/sec	Air movement from 0.15-0.25 m/sec	Air movement from 0.25-0.38 m/sec
21°C	Pigs of all ages comfortable	Pigs of all ages comfortable	Young piglets uncomfortable (1-8 weeks)
18°C	Pigs below 1 week uncomfortable	Pigs below 5 weeks uncomfortable	Pigs below 12 weeks uncomfortable
15°C	Pigs below 10 days uncomfortable	Young piglets (c.1-3 weeks old) uncomfortable	Pigs below 12 weeks uncomfortable
13°C	Pigs below 8 weeks uncomfortable	Pigs below 12 weeks uncomfortable	Pigs below 14 weeks uncomfortable
10°C	Pigs below 15 weeks uncomfortable	Pigs below c.16 weeks uncomfortable	Pigs below 16 weeks uncomfortable
7°C	Pigs below 20 weeks uncomfortable	Pigs below 14 weeks uncomfortable	Pigs below 20 weeks uncomfortable
4°C	Pigs below 20 weeks uncomfortable	Pigs below 20 weeks uncomfortable	Pigs below 20 weeks uncomfortable
2°C	All fattening pigs uncomfortable		

Fig. 3.4 The combined effect of ambient temperature and air movement on the comfort of pigs.

Growers and fatteners

Classical work on fattening pigs studied the effect of temperatures between 4 and 42°C with a relative humidity of about 50 per cent and constant air velocity of 0.13–0.18 m/s. The daily gain reached a maximum at 23°C for 45 kg pigs, reducing to 18°C approximately at 90–94 kg (bacon weight). The rate of gain was severely reduced when air temperature varied from the optimum, with the most rapid reduction occurring with the air temperature above the optimum. When air temperature was 38°C, all pigs at 67 kg or over lost weight. The daily rate of gain of any size of pig tested was 900 g or more at the optimum temperature. It was also found that at the temperature at which the maximum weight gain took place, the food was converted at its maximum efficiency (Fig. 3.5).

Although these data are reliable, there are a number of conflicting reports that suggest that in practice the range may be wider than indicated above. For animals penned in groups, as opposed to being penned separately, can thrive at lower house temperatures owing to the effects of huddling and the reduction of radiation loss.

Data from Scandinavia show that *with adequate bedding* pigs may do as well between 4 and 10°C as between 16 and 21°C, while from Northern Ireland we find a temperature range of 27–29°C favoured, although most data suggest that above 24°C feed consumption begins to decline.[15]

Whether the temperature for the fattener is constant or fluctuating ('cycling') seems to make little difference provided that the mean of the cycling temperature is about the same as that of a constant temperature, and variation above or below this mean does not exceed approximately 6°C (12°C total) in a 24 hour period.[16]

Moustgaard et al.[17] suggested that the optimum temperature of fatteners lies between 11 and 20°C, which is midway between the recommendation of the Californian and Ulster workers on the one hand, and the Swedish evidence on the other. Essentially, their work shows a considerable tolerance and acclimatization of pigs to various temperatures, but it does not indicate that temperatures

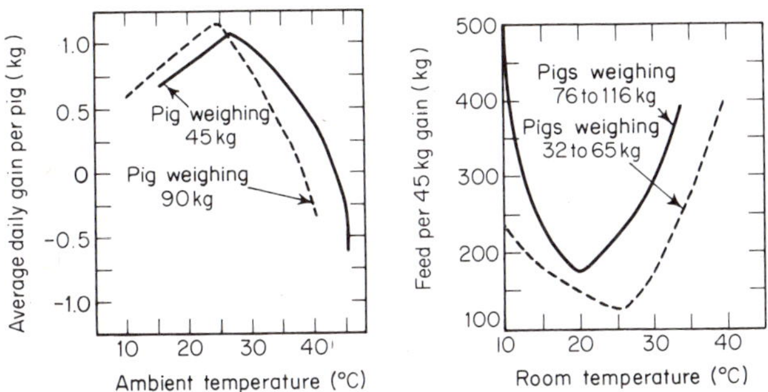

Fig. 3.5 The relationship between ambient (air) temperature and the live-weight gain and feed conversion efficiency of pigs.

should be allowed to vary greatly diurnally. Food consumption also may not be too adversely affected, provided that the pig is given time to acclimatize to the temperature regimen imposed upon it. How the control temperature shifts as pigs get older and how much food is wasted if the temperature is too low is shown in Table 3.3 which is reproduced from the work of Dr Close of the ARC Institute of Animal Physiology at Babraham, Cambridge.

Temperature *per se* is not a good indicator of the environmental requirements for keeping fattening pigs, any more than it is for piglets, and full consideration must also be given to air movement, humidity and radiation from surrounding surfaces.

Some mention should be made of the 'Turkish bath' atmosphere that has been found successful in Northern Ireland and described graphically by Gordon.[18] The temperature is kept at about 24–29°C and the relative humidity approaches 100 per cent. The moist climate has physiological advantages in the prevention and alleviation of respiratory infections and the high ventilation and 'sedimentation' rates produced by the humidity lead to a good degree of air purity in the atmosphere. Gordon found that the bacteria-carrying particles in 'Turkish bath' houses tend to be much fewer in number and larger in size than

Table 3.3 *Temperature requirements for pigs*

(a) The relation between body-weight, food intake and critical temperature for groups of pigs at levels of intake normally applied in practice

Body wt (kg)	Food intake (kg/day) 0.5	1.0	1.5	2.0	2.5	3.0	3.5
	Critical temperature (°C)						
20	21	14					
40		20	14	8			
60			18	13	8		
80				16	11	7	
100				18	13	9	
120					15	11	8

(b) The additional food requirements necessary to maintain optimum growth rates at environmental temperatures below the optimum

Body wt (kg)	Range of optimum temps (°C)	Range of food intakes equivalent to ranges of critical temperature (kg/day)	Decrease in temperature below optimum (°C) −2	−4	−6	−8	−10
			Additional food requirements (g/day)				
20	20–14	0.5–1.0	25	50	75	100	125
40	20–8	1.0–2.0	31	62	92	123	154
60	18–8	1.5–2.5	36	72	108	145	181
80	16–7	2.0–3.0	42	83	125	166	208
100	18–9	2.0–3.0	47	94	141	188	235
120	15–8	2.5–3.5	53	105	158	210	263

in normal piggeries. Thus they are more effectively trapped in the nose, which in part explains the low incidence of coughing and pneumonia. The success of this system can therefore be attributed to its environment, which is highly antagonistic to disease-causing agents, allied to the skill of the stockman in controlling these conditions so that they do not become lethal to the pigs.

This has been confirmed in some interesting comparative studies of housing systems by O'Grady[19] in Ireland where it was found that high humidities reduced the incidence of pneumonia. However, although it is apparent that there can be benefits to the pig from the maintenance of carefully controlled high humidity and warm temperatures, a practical warning must be given that excessively high values of either can be dangerous.

Environment and carcase quality

In the work of Moustgaard et al. already referred to, it was found that the hightest protein deposition took place in an approximate range of 15–23°C, which was the temperature giving fastest growth and lowest food conversion rates. Fuller[20], with single pigs, in contrast to Moustgaard's groups of pigs, found that nitrogen retention was highest at 25°C and lowest at 10 and 30°C, which is in good agreement with Moustgaard's studies, bearing in mind that single pigs will lose heat more readily and thus require a higher temperature.[20]

Referring to carcase quality, it has been shown that at low air temperatures the nitrogen retention was reduced relatively more than the rate of gain, so that the carcase became fatter. It seems from this work that the least fatty carcase is produced at about 16°C with 70 per cent RH. Both lower and higher temperatures and higher humidities tended to give fatter carcases. Holme and Coey[21] found that baconers penned individually did better and had better carcase length at a temperature of 21°C over the weight range 18–90 kg than at 12°C, while Smith and Tonks[42] with ad lib-fed pigs between 23 and 90 kg compared 28°C and 92 per cent RH with 21°C and 70 per cent RH. No effect resulted on the dressing-out percentage, carcase length, depth of back-fat, colour and pH of eye muscle. There was, however, a 27 per cent slower growth rate at the higher temperature and humidity.

Lighting needs of pigs

Braude et al.[22] investigated the effect of light on fattening pigs. They tried the following regimes: continuous darkness – that is, 24 hours' total darkness; periods of 14 hours' light and 10 hours' darkness; 10 hours' light and 14 hours' darkness; and 24 hours' light. In terms of weight gain or feed per kg gain, there were no significant differences in any treatment. There is thus much to be said for keeping fattening pigs in fairly dim conditions, provided that there is sufficient light for management, feeding and the maintenance of clean habits. The absence of windows prevents heat loss through bad insulation of glass and simplifies the construction of the house.

Similarly negative findings on the effect of light on pigs have been recorded by other workers, although Scholz[23] did find a slightly favourable effect by darkening the pens: feed conversion was improved by 3 per cent and liveweight gain by 4 per cent.

More recently Russian workers have shown the importance of the length of lighting period for breeding females. Their work showed that when gilts were given an 18-hour light period per day, they produced a stronger, longer and more regular oestrus than gilts exposed to a 6-hour lighting period. They also compared the effects on gilts of 17 hours' continuous and natural lighting conditions, the last being not dissimilar from the northern parts of Britain in winter. The Russian investigators found that gilts exposed to the longer periods produced from 0.8 to 2.7 more piglets in their first litter compared to the controls, so that it can be recommended that 17 hours' illumination be given to gilts for 10–20 days before mating and during gestation.

There is no doubt of the practical implications of this work, because in recent years breeding sows have often been kept under dim conditions most of the time. While the Russians have not found definite evidence of the effect on sows, as opposed to gilts, there is a possibility that some of the breeding troubles in intensively-kept sows may be due to the poor attention given to lighting. A longer and brighter period of light should be given during suckling and for at least 25 days after service.[24]

Summarizing, it would seem that while the temperature requirements of the grower are well defined for the individually housed pig without bedding, a wider tolerance is acceptable in practice, where acclimatization, grouping effects and bedding can alter the picture considerably. Nevertheless the limits are reasonably well known for temperature, but this is not the case with air movement and humidity, on which much less work has been done.

The effects of humidity appear to be associated more with an indirect one of disease, but a more accurate definition of these effects is needed. A great deal more study is also required on the use of supplementary heating, where the picture is confusing in terms of both the type of heat required and the prime *economic* temperature to maintain.

Breeding pigs

Most of the investigation done on sows has been concerned with the ill-effects of high temperatures. Even though sows exposed to temperatures as high as 37°C for periods of about eight days could still generally produce normal litters, it seemed however that in-pig sows showed more stress than empty ones owing to the increased metabolic load. The best temperature for the sow is not the best for the piglet, the litter thriving best at 27°C and the sow at approximately 16°C. Where temperatures habitually stay above 29°C the provision of cooling devices such as sprinklers, sprays and wallows is justified, in addition to shade. Many reports from warm regions confirm this.[25,26] For example, Whatley in Oklahoma farrowed an average of 2.35 more live piglets per litter by sprinkling a group of pregnant sows, in comparison with an untreated group. The average maximum daily temperature was 36°C. However, to the farmer in temperate climates, the problems of high summer temperatures are acute only under exceptional circumstances and much work remains to be done on the climatic needs of the breeding pig. For example, the special needs of the pregnant sow under the less generous rationing systems now advised, or the relatively immobile conditions of the sow stall. It is reasonable to assume that such animals would require higher temperatures than those kept, for example, in deeply strawed yards or kennels under traditional feeding programmes. There is also no clear definition of the first few days after farrowing, when it is known that the sow's metabolic rate is much reduced and therefore its susceptibility to chilling may be increased.

Stocking rates

It is important to stock a building to its maximum capacity; a full pen of pigs is usually the cleanest and most comfortable group. Nevertheless there is some evidence to show that one should at least proceed with caution in packing pigs in tightly. Results of extensive trials with pigs stocked at 0.46, 0.92 and 1.8 m^2 per head are shown in Table 3.4.[27] These show strikingly the bad effect of over-stocking, though obviously economic considerations have to be considered to balance the final decision.

Investigations on the effect of numbers of pigs per pen were conducted by the same investigators and are shown in Table 3.5.

It is apparent from this work that fatteners benefit quite markedly from plenty of space and small pen size. This is supported by the work of Gehlbach et al.[28] who conducted experiments with 600 fatteners fed ad lib on different types of floor in groups of up to 16 pigs at different stocking densities. They found that group size affected level of performance and that the best group size was governed by the size and weight of the pig and by the environment. A lower rate of gain took place at the higher stocking densities, which it was believed was due to lower food consumption due to heat stress. The feed conversion was not affected by the stocking density in these experiments, although this is not a general finding.

Scholz studied fatteners in groups of 1, 10, 25, 90, 210 and 530 pigs.[23] He found that with restricted feeding regimens 30 pigs are a maximum, and for ad lib feeding not more than 90. He found the best results of all were when groups

Table 3.4 *Stocking rates for pigs*

m^2 per pig	Gain in wt during experiment (lg)	Average daily feed (kg)	Feed per unit gain (kg)
0.46	40.4	2.4	4.09
0.92	42.0	2.37	3.86
1.8	45.0	2.36	3.69

Table 3.5 *Weight gain effects from stocking rates*

No. of pigs per pen	Gain (kg)	Average daily gain (kg)	Feed per unit gain (kg)
3	42.7	2.56	4.15
6	42.5	2.32	3.79
12	42.2	2.26	3.71

stayed in the same pen throughout the fattening period with the pen size restricted by sliding sides. It is interesting that Scholz recommends very high stocking rates: 0.18 m^2 per pig to 41 kg, 0.28 m^2 from 41 to 59 kg, 0.37 m^2 from 59 to 79 kg, and 0.46 m^2 up to 109 kg; but with high air movement rates in the pens of 0.5 m/s, which is about twice the usual rate in the lying area.

The harmful effects of heavy stocking seem sufficiently pronounced at least to be noted carefully by the designer and farmer. About 12–20 pigs per pen is probably the ideal number and is unlikely ever to be an unwise or an uneconomic choice; extremely dense stocking may, however, retard the growth of pigs unless the environmental conditions are carefully maintained at the optimum.

POULTRY

The most widely used method of brooding chicks is to arrange in a limited area of a house a source of warmth of about 35°C (95°F) at one day old and then subsequently reduce this by 3°C (5°F) a week. In conventional brooding systems there is a tendency to place too large groups of chicks under a source of heat with a ring of food and water outside this hottest area. This makes it difficult for the chicks in the centre of the group to reach food and water. As chick-crumbs or mini-pellets are placed for easy access on the floor on paper or cardboard it may be that the water is the most difficult facility for the chicks to find. It is absolutely essential that chick water containers are placed close enough to each other that as a chick moves, it cannot possibly avoid contacting them.

Brooding systems with large warmed areas have considerable merit. They enable a wider distribution of birds in environmentally suitable areas with more space available, factors which are known to improve growth and reduce the likelihood of disease. To ensure a good use of the house, the ambient temperature is at least as important as the brooder temperature, a range of 25–30°C (75–85°F) being associated with the best all-round performance. Below and above this range, weight gains and food conversion efficiencies are reduced. The best performance will probably be obtained if the house temperature is reduced from 30°C (86°F) during the first week to 27°C (81°F) in the second, and 24°C (65°F) in the third (Fig. 3.6).

The worst results are associated with correct brooder temperatures and low house temperatures, i.e. below 20°C (68°F), when the chicks are reluctant to venture away from the heat to find food and water. On the other hand, too

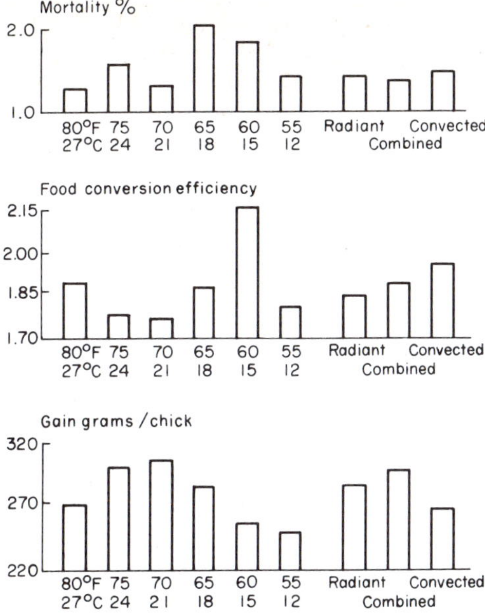

Fig. 3.6 Mortality, food conversion and gain at various temperatures, and with different types of brooders.

high a house temperature depresses appetite and retards activity and growth. The heat source from the brooder and space heater should be capable of reaching a maximum of at least 4 kW per 1000 chicks to provide these conditions in well-constructed houses and a maximum availability of up to 6 kw is preferable.

If the chicks are to be evenly distributed within the brooding area the temperature must be uniform and draughts at floor level avoided. The conventional but now rather old-fashioned arrangement of having solid brooder surrounds about 1 m high is generally satisfactory in achieving this and still has a place in poor buildings but it has been superseded by warming a large area and reducing air velocities over the whole house. Overhead, largely radiant sources of heat give the most satisfactory results since their fine thermostat control and adjustable height offer flexibility. They also serve the dual purpose of brooding and space heating (Fig. 3.7). As an alternative, however, blown hot air has its advocates because of its simplicity, low running costs and good space heating qualities. An initial tempeature of 31°C (88°F) is recommended. This represents something of a compromise between the ideal and house temperature. There should be a reduction of about 0.5°C (1°F) daily until a level of 18–21°C (65–70°F) is reached. All changes should be made steadily and regularly to avoid stress to the birds. Sometimes attempts are made to blow air great distances from one end of the house to the other which creates considerable draughts and uneven air temperatures. To compensate for this it is necessary to lift the temperature several degrees. This can be both costly and unsatisfactory for productivity and the health of the chicks. The correct procedure is to avoid this

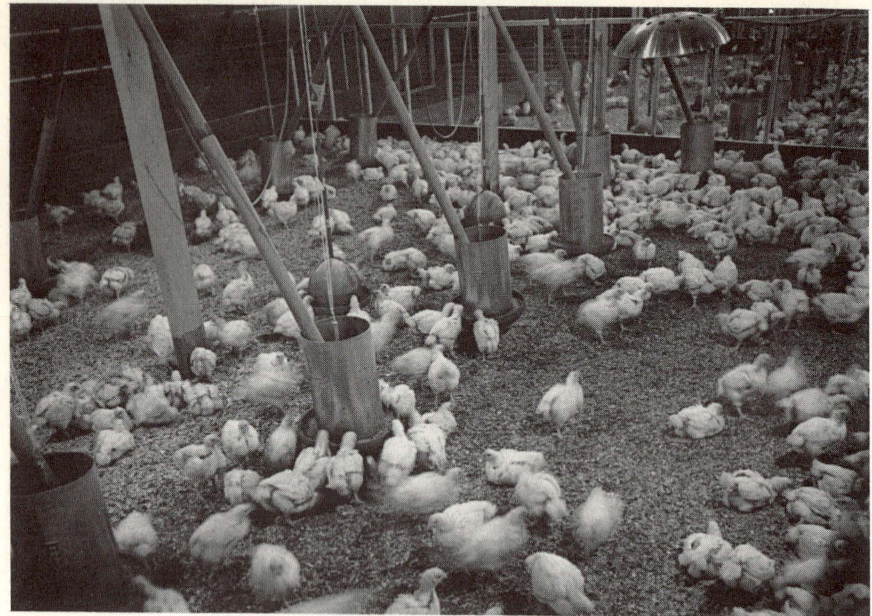

Fig. 3.7 Chicks at approximately four weeks of age, well spread out under the warmth of the heater but still with numerous drinkers and feeders.

set of circumstances altogether, either by ducting the hot air along the length or width of the house, or so integrating with the ventilation system that the incoming air is heated as it comes into the house, perhaps through a central intake duct under the ridge taking a mixture of hot and fresh air combined. The very dry air conditions produced by hot-air systems are not entirely favourable to the bird's health and well-being (see p. 55).

Post-brooding temperatures[29]

From the age of three weeks some further reductions in temperature are justified. In the case of broilers, the house temperature should be in the range 18–21°C (65–70°F) with a definite tendency to the upper figure if there is any danger of the temperature dropping below 18°C (65°F) owing to external conditions (Fig. 3.8). Under ideal conditions the best growth takes place between 18–21°C (65–70°F) and certain broiler growers are already achieving this by taking great care that reductions to this range are made very gradually, as already mentioned, so that the change is almost imperceptible to the birds and at the same time ventilation is maintained without draughts. However, in many cases the heat source does not allow the poultryman to adjust the temperature so finely or gradually whilst sometimes the ventilation arrangements are inadequate with the higher air velocities demanding a higher temperature to compensate for the

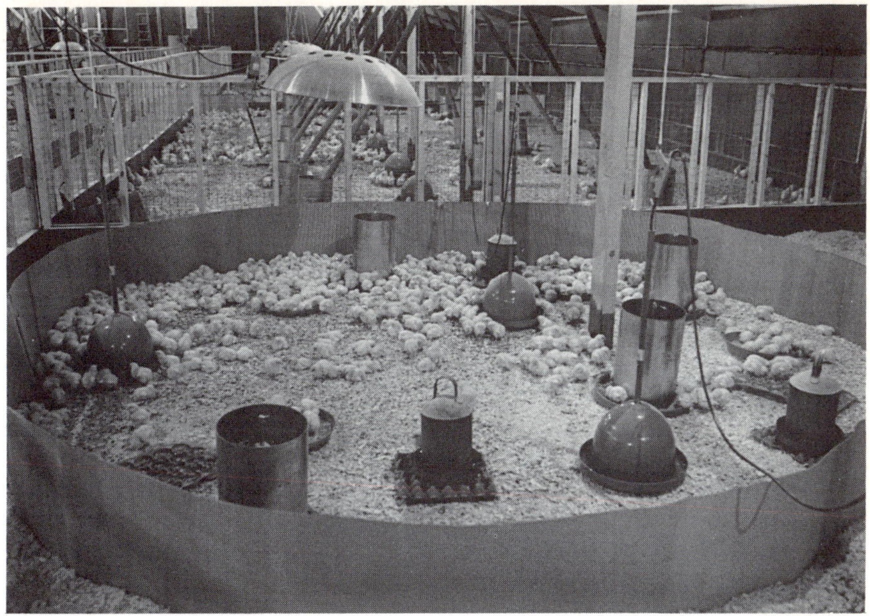

Fig. 3.8 Chicks in the early stages of brooding. Note the overhead gas heaters and numerous drinkers and feeders on wood-shaving litter.

cooling effect. Nevertheless, if the ventilation conditions can be maintained satisfactorily, a reduction of some 6°C (11°F) between three and nine weeks, giving an eventual temperature of 13–16°C (55–60°F), is desirable for optimum growth. These temperatures tend to be somewhat lower than those in common practice but their maintenance has important repercussions in reducing heating and ventilation costs and cutting down the effect and incidence of respiratory disease. Obviously low temperatures cannot be maintained in summer but this is compensated for to some extent by increasing the ventilation and air velocity, if the fans have the capacity to achieve it.

Temperature for layers[29]

For intensively kept birds, the optimal temperature is high – about 21°C (70°F). At temperatures below this there is a depression of about $\frac{1}{2}$ egg per hen housed per year for each 0.5°C (1°F). Feed intake will be reduced by about 7 g per bird per day for a rise of 15–21°C (60–70°F). On the debit side, there is some depression in egg weight, estimated to be about 1 g per egg per 3°C (6°F) rise over 15°C (60°F) but this is far outweighed by the benefits. It is estimated that if a house is kept at 21°C (70°F) rather than 15°C (60°F), then the potential saving in terms of profit margins could be as much as a 20–30 per cent increase in profit.

It should be emphasized that the hen is reasonably adaptable and tolerant to environmental changes and there is a wide range within which it can produce economically even if not at an optimal rate. The range is about 5–24°C (40–75°F). However, this does not mean that the temperature can fluctuate rapidly between these two extremes since rapid changes of any sort are undesirable. Rather, it represents the seasonal extremes one should aim for at the outset in designing the housing in the case of less intensive systems than the battery, such as deep litter and the straw yard. Provided the changes take place gradually birds can acclimatize themselves. For short-term variation, as between day and night, a maximum of 6°C (11°F) is a good target.

If the temperature rises above 24°C (75°F) for long periods the total number of eggs laid and their weight and quality will certainly suffer. Appetite will also fall. Below 5°C (40°F) the chief effect will be a sharply rising appetite, though egg weight and quality can benefit slightly. It may be possible to compensate for the depressed appetite at high temperatures by increasing the essential nutrients in the ration and so producing as many eggs of almost as good quality on a reduced – and hence more economical – quality of food. At present, however, most compounders' rations are geared to the 5–24°C (40–75°F) range.

The humidity of the air

There is no reason to have a rigid range for the humidity of the air though in practice the aim in winter will be to keep the relative humidity below about 80 per cent of saturation and preferably nearer to a maximum of 75 per cent. If the advice given in the section on thermal insulation and ventilation rates is followed, this should be possible. In the normal way there need be no problems with chicken if the relative humidity is low, but this does not hold if the birds are suffering from respiratory disease, and thus the evidence is that humidities below 50 per cent to some extent, and especially if they go as low as 30 per cent, may aggravate infection and help contagion.

Water cooling

Problems sometimes occur in temperate climates, and often in hot climates, of buildings becoming overheated either briefly or for quite long periods. This may sometimes arise from poor thermal insulation of the building, or there may be insufficient fans or these may be operating inefficiently. If these obvious faults cannot be corrected, or in cases where after correction it is still too warm, there are several ways of using water to cool the building.

A simple device is to spray water on the roof and walls, thereby effecting cooling by evaporation. In some cases a perforated waterpipe is placed along the roof ridge to discharge water uniformly along the length of the roof. A more common method is to draw the incoming air through wet pads. The pads may consist of a wooden frame filled with absorbent wood fibres with water running through from top to bottom. Surplus water has to be collected and recirculated for economy and the pads must be kept clean if they are to function successfully.

A still better way is to install spray nozzles which produce a very fine mist. They do, however, need a pump and run-off for surplus water.

Perhaps the best of all methods consists of a metal disc revolving at high speed which throws off water on to an atomizing plate. This sets up a very fine mist taken up by the air stream. Good control is achievable by a solenoid valve activated by a humidistat.

Lighting requirements[30]

In nature, the development of the reproductive (egg-laying) organ is stimulated by increasing amounts of daylight, as in spring, but is depressed when this is reduced, as in autumn. The modern genetically-improved layer, under the stimulus of spring-like conditions, will lay before sufficient bodily development has taken place fully to support egg production; it will not be able to lay either the number of eggs or the larger sizes of which it will later be capable. An autumn-like pattern, or even a constant day length, will allow the body to develop properly before the bird starts laying. Thereafter, to stimulate maximum production, the procedure is to give a weekly increase of light duration of about 20 minutes up to a maximum of 16–18 hours. Artificial lighting is, of course, essential if this is to be achieved in all seasons, though by rearing chicks in the autumn, the natural advantage of seasonal changes can be used.

There are a number of techniques available to achieve the most favourable response. Each breeder will suggest something different for his own stock, based on his sound, practical experience. Two programmes are given below for a well-known commercial hybrid. It is noteworthy that the maximum amount of light in one day is 18 hours. However, many poultrymen prefer to go no further than 16 hours so they can give an extra boost if egg production for any reason shows signs of tailing-off.

A suggested lighting programme for commercial hybrid layers is:

0–1 week	18 hours' light, 6 hours' darkness.
2–18 weeks	6 hours' light, 18 hours' darkness.
19–22 weeks	Increase light by 45 minutes per week to give a good stimulus at the first period of laying.
23–49 weeks	Increase light by 20 minutes per week.
49 weeks onwards	The lighting is kept steady at 18 hours light per day.

Those retailing eggs and seeking especially large eggs can follow the following variant:

0–1 week	23 hours' light.
2–18 weeks	Decrease by 45 minutes per week.
19–22 weeks	Increase by 45 minutes per week.
23–48 weeks	Increase by 20 minutes per week.
49 weeks onwards	Retain at 18 hours of light.

A new lighting technique that has recently been developed is the use of ahemeral lighting cycles. These are daily light cycles greater or less than 24 hours. These are not capable of modifying egg output but they can improve egg weight and shell strength so that there can be economic advantages to the farmer if prices for larger eggs are favourable. The number of second-quality eggs can also be reduced. A 28-hour light cycle which uses bright and then dimmed lights has real advantages. The dim lights enable egg collection and stock inspection at any time even during the birds' 'night' period; the bright lights have 30 times more intensity than the dim and thus simulate 'day' (bright) and 'night' (dim). A suitable ahemeral lighting programme as devised by the Poultry Department of the North of Scotland College of Agriculture is shown in Fig. 3.9.

For broilers the usual pattern throughout most of the industry is to have 23 hours' lighting and 1 hour's darkness in each 24 hours, the latter being necessary to accustom the birds to darkness. If this is not done and the light is suddenly withdrawn for any reason, a pile-up is a likely consequence, the birds tending to crowd into corners and suffocate.

There is, however, an increasing interest now in growing broilers on the intermittent lighting patterns which were once popular, as they appear capable of some improvement in growth rate but more particularly in the food conversion ratio. They are capable of improving digestion with suitable rest periods and decreasing activity. There will be a reduction in electricity usage which will result in at least a marginal saving.

A suitable lighting pattern would be as follows:

0–3 weeks	Continuous lighting (with 1 hour off in 24)
3–5 week cycle	3 hours on, 1 hour off
5–7 week cycle	2 hours on, 2 hours off
7 weeks onwards cycle	1 hour on, 3 hours off

If intermittent lighting programmes are used it is vital that the highest amount

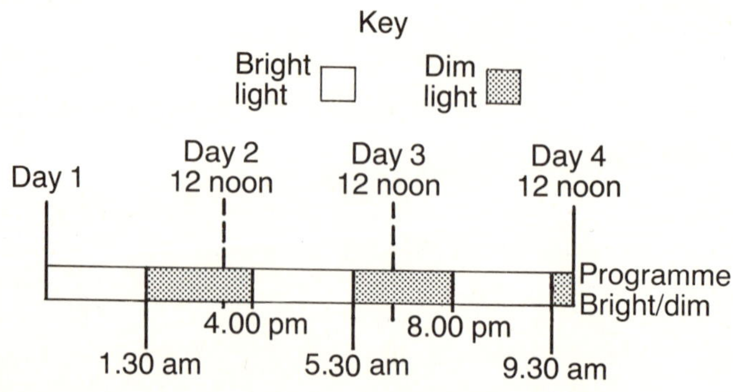

Fig. 3.9 Lighting programme for the 28-hour ahemeral light cycles.

of feeder and drinker space availability be provided as the pressure will be much greater on both than with continuous programmes.

Continuous lighting for broilers can be with a light intensity as low as 0.2 lux, which is about as low as the 'off' phase in a controlled environment house in the daytime.

The lighting procedure

For proper artificial control of lighting, exclusion of all natural light must be complete. Fully efficient baffles under fan shafts or in air inlet hoods and around the edges of the ventilators are essential. Various techniques are shown in the chapter on ventilation (Chapter 5) and it is pertinent to stress that methods used to baffle light entry also serve as draught and wind baffles, and vice versa. The insides of the ventilators should be painted black. The maximum safe level of intensity of extraneous light entering houses which are supposed to be blacked out is 0.4 lux and it is advisable, if there are any doubts on this score, to check the intensity on a light meter. To stimulate layers, the light intensity should be 10–16 lux: there is no advantage in raising the level above this.

If light intensity is uneven in the house, with bright and dark areas, the birds will favour and concentrate in certain areas. This may cause the development of vices and diseases, particularly respiratory ones. In every poultry house lighting circuit a dimming device is necessary, so that light intensity can be lowered easily should there be an outbreak of cannibalism. If birds are to receive sufficient and even light intensity, the disposition of the lights must be uniform. This uniformity is usually obtained by suspending ordinary tungsten bulbs at about 3 m (10 ft) centres along and across the house. A reflector over the bulb will assist in maintaining an even intensity and will help to keep the bulbs free of settled dust.

Suitable systems of lighting are now marketed which utilize fluorescent lighting tubes with dimming arrangements and whilst the capital cost of these is somewhat greater than tungsten bulbs, their increased efficiency enables a substantial saving in running costs which can soon recoup the higher initial charge.

ENVIRONMENTAL FACTORS AFFECTING SUSCEPTIBILITY TO DISEASE

In recent years there have been profound changes in the health status of the farm livestock population. By several processes many of the well-known diseases caused by single disease agents have been eliminated or brought under control. Often this has been done by slaughtering all infected animals following the development of good diagnostic tests. By this method diseases such as tuberculosis, foot-and-mouth disease, swine fever, Newcastle disease and sheep scab have been eliminated from many parts of the world. Now, with great energy being spent on their total elimination the prospects of this being achieved are good. Other diseases are controlled very effectively by the use of vaccines which may be the first step towards their eventual elimination. Examples of these conditions are the clostridial infections of the bovine and ovine species, swine erysipelas, infectious bursal disease of poultry and certain forms of salmonellosis. In addition, control of many diseases is effected by the use of antibiotics and chemotherapeutic drugs, but this method used on the livestock farm tends to suppress the effects but not eliminate the infection, so that variants of the pathogenic organism subsequently develop which are resistant to the drugs used and possibly a wide spectrum of other similar drugs. The disease may persist with strains of the organism that are resistant to many antibiotics now taking over.

Thus, in the place of the reasonably well-defined overt disease conditions that were experienced in the past, we are now faced with a totally different set of circumstances, where the effects of pathogens may be just as serious but the farmer may not even be aware that his animals are infected. For many of the organisms that cause ill-health in the intensive livestock unit are normally present in the animals and the environment and it is the environmental stress that acts as a trigger inducing their multiplication to such an extent that clinically obvious disease breaks out. There are numerous examples, such as pneumonia and mastitis in the bovine animals, diarrhoea in the lamb, rhinitis and dysentery in the pig, and septicaemia, gangrenous dermatitis and air sac infection in the chicken. Whilst these diseases may always become obvious in the long run there may be a lengthy period when their effects are limited to poor growth or productivity and an inefficient conversion of feed by the animal. It is an essential feature of a farmer's recording system that he keeps records of productivity which will enable him to detect when results are beginning to deteriorate. This can well be a warning that urgent action is needed to stop a slide in results leading eventually to disease. Most of the conditions of this nature are insidious, chronic and difficult to diagnose by any of the popular methods that are so effective with the well-described diseases. Little use can be made of vaccinations or antisera, nor are antibiotics or drugs an answer. The only effective way is to attend to the animal's whole environment with those methods that are known to reduce the risk of disease.

The main environmental factors, other than those which are concerned with the microclimate, can be listed as follows: cleanliness of the environment and methods of disinfection; limitation of the gross size of the site containing the livestock; the separation by pens and sub-divisions of the stock; depopulation; segregation of age groups; ventilation and air flow; bedding and flooring in general; heating; management of the sick.

The microclimate: factors affecting the dispersal, survival and deposition of pathogens in livestock

Animals live with many potentially pathogenic microorganisms – the major enteric and respiratory diseases are asociated with a multiplicity of agents and it is extremely difficult to reproduce clinical disease by experimental infections even when huge doses of mixed organisms are used.[30] Whether or not an animal becomes clinically affected depends on non-specific factors of climate, housing and husbandry which together form the total environment which is considered in this chapter. Above all it should be made clear that the state of health of the animals can transcend all other factors in determining the economic viability of a livestock enterprise. Disease at its worst kills the animal, but even in sub-lethal infections seriously affects productivity.

The factors influencing the dispersal, survival and deposition of airborne pathogens in farm animals have been reviewed comprehensively by Donaldson (1978).[31] Droplet nuclei are the primary mode of spread of a variety of contagious diseases and many pathogens have been shown to have been spread in this way, via the animal's breath and also from secretions and excretions of the infected animal.

Referring specifically to virus particles, the ambient temperature has little effect on their survival in an animal house but a general trend is that high temperatures are more harmful to their survival than low ones.[32] In fact, it has been suggested that the inactivation of viruses immediately after exhalation and aerosol formation is dependent on the relative humidity; any temperature effect occurs secondarily.[33] The effect of relative humidity on viruses in general is that viruses with a lipoprotein envelope survive best at a low relative humidity, whereas non-enveloped viruses are unstable in dry conditions but survive best at a high relative humidity.[34] Rhinoviruses appear to survive better at high humidities but IBR and P13 viruses at low humidities. In these last examples the differences in survival time reflect the association between seasonal patterns of RH and disease incidence. There is the further possibility that at high RH there is accelerated sedimentation of airborne pathogens in large aerosols. Mycoplasms on the other hand tend to be stable at very low and at high relative humidities, but sensitive to mid-range RH.[35]

So far as bacteria are concerned, a rise in temperature produces an increasing destruction of bacteria, but airborne spores are highly resistant[36] *E. coli* survives and multiplies best at about 15°C, as also do mycoplasms. Bacteria tend to be resistant to low and high RH but sensitive to mid-range RH[37] but bacterial spores are almost totally resistant to RH effects.

It is important to be aware that in airborne infections the size of the infecting dose will determine whether or not disease will result and also its severity[38] and the likelihood of infection making headway will depend on the animal's overall resistance; for example, chilling can markedly lower an animal's resistance to inhaled pathogens by depressing lung clearance mechanisms.[39]

Systems in which the air is recirculated are being favoured as a means of reducing heating costs but in such systems some form of air cleansing (e.g. filtration) may be necessary to avoid a build-up of pathogens.[40]

It is known from the work of Honey and McQuitty (1976)[41] that animal buildings are often very dusty but the factors affecting dust production are ill-defined. Small changes in relative humidity have been found to have significant effects on settled dust; lower humidites result in more settled dust. There is, however, no clear evidence that dust is associated with the passage of pathogens or of disease.

The disposal of large accumulations of animal excrement, bedding and litter is a further problem and can, in some instances, be the limiting factor in determining the size of unit. It is common practice to dilute the effluent from farm buildings into a slurry and then spray it over farmland as a fertilizer. The hazard from the dissemination of slurry-associated pathogens over a wide area in this way can be considerable, particularly in windy weather. A dairy herd of 50 cows plus 50 sows and their litters cause a potential pollution load as large as that of a village of 1000 people, yet frequently the manure is carelessly disposed of without thought of its potential dangers to man or animal.

Intensification and immunity

There are some underlying truths related to disease and immunity which need to be explained as they have a close bearing on the incidence of disease and its relationship to the environment.

An animal at birth has a degree of passive immunity to local disease, which is passed from the dam to the offspring, partly *in utero* and partly from the colostrum or first milk. Such immunity is, however, only practically effective to local infections to which the dam has been challenged. If the birth takes place in a 'foreign' environment, then the young may have little or no passive immunity to the infective organisms in their new local environment. In many cases the young are housed in their youngest stages in such a 'foreign' environment and it is therefore most important that the challenge of disease-causing organisms is reduced to a minimum – all this being done in a variety of ways which are dealt with in this chapter.

Perhaps the most important of these is by the processes of depopulation, and cleansing and disinfection. This is most readily understood in the case of the younger animal which has a poor or uncertain resistance to disease. Whilst it can never be said to be other than advantageous, it is most important on sites which have a large population of animals in an area where there are substantial numbers of animals since many diseases, especially viral ones, can travel a great distance by the airborne route. Whilst small infective particles can be carried directly by dust particles moved by the wind, other pathogens are carried indirectly by vectors, especially birds. It is most unfortunate, from the point of view of disease, that farm animal populations tend to be concentrated in limited areas so that cross-infection between sites can take place much more easily than if the animal population was spread over a country or region more uniformly. As the animal grows, however, there will tend to be an acquired active immunity to local infections so the adult is normally at much less risk.

Disinfection and disease prevention

Animals reared intensively cannot avoid receiving a degree of challenge from potentially pathogenic organisms. A major way of reducing this challenge is by instituting a thorough process of cleansing and disinfection of buildings between batches of animals.

Recently there has been a new condition affecting chiefly broiler chickens, known as the runting and stunting syndrome, which seems to be due to a multiple viral infection the nature of which remains uncertain. Field experience has shown clearly that transverse infection from one crop to a succeeding one allows infection to persist on-site when there may be little problem of vertical infection from breeder to chick. There are many other examples of this phenomenon and disinfection has a vital part to play in arresting the occurrence of persistent infection on the site.

The greatest value this procedure offers is with the young animal which has yet to gain a satisfactory immunity to infection. Disinfection, however, has to be achieved by a thorough and comprehensive procedure if it is to be effective. First, the building must be cleaned as thoroughly as possible of all organic matter. It is even more satisfactory if the building–or preferably whole site–can be depopulated of all the animal population at the same time. If only one animal remains there is a potential reservoir of infection that is capable of undoing much of the value of the disinfection. Also the retention of any animals in the building to be cleaned and disinfected eliminates the possibility of using fumigants as part of the disinfectant process.

Thus the process ideally consists of the following. All the animals are cleared from the building. The buildings and their environs are then cleared of all organic matter which should be removed far from the site. At this stage the building is best cleaned with a pressure hose using a detergent and disinfectant in the water. After this, the house can have an application of any special fumigation and disinfection procedure which is indicated by the type of infection most likely to be harboured by the stock or building in question – for example, glutaraldehyde for viruses, phenolic disinfectants for bacterial spores or organo-phosphorus compounds for parasites. After such a thorough process there is nothing to be gained in leaving the building unused and as soon as it has dried out, and no harmful residues remain, it can be restocked.

Attention should be drawn to the fact that in controlled environment houses with cavities within the structure, especially the insulation of the building, insects may be harboured that can transfer disease from one crop of livestock to another unless they too are destroyed by penetrating fumigation techniques. There are also special dangers of animal accommodation with earth or soil floors. Few disinfectants have very much penetrative power in the presence of soil, though a useful technique is to mix a suitable disinfectant (often a synthetic phenol) with an oil which will soak into the soil and then cover this with tarred paper or polythene before placing the litter or bedding in position. This will separate the next batch of animals from the contaminated soil for some time, during which there will be continuing action by the disinfectant.

REFERENCES

1 Findlay, J. D. and Beakley, W. R. (1954) In *The Physiology of Farm Animals*. London: Butterworth.
2 Brody, S. (1945) *Bioenergetics and Growth*. New York: Reinhold.
3 Webster, A. J. F. (1981) Optimal housing criteria for ruminants. In *Environmental Aspects of Housing for Animal Production*. (Ed: Clark, J. A.) p. 217. London: Butterworth.
4 Brody, S. (1955) Climatic physiology of cattle. *Missouri Agric. Exp. Stn. J.*, Series 1607.
5 Lee, D. H. K. (1959) The status of animal climatology with special reference to hot conditions. *Anim. Breed. Abstr.*, **27**, 1–14.
6 Rusoff, L. L., Miller, H. D. and Frye, J. B. (1955) The effect of cooling on dairy cattle. *La.Agric. Exp. Stn. Bull.*, 497.
7 Murphy, P. (1978) Paper presented at a symposium on *'Injuries to Animals due to Floor Surfaces'*. Cement & Concrete Assoc., Slough, Nov. 1978.
8 Newland, H. W., McMillen, W. N. and Reineke, E. P. (1952) Temperature adaptation in the baby pig. *J. Anim. Sci.*, **11**, 118.
9 Cairne, A. B. and Puller, J. D. (1957) The metabolism of the young pig. *J. Physiol.*, **139**, 15.
10 Mount, L. E. (1966) Heat loss from young pigs. *Report Inst. Anim. Physiol.*, Babraham. 1966, p. 46.
11 Mount, L. E., Fuller, M. F., Hosie, K. F. and Ingram, D. L. (1961) Climatic studies on pigs. *Report Inst. Anim. Physiol.*, Babraham. 1960–61. p. 23.
12 Mount, L. E. (1968). *The Climatic Physiology of the Pig*, pp. 167–195. London: Edward Arnold.
13 Heitman, H. and Hughes, E. H. (1949) The effects of air temperature and relative humidity on the physiological well-being of swine. *J. Anim. Sci.*, **8**, 171–81.
14 Heitman, H., Kelly, C. F. and Bond, T. E. (1958) The relation of ambient temperature to weight gain in swine. *J. Anim. Sci.*, **17**, 62.
15 Hellberg, A. (1961) The reaction of pigs to low temperature. *Festschr. 8th Int. Tierzuchtkrongr.* 106–107. Hamburg.
16 Sorenson, P. H. (1961) The influence of the piggery climate on the growth, food utilisation and carcase quality of pigs. *Aarsberetn. Inst. Sterilitetsforskn. Kgl. Vet. og. Landbokojsk*, 185–201.
17 Moustgaard, J., Brauner, N. and Sorenson, P. (1960) Influence of environmental temperature and humidity on growth, feed utilisation, and bacon quality of pigs. *Landlr. Bygg. Bygg-forskn-Inst. Kbh.* **18**.
18 Gordon, W. A. M. (1980) *Environmental Studies in Pig Housing*. Doctoral Thesis. Queen's University, Belfast.
19 O'Grady, J. F., Tuite, P. J., O'Brien, J. J. and Attwood, E. A. (1966) *Pig Farming*, **14**, 1.
20 Fuller, M. F. (1964). Ph. D. Thesis, University of Cambridge.
21 Holme, F. W. and Coey, W. E. (1966) Proceedings of the 44th meeting of the British Society of Animal Production.
22 Braude, R., Mitchell, K. G. Finn-Kelsey, P. and Lowen, V. H. (1958) The effect of light on fattening pigs. *Proc. Nutri. Soc.*, **17**, 38.
23 Scholz, K. (1966) Proceedings of C.I.G.R. Second Section Seminar.
24 Pointer, C. G. (1972) Do gilts and sows need supplementary lighting? *Pig International*, Jan. 1972, 23–24.
25 Kelly, C., Heitman, H. and Hughes, E. (1951) Effect of elevated ambient temperature on pregnant sows. *J. Anim. Sci.*, **10**, 907–915.
26 Whatley, J., Palmer, J., Chambers, D. and Stephens, D. (1957) The value of water sprinklers for cooling pregnant sows. *Misc. Publ. Okla. Agric. Exp. Sta.*, No. 48, 2–4.

27 Bond, T. E., Heitman, H., Hahn, L. and Kelly, C. F. (1962) *California Agric.* 1962, 9–11.
28 Gehlbach, G. D., Becher, D. E., Coss, J. L., Harmon, B. G. and Jensen, A. H. (1966) *J. Anim. Sci.*, **25**, 386–391.
29 Charles, D. R. (1981) Practical ventilation and temperature control for poultry, pp. 183–196. In *Environmental Aspects of Housing for Animal Production* (Ed. J. A. Clark). London: Butterworths.
30 Morris, T. R. (1981) The influence of photoperiod on reproduction in farm animals, pp. 85–102. In *Environmental Aspects of Housing for Animal Production* (Ed. J. A. Clark), London: Butterworths.
31 Donaldson, A. I. (1978) Factors influencing the dispersal, survival and deposition of airborne pathogens of farm animals. *Veterinary Bulletin*, **48**, 83–94.
32 Songer, J. R. (1967) Influence of relative humidity on the survival of some airborne viruses. *Applied Microbiology*, **15**, 35–42.
33 Donaldson, A. I. and Ferris, N. P. (1976) The survival of some airborne animal viruses in relation to relative humidity. *Veterinary Microbiology*, **1**, 413–420.
34 Akers, T. G. (1969) Survival of airborne virus, phage and other minute microbes. In R. L. Dimmock and A. B. Akers (eds). *Introduction to Experimental Aerobiology*, pp. 296–339. New York: Wiley.
35 Wright, D. N., Bailey, G. D. and Hatch, M. T. (1968) Survival of airborne mycoplasma as affected by relative humidity. *J. Bacteriology*, **95**, 251–252.
36 Ehrlich, R. (1970) Relationship between environmental temperature and the survival of airborne bacteria. In I. H. Silver (ed.), *Aerobiology*, p. 209. Proc. 3rd Int. Symposium. London & New York: Academic Press.
37 Hatch, M. T. and Walochow, H. (1969) Bacterial survival: consequences of the airborne state. In R. L. Dimmock and A. B. Akers (eds), pp. 267–295. *An Introduction to Experimental Aerobiology*. New York: Wiley.
38 Robertson, O. K. (1943) Air-borne infection. *Science*, **97**, 495–502.
39 Whittlestone, P. (1976) Effect of climatic conditions on enzootic pneumonia in pigs. *International Journal of Biometerology*, **20**, 42–48.
40 Strauch, D., Kösters, J., Müller, W. and Weyers, H. (1968) Das Abfallproblem in der landwirtschaftlichen Nutztierhaltung. *Berl. Munch. tierärztl. Wschr.*, **81**, 209–212.
41 Honey, H. F. and McQuitty, J. B. (1976) *Dust in the Animal Environment*. Monograph published by Dept. of Agricultural Engineering, University of Alberta, Canada.
42 Smith, W. C. and Tonks, H. M. (1966) Proceedings of 9th International Conference of Animal Production.

4

Livestock Welfare and Animal Health

Recently there has been widespread disquiet voiced about the humanity of some of the modern and intensive methods of rearing livestock. Under critical attack from a number of animal welfare groups have been certain systems, especially chickens kept in battery cages, calves housed in crates for the production of veal, sows closely confined or tethered during pregnancy, and any animals kept on totally slatted or perforated floors. Whilst so far there is little absolute evidence to prove the position on these major issues one way or another, the dispute has probably been beneficial since it has thrown a sharp light on husbandry methods and forced everyone involved to think carefully about what they are doing. It is now leading, rather belatedly, to considerable active research and investigation which may answer some of our doubts.

Animal welfare is defined as the provision of a husbandry system appropriate to the health and, so far as is practicable, the behavioural needs of the animals, together with a high standard of stockmanship.[1] Most of these needs, listed below, are straightforward to follow but some are more difficult:

1. Comfort and shelter.
2. Readily accessible fresh water and a diet to maintain the animals in full health and vigour.
3. Freedom of movement. This is further defined as allowing the animal to stand, lie down, turn, stretch, and preen, groom and scratch itself.
4. The company of other animals, particularly of like kind.
5. The opportunity to exercise most normal patterns of behaviour.
6. Light during hours of daylight and lighting readily available to enable the animals to be inspected at any time.
7. Flooring which neither harms the animals nor causes undue strain.
8. The prevention and rapid diagnosis and treatment of vice, injury, parasitic infection and disease.
9. The evidence of unnecessary mutilation.
10. Emergency arrangements to cover outbreaks of fire, the breakdown of essential mechanical services and the disruption of supplies.

'Stockmanship' is difficult to define but is certainly a key factor because no matter how acceptable a system may be in principle, without competent, diligent stockmanship the welfare of the animals cannot be adequately catered for. We all have our own ideas of what stockmanship means. What is clear is that good training is essential. Modern intensive husbandry relies on sophisticated equipment and methods so training is vital if they are to be properly used, in addition to the caring and understanding required in any good stockman.

INTENSIVE MANAGEMENT AND WELFARE

The great majority of the foregoing list of needs for the good welfare of animals are easy to provide and are in fact no more than good husbandry. The really difficult problems only arise, critically, with certain environmental and management techniques – those that severely limit freedom of movement, or provide little or no exercise, or deny the animal a comfortable floor or bedding. It should be stressed too that, allied to the welfare problems, are the fears in the public mind of the dangers that may occur from the consumption of animal products which have received considerable quantities of drugs, antibiotics and growth promoters. There have been claims that residues in meat, eggs or milk may be harmful; also that the use of such substances continually will lead to the development of resistant strains of pathogenic organisms. There is also the nagging doubt that it is wrong to practise husbandry systems and housing methods that do not function without the aid of drugs. That this is so is generally agreed but it may have no direct bearing on livestock welfare. It does, however, have an indirect connection in so far as it is a generally expressed truism that any livestock system which requires the permanent use of artificial aids in the form of antibiotics or drugs will fail, and in the process will be liable to cause widespread disease – which is certainly avoidable pain and distress.

Animal welfare and health

Animal welfare in all cases is very pertinent to the question of health since there is no doubt that one of the essential criteria for the provision of good welfare is the maintenance of health in the animals. It has also become apparent from recent research that the eventual goal of establishing good welfare scientifically is going to be very difficult indeed, if not impossible. Thus we shall have to continue to rely, at least in the foreseeable future, on the overall knowledge, expertise and even instinct of the persons concerned with the management and care of animals – farmers, stockmen and husbandry and veterinary advisers. It is essential to keep in the forefront of one's mind the overriding importance of welfare and humanity to animals on all occasions. Anyone who has closely observed sick animals understands what constitutes 'misery' in the animal kingdom and will contrast this with the alert and buoyant appearance of an animal in good health.

An especially beneficial feature of this controversial field is the way in which it has forced us to question whether it is necessary to house animals using

Table 4.1 *The essentials of welfare*

1	Enough space for the animals to move around freely and stretch their limbs or wings, and to turn round and groom or preen themselves.
2	All surfaces, especially the flooring, must be comfortable and unlikely to cause injury.
3	A suitable microclimate to be provided, that is, appropriate ambient temperatures, humidities, air movement and ventilation.
4	All measures must be taken to ensure healthy stock.
5	A balanced ration should be available in sufficient quantity and of a suitable consistency for the animal's digestive system. Clean water should always be available.
6	Groups of animals should be evenly matched. If animals are kept individually they should have sight of others.
7	All sick animals and 'bullies' must be removed and the former should be isolated from healthy stock.
8	There should be adequate provision to cope with emergencies such as fire and electrical or mechanical failures.
9	Wherever possible, and especially with young animals, bedding such as clean straw or wood shavings should be provided.
10	Mutilation of animals, such as beak-trimming of birds, or de-tailing of pigs, should not be undertaken except under exceptional circumstances when more suffering might result if it were not done. Alternative husbandry systems which do not require mutilation should be considered.
11	Lighting should be generous for the management of the animals and adequate at all other times.

methods which involve an abnormal degree of restriction in their movement. This has resulted in a search for alternatives which has been fruitful in that it appears to indicate that there may be less need for the extremes of intensification and indeed it may be cost-efficient to have systems which are more in harmony with the overall agricultural scene.

Very large and intensive livestock enterprises have often been unsuccessful and even catastrophic. First, the management of large numbers of *living beings* is not easily organized on a large scale. Stockmanship is partly science and partly art, and art must rely heavily on the individual. If only one small item goes wrong or is overlooked, it can lead to a very serious chain of events. Second, disease is much more likely to have a disastrous effect in the large unit whether in sub-clinical or clinical forms. The failure of many units can be ascribed to their inability to control disease so that the economic viability of the unit has been totally destroyed. Third are the heavy costs of buying or bringing in fodder and moving out the muck in such enterprises. It is common for the highly intensive unit to be totally dependent on food from outside the farm or the locality. And it is faced with great difficulty in disposing of all the waste products. In smaller units home-produced crops can be used to feed the livestock and the muck they generate is of great value to the land; energy is conserved and the result is agriculture of a totally balanced sort.

The welfare standards that are gradually emerging across the world are based on evidence which, as far as is possible, does not conflict with sound economics. For example, if animals are housed at concentrations and intensities above those recommended or allowed, it is most likely that their productivity will fall. Particularly so when it comes to stocking density and its relation to growth, production and the efficiency of food utilization. Good welfare standards can be used, therefore, as good husbandry standards with some confidence.

Table 4.1 summarizes the essentials of livestock welfare.

REFERENCES

1 *Codes of Recommendations for the Welfare of Livestock (1978–83)*. London, Ministry of Agriculture, Fisheries and Food.

5

Ventilation

There are few topics in animal husbandry where there have been more totally erroneous statements made than on the reasons why housed livestock require ventilation or 'air change'. For example, for many years it was accepted that the principal harmful effects of having too little ventilation were due to the build-up of harmful concentrations of the gaseous products of respiration and in particular carbon dioxide, combined with a depletion in the oxygen content of the air. It is now known that this is far too simple and usually a quite incorrect hypothesis.

UNDERLYING PRINCIPLES AND CALCULATIONS

In any seriously under-ventilated building the stagnant air gradually becomes warmer and more humid and there is a rising concentration of dust, other particulate matter, ammonia and other gases and any pathogenic micro-organisms the livestock may be carrying. The end-result is that the animals suffer from 'heat stagnation', exposing them to a susceptibility to chilling. Along with this will go poor productivity and a likelihood of disease – particularly respiratory diseases – which experience shows to be the greatest danger in intensive forms of housing. However, it is not just respiratory disease that may result from poor ventilation.

In a badly ventilated building, condensation on the surface often occurs and bedding and floors may become wet and the animals uncomfortable. This leads to an uneven distribution of the stock in the building, which in turn will have harmful effects, especially due to the consequent unequal concentration of excreta and expired air. These will tend to exacerbate any respiratory or enteric diseases, or infections such as mastitis. It should be emphasized that the combination of high humidity and low temperature, common in winter in badly constructed and ill-ventilated housing, is especially favourable to the viability and infectivity of many pathogenic microorganisms. Then in recent years, a new hazard to livestock and their attendants has been the risk of gaseous intoxication of livestock due to the gases arising from slurry pits or channels beneath the animals. The risk is very great and has caused the death of many animals and several stockmen. This is given detailed consideration on p. 172.

The object of ventilation is, therefore, to remove the stale air in a building, and replace it with fresh air thereby removing the danger of toxic gases. But while too little ventilation is obviously serious, so also is too much. In cold weather much valuable animal heat will be wasted. Further, over-ventilation may be accompanied by draughts. Draughts are themselves responsible for causing many deaths by direct chilling and they may also act indirectly by lowering the animals' resistance to disease-producing organisms. Particularly vulnerable are unprotected newborn stock such as piglets and chicks.

In planning a ventilation system allowance has to be made for all the factors that can influence the necessary ventilation – type, age and number of livestock, their management, the construction and locality of the house, and finally the weather conditions. The practical difficulties associated with these demands are considerable and few scientific data are available to show what constitutes the optimal level of ventilation for the different species. It is important to appreciate that sweeping generalizations on the ventilation of animal houses can never be justified. One has only to consider the 'open' ventilation of the climatic house, such as the cattle yard, and compare it with the very careful control that is necessary in a controlled environment building, such as a fattening piggery, or the almost infinitesimal requirements in a brooder house for chicks. In practice the ventilation of the open shelter may present few problems unless construction is very bad and as long as lower temperatures are acceptable in the winter. Ample air flow in these buildings promotes hardiness and a good growth of the coat of the stock and prevents accumulation of animal waste products in the air.

The main difficulty here is to avoid through-draughts, particularly at ground level, and to ensure that the open side or sides of the yard face in the most favourable direction, which is generally towards the south. Another form of sheltering relatively easy to ventilate is one which houses only a small head of stock, for instance, the many forms of kennel accommodation. In this case there is usually little trouble because the actual demands are so small and by-products from the animals are minimal, being outside the sleeping or lying area.

TOTALLY ENCLOSED INTENSIVE HOUSING

Ventilation is nearly always a major problem in the large enclosed house in which many animals or birds are kept under one roof. We meet the problem in one of the mildest forms in cow accommodation, such as a cubicle house, since adult cattle thrive at low temperatures and a simple free circulation of air is sufficient. A fixed open ridge for stale air outlets and plenty of opening window space or wall ventilators form the basis of good air flow (Fig. 5.1).

The problem may become acute in the case of calf houses, intensive piggeries, deep litter and cage-laying houses and broiler chicken accommodation. In every case a good circulation of air is needed in hot weather, but in winter no more must be allowed than is necessary to keep the atmosphere healthy. This means that tremendous variations are necessary, from the minimal winter needs with

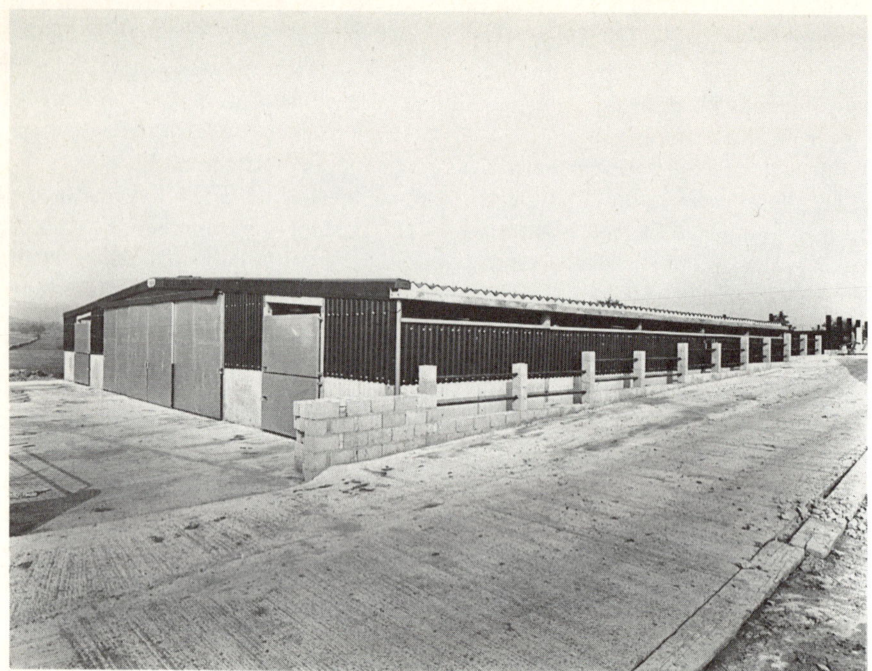

Fig. 5.1 A shallow pitched cubicle house with good ventilation at the eaves. A satisfactory arrangement used with a 'breathing' roof.

a low density of young stock, to the maximum requirements in hot weather with a full complement of mature animals. For example, a broiler chicken needs no more than about 0.17 m^3/h of ventilation in its early days but may need as much as 7 m^3/h at full weight in summer, a variation in air change rates under normal housing conditions from well under one air change per hour to 30 or 40 changes (Figs. 5.2 and 5.3). To achieve this we have to choose between natural ventilation, using wall and roof ventilators or cowls and windows, or artificial systems using electric fans, sometimes assisted by ducts to distribute the air evenly.

NATURAL VENTILATION

If natural ventilation is to be effective, it must function well in all weathers. To avoid too great a dependence on external wind and weather, it is best to make use of the so-called 'stack effect' as its foundation. As the warm stale air around the body of the animal is lighter than cold fresh air, it rises to the top of the building. Outlet ventilation is therefore provided at a suitable point or points in the ceiling or roof. The greater the difference between inside and outside temperatures, and the greater the distance between inlets and outlets, the greater

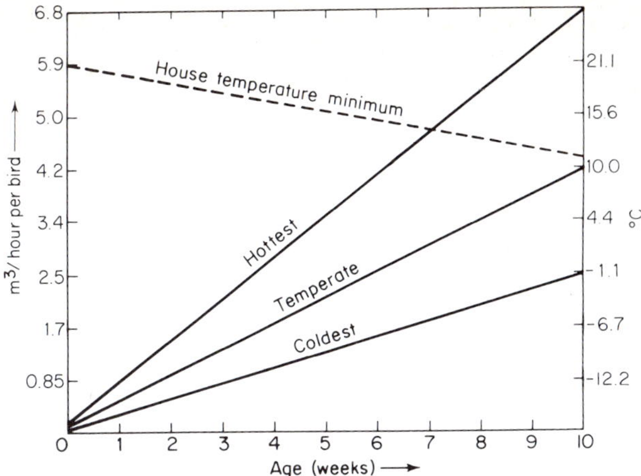

Fig. 5.2 Suggested ventilation scheme for broilers.

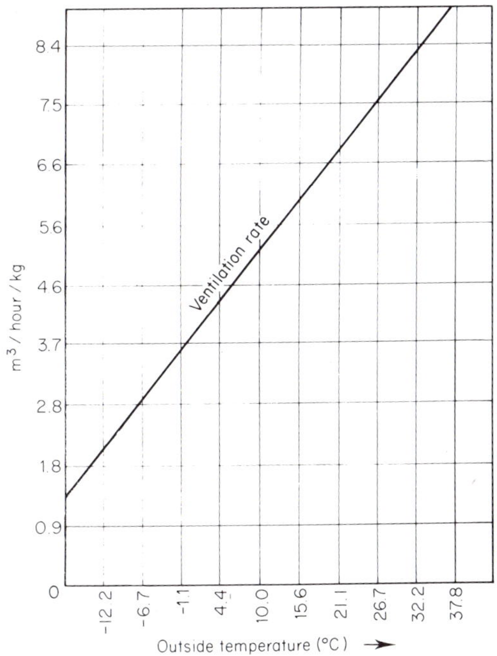

Fig. 5.3 Ventilation rates for adult birds.

the stack effect. If, therefore, an area of outlet ventilation is provided to cope with difficult conditions (that is, a small difference between inside and outside temperatures) it can easily be restricted when temperature differences are greater or appreciable winds help in the ventilation. As mentioned, in houses where no great control is necessary, such as climatic housing for cattle, a fixed open ridge with a protective cap may be sufficient. But in other controlled climate accommodation far more control is needed and down-draughts, which can be common with the fixed open ridge, must be avoided (Fig. 5.4). Experience has shown that for the latter good results are obtained by the use of a limited area of controlled outlet ventilation, and for this purpose a simple chimney type of insulated 'flue' is satisfactory (Fig. 5.5). It is good practice to have one or a few outlets, but a much larger number of smaller air inlets as the fresh air should come in slowly all round the building diffusely and carefully baffled. The basis of a useful inlet system consists of hopper-type windows, fitted with gussets to prevent direct draughts, serving as principal inlets, and small baffled openings between the windows which alone are left open during cold or windy weather (Figs. 5.6 and 5.7). Since cold air coming into the building falls naturally towards

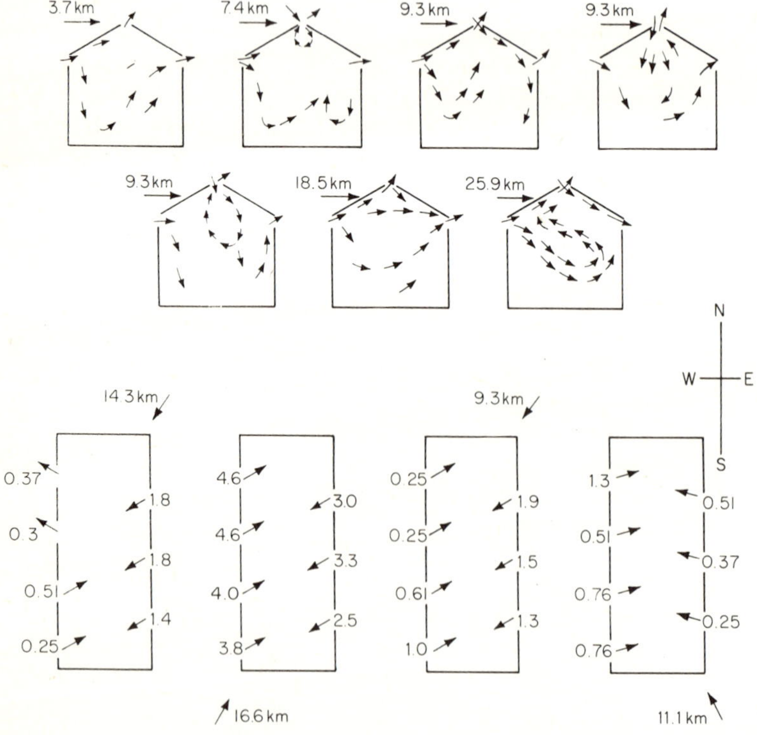

Fig. 5.4 (a) Air circulated in a piggery with open eaves and ridge ventilation under different wind conditions. Note the frequent occurrence of down draughts. (b) The pattern of air entry through the side ventilation of a piggery at different wind speeds. Wind speeds in km/h. Air velocity through vents in m/s.

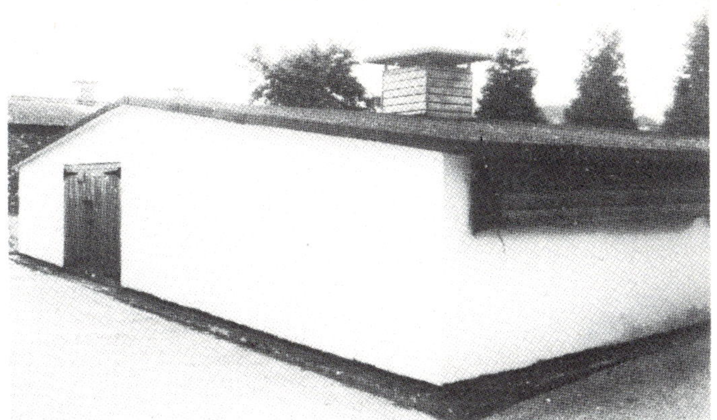

Fig. 5.5 Insulated air outlet flue.

the floor, there is no necessity to site inlets at floor level, where the danger of chilling draught is considerable.

The arrangement detailed here is widely used in temperate climates, but with increasing complexities in housing and greater intensity of stocking more sophisticated arrangements must be used, which are given; the principle remains the same.

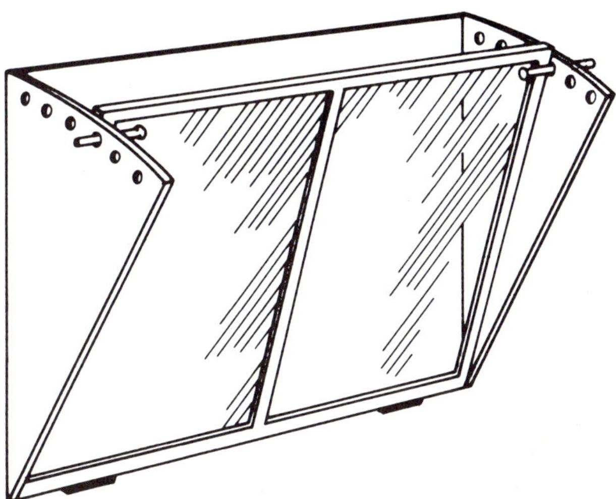

Fig. 5.6 Hopper-type window used as air inlet with side cheeks to prevent draughts. Double glazing is well worthwhile.

Calculation of stack effect ventilation

The air flow actually arising from the stack effect is given by the following equation:

$$Q = \mathrm{Kh} A_1 \sqrt{(h \times \theta)}$$

where Q = rate of air flow (m^3/h);
A_1 = area of inlets (m^2);
h = height difference between inlets and outlets (m);
θ = difference between mean internal and external temperature (°C); and
Kh is a constant which depends on the ratio of outlet to area of inlet (R) and can be calculated for any value of R as follows:

$$\mathrm{Kh} = \frac{565.2R}{1 + R^2}$$

Some values of R and Kh are as follows:

R	Kh
$\frac{1}{4}$	136.8
$\frac{1}{2}$	232.0
$\frac{3}{4}$	338.4
1	339.6
2	504.0
3	532.8
4	547.2
5	550.8

From this it is apparent that if the inlet/outlet ratio is high – for example, 2:1 or more – the stack effect will function most efficiently.

Air flows required per head of stock can be obtained from Table 5.1 or can be calculated on the lines mentioned in the section on ventilation rates. This formula will be mostly used to calculate the outlet area required in a naturally ventilated building when the design is otherwise generally established and stocking densities are decided. It will also be useful for checking that the outlet area is sufficient in an existing building.

In practical terms planning a building will be done as follows. The rates of air flow required for the animals within the building are known (see Table 5.1) and the height of inlets below outlets will be decided in the basic design. Likewise the area ratio can be suggested between them. The internal and external temperatures can also be calculated by using the procedure given on p. 77. From these data the inlet and outlet area required can be calculated, but if the result is not constructionally satisfactory, it may be possible to change the differences

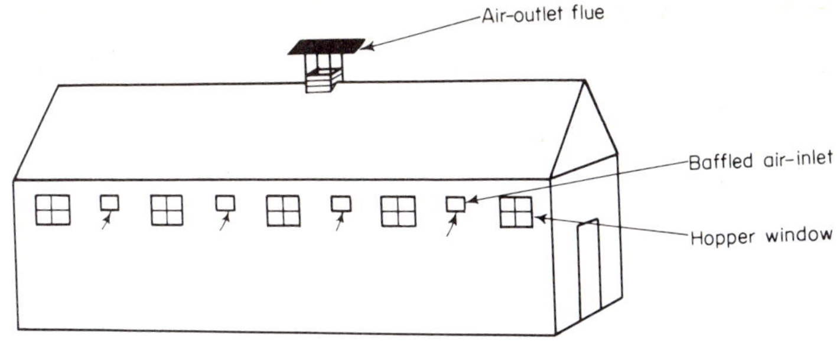

Fig. 5.7 Suggested scheme for draught-free and fully controllable ventilation.

in height, or the temperature difference (by insulation, for example) to make the result more practicable.

It may be asked how a system based on the above calculation will work out in practice. Suppose, for example, an area of outlet ventilation was built on the basis of a temperature difference of 11°C, e.g. 4°C outside and 15°C inside, such as may be typical in a piggery in January or February, and to give ventilation rates similar to those given in Table 5.1. If the weather gets colder, the stack effect will become greater and outlets can be restricted. As the outside temperature rises, however, the stack effect will become less and it might seem that the ventilation would become insufficient. However, the working of an outlet chimney is usually assisted by the action of the wind and its 'pulling' or aspirating effect as it blows across the top. When there is complete calm and the temprature is rising, it is satisfactory to open up windows gradually giving further air change by cross-ventilation. It is essential in a system such as this that all ventilators should be easily controllable, usually by hand, although some ventilators are closed by increasing wind pressure (Fig. 5.8).

Table 5.1 *Ventilation rates for varying climatic conditions in the U.K. for farm livestock*

Animal	Ventilation rate (m^3/h per kg body weight)
Winter rates	
Adult cattle	0.19
Young calf	0.38
Sow and litter	0.38
Fattening pig	0.38
Broiler chicken	0.75
Laying poultry	1.50
Summer rates	
Adult cattle	0.75–1.4
Young calf	0.94–1.9
Sow and litter	0.94–1.9
Fattening pig	0.94–1.9
Broiler chicken	2.8 –4.7
Laying poultry	5.6 –9.4

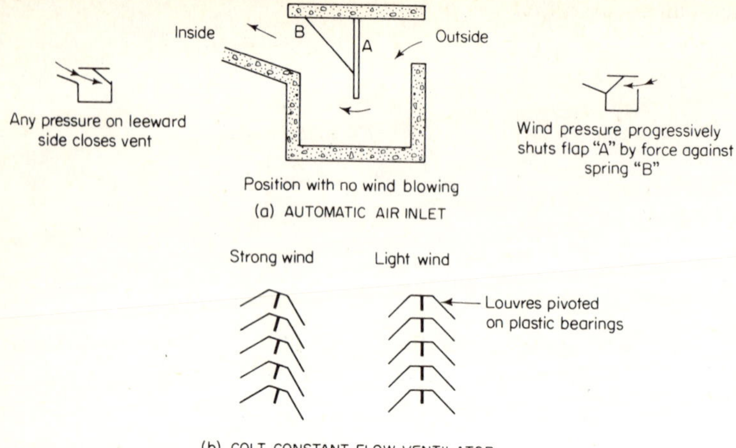

Fig. 5.8 Air inlets designed for constant air flow.

Automatic control of natural ventilation (ACNV)

In fact, the most recent development with natural ventilation is to regulate the open area by automatic thermostatic means. This is achieved by linking the thermostat to a motor which progressively opens or closes the ventilator flaps, inlets or outlets, according to the temperature. This is a very useful way of dealing with natural ventilation as the stockman cannot be present at all times.

Ventilation by wind

The following equation can be used:

$$Q = \mathrm{Kw} \cdot A_1 \cdot V$$

where Q = rate of air flow (m^3/h)
A_1 = area of inlets (m^2);
V = mean wind speed (km/h); and
Kw is a constant which will depend upon R, the ratio of outlet to inlet area, according to the following equation:

$$\mathrm{Kw} = \frac{844R}{\sqrt{(1 + R^2)}}$$

Tabulated values for *R* are:

R	Kw
1	596
2	756
3	804
4	822
5	832
$\frac{3}{4}$	510
$\frac{1}{2}$	378
$\frac{1}{4}$	208

It is pertinent to point out that on exposed sites the average wind speed is about 16 km/h but on sheltered sites it will be very much lower, even down to 1 or less km/h. It is therefore important that farm buildings that are naturally ventilated are not placed in too sheltered a site. It is always possible to restrict ventilation but wind cannot be created.

Natural ventilation on these general principles functions especially well in the less intensive type of house and in small narrow-span buildings. It does, however, have some disadvantages which limit its use. Fully automatic control is impossible and manual control can be wasteful of labour. Too much is left in the hands of the stockman, who may not appreciate the importance of careful environmental control and sudden changes in the weather are always liable to cause serious fluctuations in indoor conditions. No natural system functions particularly well in very hot, airless, summer conditions or in calm 'muggy' weather. Finally, it makes light control, such as is required in the poultry house, nearly impossible.

Calculations to find inlets and outlets required for stack effect ventilation

An example is given of a calculation to determine the size of inlets and outlets require in cold weather in a pig fattening house containing 100 pigs. Applying the formula:

$$Q = \mathrm{Kh}A\sqrt{(h \times \theta)}$$

where $Q = 30\,\mathrm{m}^3/\mathrm{h}$ for a pig finishing weight in the house;
$h =$ a distance of 4 m
$\theta = 10°\mathrm{C}$; and Kh (at a ratio of 2 : 1) = 504.

Thus, $3000 = 504 \times A_1\sqrt{(4 \times 10)}$ or $A_1 = 1\mathrm{m}^2$ approximately.

Thus if the inlet area must equal 1 m^2 and the inlet : outlet ratio is 2 : 1, the outlet 'stack' will be 0.5 m^2 in area (approximately 700 × 700 mm in dimension).

Calculations relating to the design of housing for intensively maintained animals

Two simple basic criteria have been mentioned for ventilation needs, viz. the need to remove the moisture produced by the livestock as the *minimal* need and the need to minimize temperature lift in the summer as the *maximum* need. Simple and accurate calculations for these may be done as follows:

Airflow for moisture removal:

$$Q = \frac{Wa}{gi - go}$$

where Q = air flow necessary to remove moisture (m^3/h per animal);
Wa = total respiratory moisture production of animal plus added moisture from evaporation from excreta and urine (g/h per animal);
gi, go = absolute humidities of inside and outside air, respectively (g/m^3)
(See basic data on pp. 78 and 79.)

Example Minimum air flow is required for a piggery under cold conditions. The pigs average 70 kg liveweight, house temperature is 18°C and relative humidity 76 per cent. Outside temperature is −1°C and relative humidity 90 per cent.

Then moisture production of pigs = 140 g/h
moisture in air inside = 11 g/m^3
moisture in outside air = 3 g/m^3

$$Q = \frac{140}{8} = 18\ m^3/h$$
$$= 0.30\ m^3/min.$$

Maximum summer ventilation rate

For summer the aim is to limit the temperature rise to the minimum possible and a suggested practical figure is 3°C. The formula used to calculate the ventilation rate required is derived from the following:

$$\frac{K}{B + V} = Tp$$

where K = heat production of animals (kW per pig);
B = building heat loss (kW per pig per °C);
V = ventilation heat loss (kW per pig per °C).

If Tp is 3°C and $V = 20148 \times (C/10^6)$ where C = ventilation rate required, and formula is derived from Table 5.1 (p. 73),

$$\text{then } C = 50\left\{\frac{K}{Tp} - B\right\}\ m^3/\text{min per animal.}$$

Example Taking as an example a piggery with an average of 68 pigs from Table 5.2, heat production = 0.09 kW; an average building heat loss per pig would be 0.02 kW/°C per pig. Thus:

$$C = 50\ \frac{(0.09}{3} - 0.002)\ \mathrm{m^3/min\ per\ pig}$$
$$= 50\ (0.03 - 0.002) = 1.4\ \mathrm{m^3/min/pig}$$

that is, summer ventilation rate of 1.5 $\mathrm{m^3}$/min per pig (or 90 $\mathrm{m^3}$/h per pig) will ensure a temperature limit of approximately 3°C.

However, for the calculation of the full air flow, heat and moisture balances, the following is more complete.

Calculation of ventilation and heating requirements for intensively housed animals

A suggested procedure for the calculation required in any thorough design of livestock housing is as follows. As a basis:

1 It is assumed that in winter use is made of the metabolic heat of the animals to raise the general temperature level of the house as close as possible to the required value, under average winter conditions in the U.K. or similar temperate conditions.
2 The ventilation rate used is calculated to provide a relative humidity (RH) in the outgoing air, after allowance is made for moisture added to the atmosphere by the animals' respiration and a proportion of their waste products, which is low enough to prevent condensation occurring on the structure, and is of a value considered from experience to be satisfactory for the development of the stock. The choice of a suitable RH is therefore arbitrary, but it is suggested it should be between 70 and 80 per cent under average winter conditions, although it would be acceptable if, under exceptionally cold conditions, 85–90 per cent was reached for short periods. Experimental evidence suggests that these criteria are satisfactory.
3 If calculations show that the natural metabolic heat is insufficient to provide the temperature rise required at the calculated ventilation rate, then supplementary heat will correct the situation.
4 The basis of calculation for summer conditions is to limit the rise in temperature due to metabolic heat (which will in any case occur) to 2–3°C. The tendency in recent years has been to reduce this limit of temperature rise first from 6°C to 3°C and then from 3°C to 2°C. No calculation of humidity levels is usually made for summer ventilation, as it is considered that the more ventilation there is the better. It should be noted that planning for a 3°C lift instead of a 6°C lift will require virtually twice as much air continuously.

An example will illustrate how the most suitable ventilation rates can be calculated not only for average winter conditions, but also for colder and warmer winter temperatures.

Tables 5.2 and 5.3 provide for other cases than the worked example. Table 5.3 gives winter ventilation rates: Table 5.2 summer requirements. The psychometric chart (Fig. 5.9) gives data for worked examples.

Steps in calculating ventilation rates

Fan ventilation and heating are required as necessary for a pig fattening house for 560 fatteners with a weight range of 27–109 kg (average 68 kg) at any one

Table 5.2 *Estimated heat output of farm livestock at different weights under summer conditions*

Animal	Approximate age at weight given	Liveweight range (kg)	Sensible heat output per animal at 21°C (W)
Calf	birth	45	110
	12 wk	90	170
		135	210
Growing cattle		180	250
		226	270
		272	280
		317	300
		362	320
Cow		per 450	480
Fattening pig	7 wk	13.5	35
	8 wk	18	40
	9 wk	22.6	50
	10 wk	27.2	55
	13 wk	45.3	75
	15 wk	56.7	85
	17 wk	68	90
	21 wk	90	110
	26 wk	113	145
Farrowing sow		147	200
and litter of 10		193	230
Meat chicken (broiler)	day-old	0.036	0.35
	3 wk	0.27	3.1
	4 wk	0.453	3.9
	5 wk	0.60	4.6
	6 wk	0.9	5.4
	7 wk	1.225	6.5
	8 wk	1.495	7.2
	9 wk	1.723	8.3
Chicken reared for eggs	day-old	0.036	0.35
	3 wk	0.113	1.6
	8 wk	0.680	4.6
	12 wk	1.135	6.2
	16 wk	1.580	7.5
	18 wk	1.815	8.3
Laying poultry	adult	1.815	8.3
		2.268	9.9
		2.720	10.9
		3.175	12.4

Table 5.3 *Estimated heat output and moisture respiration from farm animals when housed under approximately optimum conditions in winter*

1. Animal	2. Approx. age at weight given	3. Practical critical temperature (°C)	4. Liveweight range (kg)	5. Sensible heat output per animal (W)	6. Moisture respired per animal by evaporation at critical temperature (g/h)
Calf	birth		45	120	95 0.0648
	12 wk	16	90	200	150
			135	250	192
Growing cattle		2	181	375 (290)	155 (221)
			227	390 (310)	163 (237)
			272	425 (330)	176 (251)
			318	435 (350)	180 (269)
			363	445 (370)	185 (279)
Cow		2	per 450 kg	810 (570)	385 (521)
Piglet	birth	27	1.1	4	12.6
	2–3 wk	21	4.5	10	330 21
Fattening pig	7 wk		14	37	43
	8 wk		18	45	52
	9 wk		23	55	60
	10 wk		27	60	68
	13 wk	18	45	82	94
	15 wk		57	95	109
	17 wk		68	102	117
	21 wk		90	125	144
	26 wk		113	162	185
Farrowing sow		13	135	200	176
			181	245	196
Meat chicken (broiler)	day-old	21	0.036	0.35	0.20
	3 wk		0.27	3.1	1.7
	4 wk		0.45	4.3	1.5
	5 wk		0.68	5.2	1.8
	6 wk	16	0.90	6.1	2.1
	7 wk		1.22	7.1	2.5
Chicken reared for eggs	day-old	21	0.036	0.35	0.20
	3 wk		0.11	1.6	0.91
	8 wk		0.7	5.3	1.56
	12 wk	13	1.1	7.0	2.06
	16 wk		1.6	8.7	2.52
	18 wk		1.8	9.7	2.78
Laying poultry	adult	4	1.8	10.3 (9.2)	1.58 (3.25)
			2.2	12.3 (11.0)	1.91 (3.92)
			2.7	13.6 (12.1)	2.12 (4.34)
			3.1	15.5 (13.8)	2.42 (4.92)

Notes 1. The figures in parentheses in columns 5 and 6 for growing cattle, cows and laying poultry give the sensible heat outputs and moisture respiration for these animals at 16°C.
2. Figures for moisture respiration are quantities respired through skin and lungs and exclude moisture voided in dung and urine, for which an extra allowance must be made (see text).

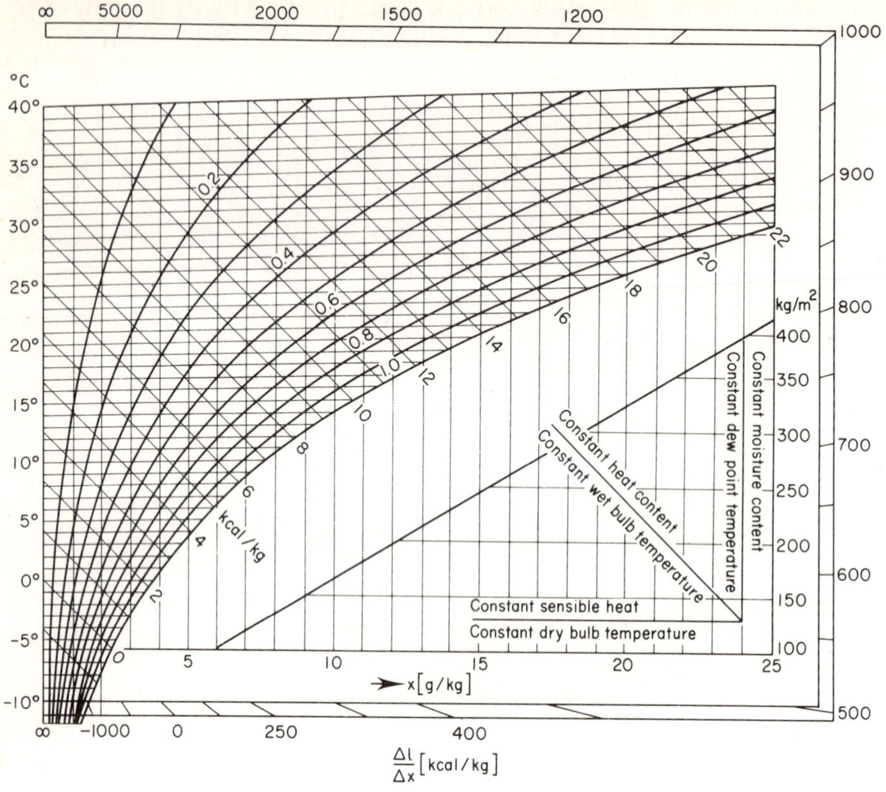

Specific gravity (kg/m³) of humid air at various temperatures (°C)						
t = °C	-5	0	10	20	30	40
kg/m³	1315	1290	1242	1195	1146	1097

Fig. 5.9 Mollier diagram (psychometric chart) for humid air.

time. The house temperature and relative humidity to be maintained are 18°C and not exceeding 76 per cent respectively. The building is 41 m long by 10 m wide, 2.0 m to the eaves, 5.4 m to the ridge, and is provided with a 12 mm fibreboard false ceiling below the roof with an overlay of 50 mm of glass fibre and corrugated asbestos for the roof covering; there is a 280 mm cavity wall with 18 windows, each 1524 × 914 mm. The floor is concrete.

The steps in the calculation are shown below:

Step 1. The building heat loss (BHL) measured in kcal/h/°C is calculated first. From this the BHL per pig is calculated (by dividing by the number of pigs) and then expressed as kw/°C per pig, by dividing BHL per pig by 860; this figure is designated *B*.

Step 2. Using the psychometric chart, the amount of moisture (in g/h) is calculated which it would be permissible to add by moisture respiration, etc. from the pigs to each m^3 of outside air, while ensuring that the internal relative humidity of the air at 18°C does not exceed 76 per cent. This calculation is made for outside temperatures from −5°C to 10°C, at intervals of 5°C, and for outside relative humidities between 88 and 92 per cent. This results in figures for the permissible g/m^3 for each outside temperature, designated ΔM.

Step 3. The average moisture respiration in g/h and the average heat production in watts for a 68 kg pig at 18°C are then estimated from Table 5.2. To the moisture respiration figure is added an amount (in this case 25 per cent) to allow for moisture added to the atmosphere from droppings, urine and free water surfaces. This figure is then converted from g/h to g/min by dividing by 60. The result is designated *P*.

The amount added depends on the circumstances in which stock are kept, and is still the subject of investigation. For beef animals kept on deep straw, for example, it would appear that an amount equivalent to twice the moisture respiration figure should be added. For poultry and pigs kept on deep litter, an amount equal to the moisture respiration figure would appear to be realistic. For poultry in batteries and pigs on concrete, where in both cases droppings and urine are removed daily, about 25–50 per cent should be added.

Step 4. Each m^3 of air can absorb up to ΔMg without the internal relative humidity exceeding 76 per cent. But *P*g of moisture are being added to each m^3 of air each minute. It follows that the minimum rate of air displacement to ensure that at 18°C the RH does not exceed 76 per cent is $p/\Delta M\ m^3/min$, designated *C*.

Step 5. Step 4 calculated for each outside temperature will give a number of ventilation rates which, at each of these temperatures, are the minima which can be used if 76 per cent RH is not to be exceeded when the internal temperature is 18°C. It is now possible to calculate for each value of *C* the ventilation heat loss per pig, which is designated *V*:

$$V = 20148\ \frac{C}{10^6}\ \text{kW/°C per pig}$$

Step 6. The total heat loss is $B + V$, and this is measured in kw/°C per pig. The temperature lift will be determined by the average rate of heat production from the pigs in the house, and for the purposes of this calculation the heat production of the average weight of pig (68 kg) is taken when it is in a temperature of 18°C. From Table 5.3 it will be seen that this is 0.1 kW (100 W approximately). This is designated K and is measured in kW per pig.

If heating occurs at the rate of KkW and the total heat loss from the building is $(B+V)$kW/°C per pig, it follows that the temperature rise due to heat K of each pig (and designated T_p°C) is equal to:

$$\frac{(K)}{(B+V)}\ {}^{\circ}\mathrm{C}$$

Thus the temperature rise above each outside air temperature considered can be found.

Step 7. By adding the temperature rise due to the pigs alone to the value of the outside temperature, the internal temperature at the minimum ventilation rate is obtained. If this should be less than 18°C, then it is evident that, to meet the required temperature and humidity conditions, artificial heat is necessary. The rate at which it will be needed may be calculated as follows.

Suppose that the temperature rise due to the pigs alone at the minimum ventilation rate is 11°C when the outside temperature is −1°C. The internal temperature will then be 10°C. There is therefore a shortfall of 8°C which has to be supplied artificially if 18°C is to be reached. The heat loss per °C is $(B+V)$ when the outside temperature is −1°. The total kW for the whole house of 560 pigs would, of course, be $(560 \times 8)\ (B+V)$, i.e. $4480\ (B+V)$ kW.

Step 8. If no heat is provided and the outside temperature is −1°C, the internal temperature is only 12°C. The relative humidity at this temperature will be much higher than at 18°C; indeed, saturation of the atmosphere and condensation may well occur. The psychometric chart can be used to determine what the conditions will be both with and without heat, and an example is worked out later.

Step 9. For summer, the aim is simply to limit the temperature rise to a minimum, in this case to 3°C. Because on average the metabolic heat from the animals will be rather less than in winter, since the house temperature will be around 21°C, Table 5.2 is used. This lists animal heat at 21°C. The formula used is:

$$\frac{K}{B+V} = Tp$$

Tp in this case being 3°C.

From Step 5, $V = 20148\ \frac{C}{10^6}$ from which it follows that for summer ventilation

$$C = 50\left(\frac{K}{Tp} - B\right)\mathrm{m^3/min\ per\ pig}$$

Table 5.4 *Metric and other conversion factors*

Definition	*To convert*	*into*	*Multiply by*
Temperature rise	deg F	deg C	0.55
	deg C	deg F	1.8
Length	in	mm	25.400
	mm	in	0.0394
	ft	m	0.3048
	m	ft	3.2808
Area	ft^2	m^2	0.0929
	m^2	ft^2	10.7639
Volume	ft^3	m^3	0.0283
	m^3	ft^3	35.3148
Velocity	ft/min	m/s	0.0051
	m/s	ft/min	196.8504
Mass	lb	kg	0.4536
	kg	lb	2.2046
Rate of thermal transmission	watts (W)	B.t.u./h	3.4121
	B.t.u./h	W	0.2931
	W	kcal/h	0.8598
	kcal/h	W	1.1630
	B.t.u./h	kcal/h	0.2520
	kcal/h	B.t.u./h	3.9680
			0.4536
			2.2044
A. Building heat loss data			
Thermal conductivity	B.t.u./h/deg F	kcal/h/deg C	0.1240
	kcal/h/deg C	B.t.u./h/deg F	8.0636
Thermal conductance and thermal transmittance	B.t.u. in/ft^2 h deg F (*K* value)	kcal/m^2 h deg C	4.8824
	kcal/m^2 h deg C	B.t.u. in/ft^2 h deg F	0.2048
Thermal resistivity	B.t.u./ft^2 h deg F (*U* value)	kcal/m^2 h deg C	8.0636
	kcal/m^2 h deg C	B.t.u./ft^2 h deg F	0.1240
Thermal resistance	ft^2 h deg F/B.t.u. in (I/*K*)	m^2 h deg C/kcal m	0.2048
	m^2 h deg C/kcal m	ft^2 h deg F/B.t.u. in	4.8824
	ft^2 h deg F/B.t.u.	m^2 h deg C/kcal	2.2044
	m^2 h deg C/kcal	ft^2 h deg F/B.t.u.	0.4536
B. Ventilation heat loss data			
Volume rate of flow	ft^3/min	m^3/h	1.699
	m^3/h	ft^3/min	0.5886
Approx. rate of thermal extraction by air	ft^3/min	W/deg F	0.317
	m^3/h	W/deg F	0.1866
	m^3/h	W/deg C	0.3358
	ft^3/min	B.t.u./h/deg F	1.08
	m^3/h	B.t.u./h/deg F	0.637
	m^3/h	kcal h/deg C	0.2886

Above figures are calculated on basis of dry air being 0.075 lb/ft^3 (1.2 kg/m^3) and specific heat of dry air of 0.24 B.t.u./lb (0.133 kcal/kg).

C. Atmospheric water vapour data			
Moisture respiration rate	grains/h (gr/h)	g/h	0.0648
	g/h	gr/h	15.432
Water vapour concentration in atmosphere by weight	gr/lb of air	g/kg of air	0.143
	g/kg of air	gr/lb of air	7.0
Water vapour concentration in atmosphere by volume	gr/ft^3 of air	g/m^3 of air	2.285
	g/m^3 of air	gr/ft^3 of air	0.437

THE TOTALLY COVERED YARD

Many problems have occurred within the environment of the modern, densely-stocked, intensive livestock yard. These are generally connected with respiratory disease and pneumonia, condensation and dampness of the litter, and poor growth and productivity, particularly in colder weather. It is hardly surprising that this has occurred, since the animals have often been housed more densely than in a piggery or even a broiler chicken house. Yet the attention to environmental control is rudimentary in the extreme – or even absent. While it is accepted that animals such as cattle from three months of age are reasonably well-endowed with protective hair and are quite hardy, it is wrong to suppose that they can be kept in grossly fluctuating or humid conditions. Nor are they able to accept with equanimity exposure to the elements, particularly draughts, to which they may have no resistance by virtue of their previously sheltered existence.

In practice the following major faults are commonly found in the construction of covered yards:

1 Either there is no ridge outlet for stale air or it is inadequate.
2 Eaves openings are either absent or, where present, uncontrollable and at the mercy of the weather, causing chilling draughts in cold weather.
3 The extreme width of many yards (20 m upwards) prevents natural ventilation functioning properly. This problem is often combined with multispan construction and low eaves and roofs, so that the flow is generally impaired.
4 The gable ends are closed and sealed.
5 There is no insulation of the roof. While insulation is not usually necessary it may be a desirable 'extra' under a few circumstances, particularly where younger stock are housed or where the roof is low and natural air flow is difficult.
6 Poor drainage under or around the yard leads to excessive straw usage and contributes to the humidity of the atmosphere.
7 Bad construction of the walls leads to excessive moisture penetration at all points.

Natural ventilation works most satisfactorily on open sites. It is always useful to have it controllable but this is not usually done. An open ridge 300 mm wide, with a flat continuous top at least 150 mm above, is a simple solution to extraction in narrow yards, and a 600 mm width in yards above 14 m width (Fig. 5.10).

A more satisfactory arrangement is to have a series of chimney-type ventilators along the ridge, allowing 0.09 m^2 per beast. A useful size of chimney is 1 m^2; that is sufficient for eleven animals. The throat can be controlled by a butterfly valve or hinged flap (Figs. 5.11 and 5.12).

There has been extensive research recently on the design of natural ventilators, the most important centre of investigation being the Scottish Farm Buildings

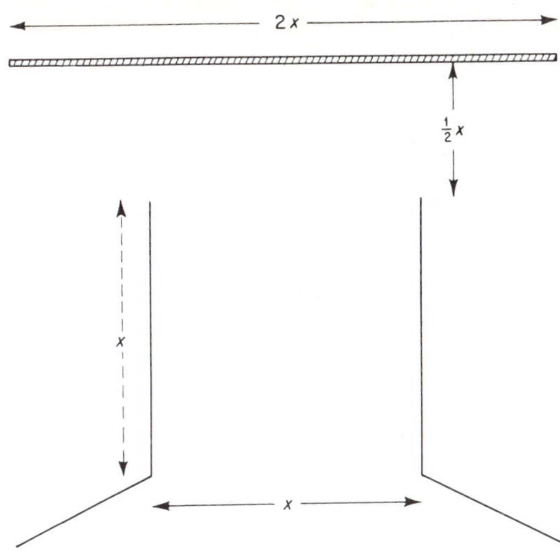

Fig. 5.10 Detail of capped ridge of cattle yard. For most yards x may be taken as 0.3–0.7 m. For farmyards up to 12 m, 0.3 m should be sufficient. For yards 12–24 m use 0.6 m widths.

Investigation Unit, where work has been pursued by Dr J. M. Bruce and Dr C. D. Mitchell. In a paper by Bruce, which reviews the evidence for design features and also reports on original work, the conclusions are that:

1 There is an increased flow resistance factor as the ridge design becomes more complex. The simpler the design the less resistance is required.
2 Upstands may help in reducing entry of precipitation through an open ridge, particularly on low-pitched roofs.
3 Caps increase the probability of entry of wind-driven precipitation and may lead to choking of the opening with snow. Caps do, however, prevent the entry of precipitation in calm weather.
4 Various ridge designs studied showed no practical advantage, one over the other.

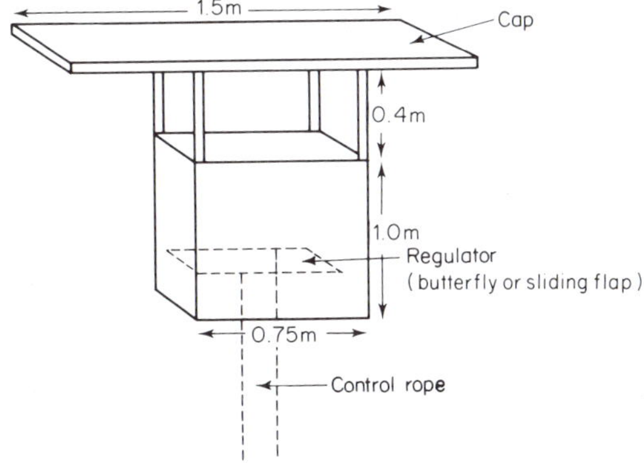

Fig. 5.11 Air outlet flue.

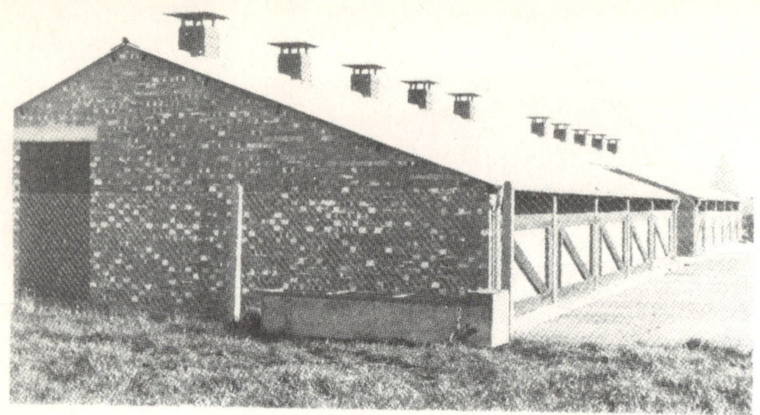

Fig. 5.12 Series of chimney trunks on piggery.

Therefore, while it may be decided to have a cap over an open ridge if the building is in a sheltered site and winds are likely to be low, this is almost contraindicated in very exposed cold areas. A suitable arrangement without a cap is shown in Fig. 5.13.

There are other ways than the open ridge of achieving good 'top' ventilation. These are as follows:

(a) Raised sheets, consisting of conventional steel or asbestos sheets fitted with a batten or washers raising the overlapping, allowing air to pass between the sheets. A spacer batten of treated timber measuring 50 × 25 mm is suitable. This is sometimes called the 'breathing roof' (Fig. 5.14).

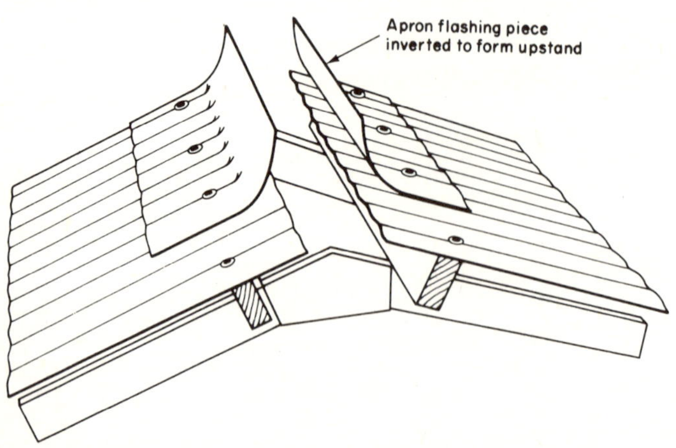

Fig. 5.13 Open ridge without cap.

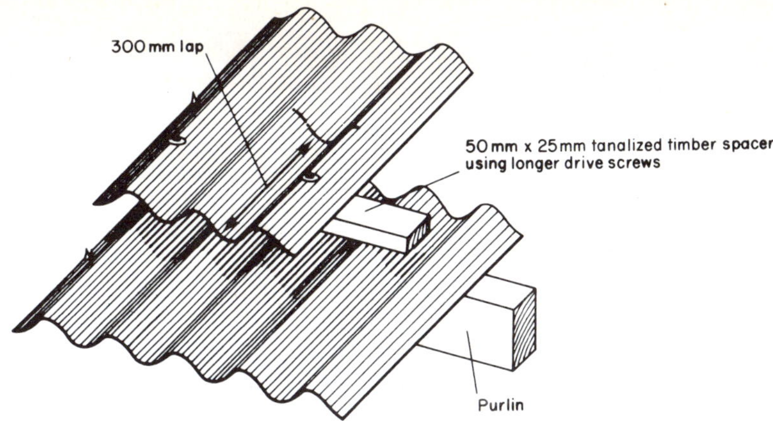

Fig. 5.14 Breathing roof.

(b) Upturned corrugated sheeting. Conventional galvanized corrugated steel sheeting is fixed upside down with a gap between each sheet, forming a Venturi slot between each sheet. Typically a 25 mm gap is used which would give 3.75 per cent opening of the roof (Fig. 5.15).

Mechanical ventilation

This has a place in some cattle yards as well as in other forms of intensively housed stock. With a system of chimney trunks, fans can be added as a complementary arrangement, since an extractor fan can be fitted at the base. If a 600 mm fan running at a maximum of 900 rev/min is fitted, 10 194 m^3/h will be extracted. A maximum allowance of 510 m^3/h per beast (or approximately 0.42 m^3/h per kg body weight) is found satisfactory, so that one fan will serve approximately 30 beef animals to slaughter.

Automatic or semi-automatic control can be achieved if a proportion ($\frac{1}{2}$–$\frac{2}{3}$) of the fans are put on thermostatic control, with a thermostat which is easily

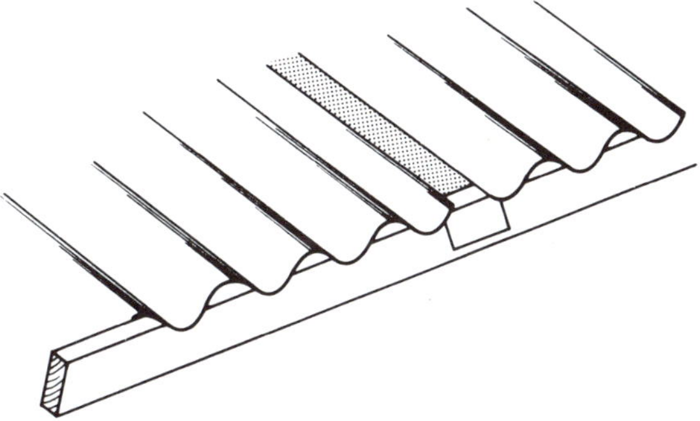

Fig. 5.15 'Upside-down' roof ventilation (corrugated metal sheets with 24 mm gaps).

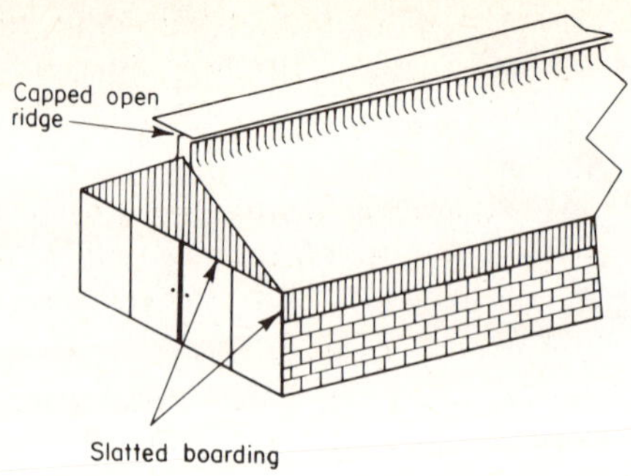

Fig. 5.16 Covered cattle yard.

seen and adjusted. Fans thus operated should have automatic anti-back-draught flaps fitted to prevent down-draughts when they are switched off. All fans should be speed-controlled. Alternatively, a system of variable fan speed on a motorized thermostat or electronic control will give full automation on all fans.

Fan ventilation halves the number of roof outlets that need to be installed. The total cost of a fan-operated system will hardly be more than £5 per animal place, an economical cost for automatic environmental control, but unfortunately running costs with inflationary electricity tariffs are a rather more daunting prospect.

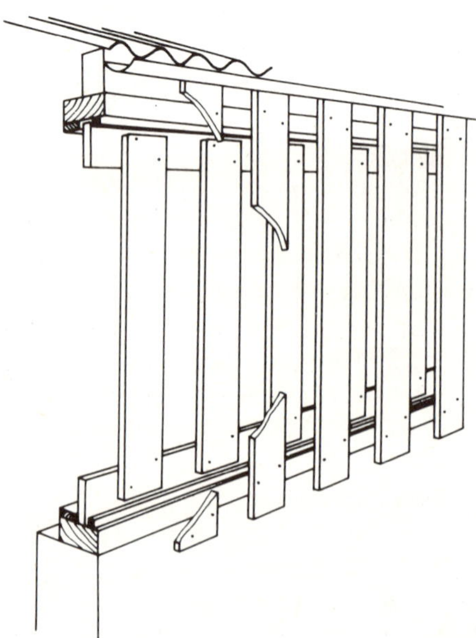

Fig. 5.17 Adjustable spaceboarding for wall cladding. Dimensions of adjustable boarding: fixed outer slats (125 × 25 mm); inner sub-panel, sliding slats (125 × 25 mm) in runner guide; slats spaced at 150 mm.

The main use of fan ventilation in cattle yards is in those cases where extremely high stocking rates are used, as with slatted floor units, or where the topography of the site or restriction of wind around the building makes natural flow all but impossible.

The inlet of fresh air is no less important, and it has been found satisfactory to provide inward-opening hopper flaps along both side walls, bottom-hung and 700–900 mm deep, with gussets and variable control through casement stays or remote control from the feeding passage. Alternatively, the hoppers may be controlled from the ends with horticultural glasshouse-type fittings. It is preferable if the inlets are not closer than 600 mm to the eaves, to prevent incoming air 'bouncing' off exposed purlins and causing an irritating down-draught on the animals. The flaps should be made so that they can be removed or hinged down flat in the summer; they should extend along at least one-half and preferably two-thirds of the wall length.

With wide-span yards over 21 m, slatted boarding (100 mm boards and 12 mm gaps or 150 mm boards and 25 mm gaps) should be fitted at the gable ends and part of this area made as hinged doors that can be opened in the summer (Fig. 5.16). This is normally not necessary, however, in narrow-span yards. In addition, there are a number of other excellent techniques for achieving good inlet ventilation for cattle and other yards.

'Space-boarding' is excellent all around a yard, at the gable ends and along the walls above animal height. It gives an opening area of about 20 per cent of the total but cannot be controlled; an alternative is to have an adjustable system with fixed outer slats and inner sliding slats. There are also various other arrangements, such as the Ventair steel sheet with patented louvres (13 per cent open); slatted hardboard with slats 5 × 25 mm giving 30 per cent opening; Netlon polypropylene mesh (45 per cent open): Ventrex steel sheet with louvres (0.7 per cent open) and a common device of a space left between the outer sheet and the wall, giving a baffled, protected inlet (Fig. 5.17).

It is in no way suggested that the systems outlined here are the only satisfactory methods of ventilating intensive cattle yards. Other mechanical means have been used, often with equal success. These do, however, often need more careful designing and management to prevent draughts and to give adequate control. The systems suggested are logical and generally understood and easily controlled by the stockman. Mechanical assistance with the designs shown are complementary to natural flow and indeed may be used as an additional stage in the development and improvement of a design. Draughts are least likely where there is the fullest control of the system. Ventilation continues to function at a reduced rate in the event of power failure with the system advocated, since natural stack effect ventilation takes over from the fans to tide the stock over this period.

If the trend towards high stocking rates continues it is inevitable that the farmer will turn increasingly to thermal insulation of the surfaces, especially the roof. Farmers who have used insulation of the roof have recorded considerable benefits in terms of liveweight gain and food conversion, but above all because it helps to solve environmental problems. A popular way of arranging the

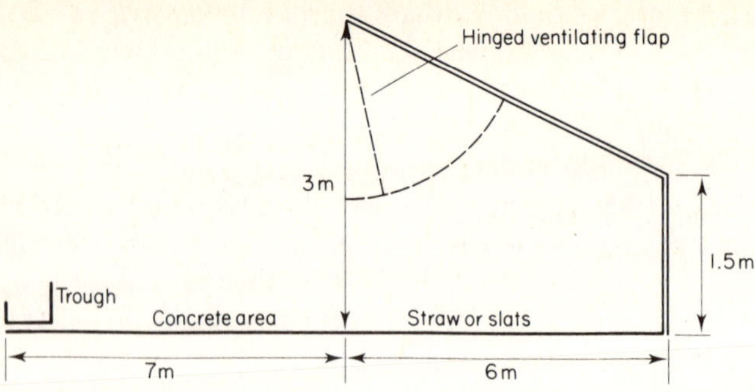

Fig. 5.18 Kennel with outside uncovered yard.

insulation is by using two skins of fibre-cement sheeting for the roof, separated by a vapour-sealed layer of mineral wool or glass wool. For the latter, a 50 mm thickness is minimal but 100 mm is very much better. A low-cost though temporary treatment for an existing uninsulated building is to build a false ceiling of wire mesh supporting vapour-sealed insulation.

It should be emphasized that each yard will have its individual requirements according to site and locality. It is one of the advantages of fan ventilation that with mechanical ventilation this is much less true, since the use of fans rules out in part the dependence on site and weather. It is generally better to have yards in exposed positions because it is easier to restrict the open area if too much air comes in then to open up the ventilation space in a sheltered site. Sometimes the proximity of other buildings makes it impossible to increase the air flow at all.

Livestock yards are now often made very wide – of the order of 40–50 m. These are invariably the most difficult units to ventilate. From the point of view of ventilation it is desirable to limit the span to some 30 m. Indeed, if the trend towards the use of thermal insulation continues, views on what constitutes an adequate cubic area may change. In an uninsulated yard a large cubic area helps to buffer the outside weather extremes. But in an insulated construction, the roofing area must be reduced to a minimum to cut costs. More economical dimensions would be a height of 3.6 m to eaves with a maximum yard span of

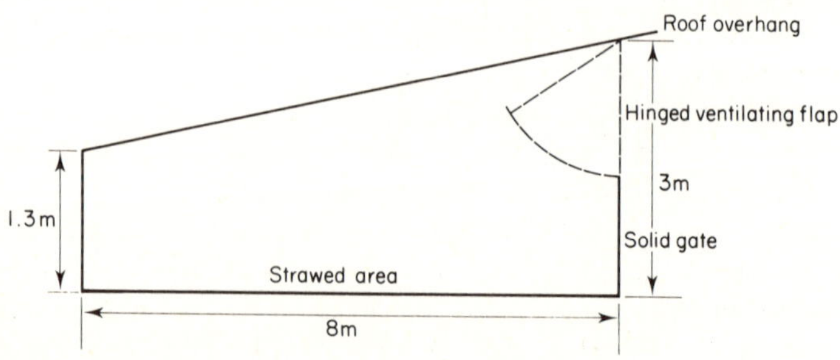

Fig. 5.19 Totally covered lean-to.

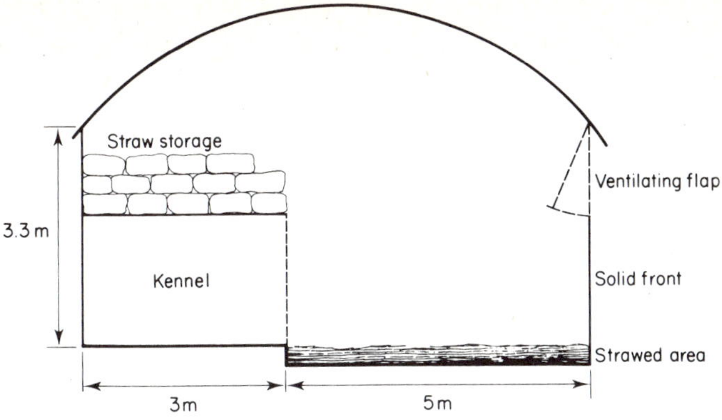

Fig. 5.20 Open-fronted yard with kennel.

21 m. These widely used recommendations for cattle buildings apply, with only minor modifications, to climatic yard accommodation generally, including that for pigs, sheep and turkeys.

OPEN-FRONTED YARDS AND KENNELS

A fundamentally different approach to climatic housing is the 'lean-to' or open-fronted yard, often called the mono-pitch building. This is attractive in several respects and continues to gain in popularity as an alternative to the span roof yard. It is usually cheaper. Also, by its very nature, it is impossible to make it very wide–a depth of 10 m being about the maximum–so the enormous problems of ventilation created by wide spans are avoided and stock concentrations in one air space are limited. Best of all, such a system gives low-cost isolation of groups by carrying vertical partitions to the roof and if necessary supporting it every 3–6 m. With an open-fronted design animals have a choice of environment, as they can go towards the lower back part in colder conditions to keep warm, or come to the front for sunlight and more fresh air in warmer weather. Control of air flow can be by simple hinged flaps on the front, and kennels can be incorporated if desired. It is most desirable that open-fronted yards face in a southerly direction only and it is preferable not to face two rows together, as there is a risk of the passageway between becoming

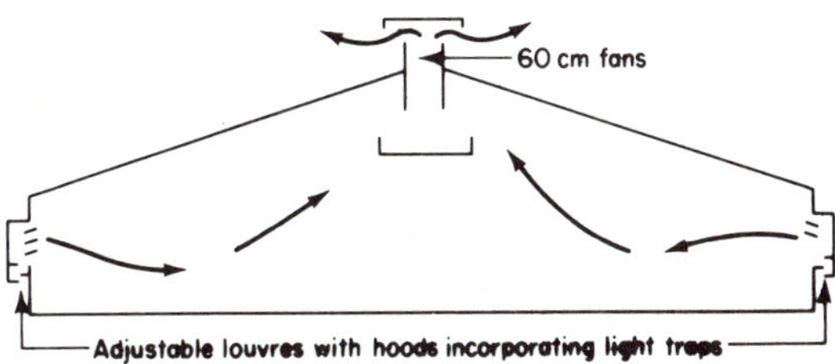

Fig. 5.21 Roof extraction with air entry through side.

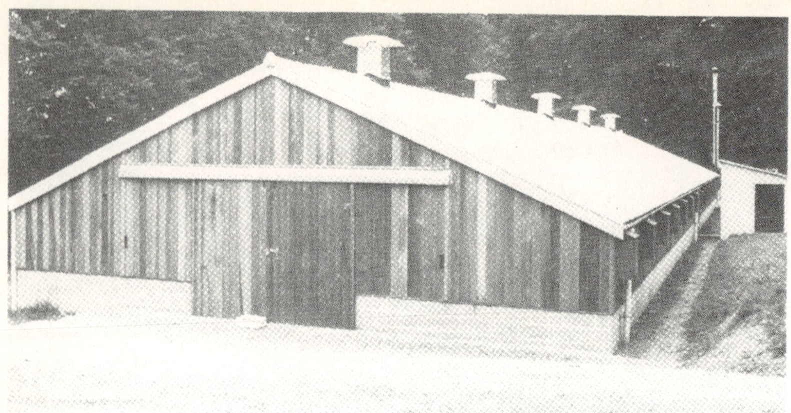

Fig. 5.22 General view of windowless broiler house with artificial ventilation. Brooding is by oil-fired boiler circulating hot water. Exterior of house in cedar wood.

a wind tunnel; further one side at least will face north or east and so may get little sun and indeed suffer from distinctly cooler conditions.

The three main developments of this system are shown in Figs 5.18–5.20. Simplest of all is the kennel with outside uncovered yard (Fig. 5.18), widely used in milder areas of the country and especially favoured for pigs. In the case of these animals, since the muck and feeding are both outside, and if the pigs are in small kennels of 10–15 only, ventilation problems are most unlikely and good health is favoured by the isolation and the freedom from any muck in the sleeping environment. For more severe climatic areas the totally covered 'lean-to' (Fig. 3.19) is favoured, or the kennel arrangement (Fig. 5.20).

CONTROLLED ENVIRONMENT VENTILATION SYSTEMS

The conventional method of ventilating a livestock building is to extract the air from a limited number of ridge fans while the air enters through baffled inlets around the wall (Figs. 5.21 and 5.22). The inlet areas should be related to the extraction rate: to each 1000 m^3/h extracted an allowance of 0.27 m^2 of inlet area can be made. This ensures, in practice, that the inlet velocity is low and the likelihood of draughts is minimized. The advantage of this system is that it is most flexible, the fans assisting or supplementing the natural flow of air. If the fans (or electricity) fail, then this natural flow offers some ventilation until they are restored (Fig. 5.23).

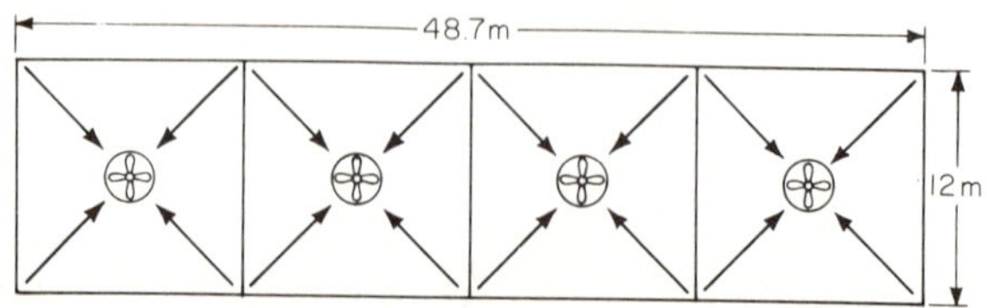

Fig. 5.23 Diagram showing the distribution of fans in a rectangular building.

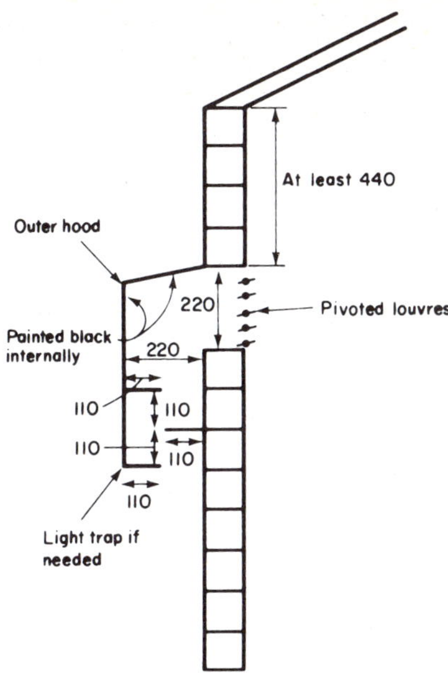

Fig. 5.24 Design of controlled fresh-air inlet incorporating light trap.

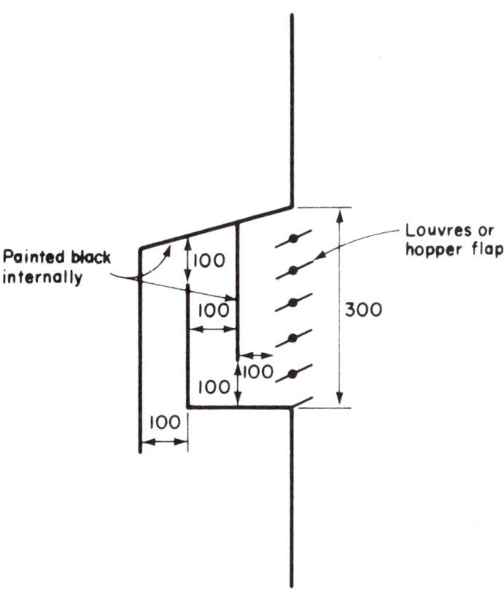

Fig. 5.25 Improved wall air inlet giving complete wind and light control.

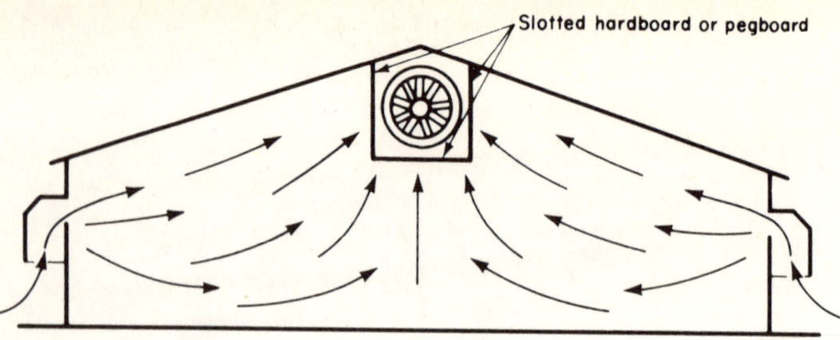

Fig. 5.26 Ducted air system exhausting through end walls with air entry through side walls.

A 'chimney' trunk may be used to take the fan and is an alternative to the manufacturer's cowl; the trunk may be placed on or just to the side of the ridge. If there is a false flat ceiling, the trunk must be extended down to it. This must also be insulated to avoid any risk of condensation. The fresh air inlets, on the other hand, should extend all around the walls and form a nearly continuous line at least 1 m above the livestock, but not less than 300 mm below the eaves; if these limits are exceeded there is a danger of draughts on the stock. The detailed design of the air inlet also needs great care. Suitable forms for normal

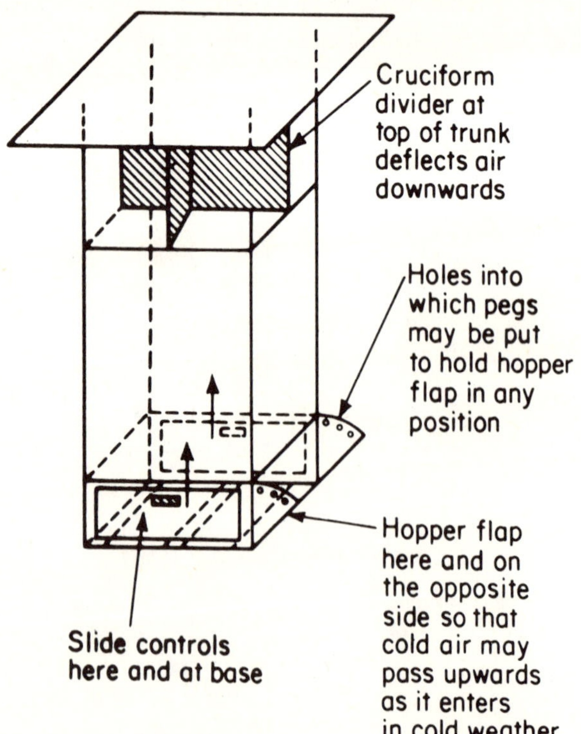

Fig. 5.27 Detailed design on chimney air inlet.

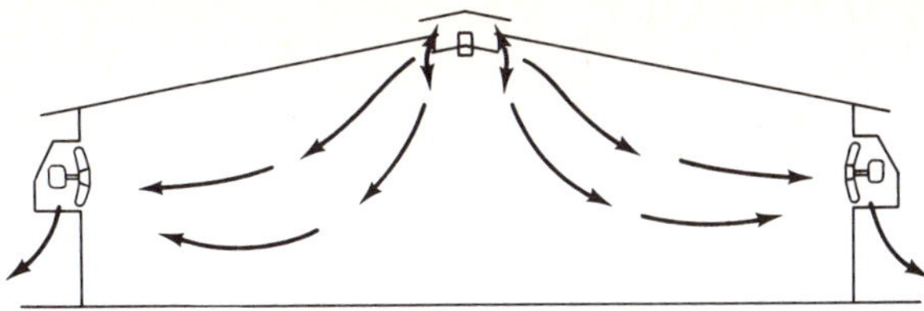

Fig. 5.28 Side wall extraction with air entry through the ridge.

sites are shown in Figs. 5.24 and 5.25. Its main features are the centrally pivoted louvres on the inside and the hood on the outside. The louvres should be controllable in stages.

It is sometimes more convenient to place the extractor fans in the gable ends, connecting them to a duct under the ridge (Fig. 5.26). This arrangement is usually only practicable in short buildings. Because quantities of dust may accumulate in the duct, the latter must be easy to dismantle and clean. In poultry house ventilation it is almost always essential to prevent entry of light through the inlets. The hood on the outside therefore requires good light baffles incorporated. Two forms are shown in Figs. 5.24 and 5.25. A baffle is placed under the outlet ventilator to prevent the entry of light at this point. Such an arrangement is suitable for most broiler, brooder and laying houses with the birds on the floor. In the case of battery houses, further problems are presented due to the birds being kept at various heights within the house and to the difficulty of bringing fresh air into the central cages when three or more lines of cages are installed. There are two methods of overcoming these problems: (1) install two lines of inlets, one 300 mm below the eaves and the other 760 mm from the floor; and (2) use underfloor ducting to bring the correct percentage of air to the central cages.

With four rows of cages the underfloor ducts are usually made about 600 mm wide and 300 mm deep, running transversely across the building at 3 m centres. The precise shape and size will depend on the number of birds housed, the aim being to bring the air in at not more than 2.5 m/s. Some of the alternative systems listed below are also suitable for battery houses and in particular, the arrangement with ridge air entry and side wall extraction is often favoured and is detailed later.

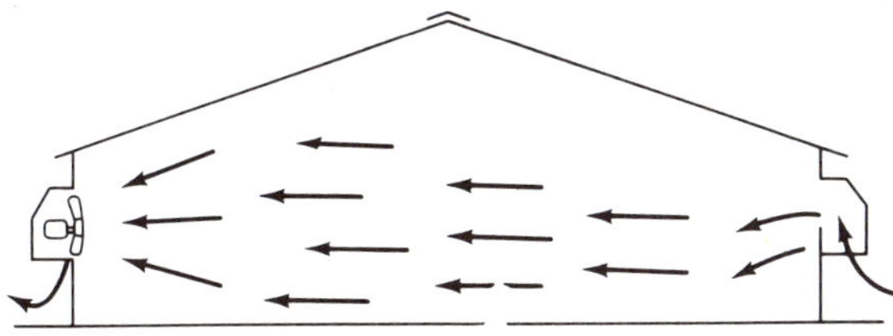

Fig. 5.29 Cross ventilation with air entry through side wall and fan extraction through opposite side.

The conventional system described is suitable for many forms of livestock building. There are however a number of useful alternatives which are gaining in popularity.

Extraction from side walls

The majority of the most unpleasant effusions in a piggery arise in the dunging area and it has become popular in those piggeries with dunging passages along the outer walls to extract the stale air from this point and bring the fresh air in at or near the ridge. This is a particularly appropriate system for the Danish-type or other piggery with screened-off dunging passages. Multiple fan units are used in the dung passage walls and the air is brought into the piggery either through chimney-type ventilators on the ridge or through a continuously open ridge.

The detailed design of the inlet is of supreme importance in the correct functioning of such a system. Where a chimney-type inlet is used (Fig. 5.27) the open area at the top immediately under the cap should have a cruciform-shaped divider to deflect the wind and fresh air down the chimney. At the base of the chimney control flaps give directional flow of air. This is done by blocking the base of the chimney and allowing the air to enter the piggery through control flaps in the side. With these flaps the air can be directed away from the pigs in the colder weather and towards the pigs in hot summer conditions. If a continuous open ridge is used (Fig. 5.28) the volume and direction of the air entering is controlled by centrally hinged flaps regulated remotely at the ends of the house.

Cross- and end-to-end ventilation

With buildings of moderate width (less than 12 m) a simple system is to ventilate across the span. This principle can also be applied along the length of a building provided that it is not more than about 30 m long. Fig. 5.29 shows a typical arrangement of cross-ventilation. It is apparent that, depending on the length of the house, a number of fans may be needed in one side wall. This means that in some cases a smaller number of fans can be employed in comparison with side wall extraction. A disadvantage, however, is that in the event of a supply interruption there is no provision for natural ventilation to take over so automatically controlled stand-by generators are essential. With the end-to-end system, which has mainly been used for battery houses, good air distribution between and among the rows of cages is achieved but it is usually a few degrees warmer at the fan extraction end than the inlet end since animal heat is being picked up.

Ventilation of wide-span buildings

Modern practice frequently favours a wide-span house of 14–22 m. With the conventional extraction arrangement there may be a tendency for variations to exist between the temperature of the incoming fresh air at the side of the house and the stale air at the centre of such a wide building. If the stock is on the floor, this can result in poor distribution, leading to overcrowding in some areas, which can have harmful effects on productivity and the incidence of disease.

One method of improving air distribution in the house is to diffuse the incoming air by means of a filter of glass-fibre or hessian. Whilst this is certainly effective, it should be borne in mind that in use fine filters tend to clog with dust and so the fans will eventually draw less air through the house. It is then necessary to replace or clean the filters. Possibly more successful is the use of peg board or slotted hardboard as 'diffusing' agents.

The introduction of air through low walls presents particular problems as it may be almost impossible to avoid draughts at floor level. In such cases a satisfactory solution is to bring air in under the ridge and place extraction fans in opposite walls (Figs. 5.30 and 5.31) This system functions in the following way:

1 Multiple extracting fans are placed in the side walls with external baffles to prevent wind pressure effects and light entry.
2 A large central duct is placed under the ridge of the building and is designed to be of such an area that the air velocity along its length is not in excess of 300 m/min.
3 The duct of perforated hardboard is opened at each end to the atmosphere; controllable louvres allow sufficient free fresh air entry, but protect the duct from rain or snow.
4 Heating may be applied to the incoming air either inside or outside the duct. The most common arrangement is to heat the air at one or both ends of the duct.

This system has been used to provide 'whole house' heating for broilers. In this case a large centrally-mounted duct of slotted hardboard is fixed along the full length of the house and a heater introduces warm air to mix with incoming cold air into the duct. While this system has been effective in raising the house temperature to the required value of 27–29°C and chicks have been successfully brooded on the floor, a very low humidity value in the house results. There have ben examples of respiratory infection which may have been encouraged by this condition. In such cases humidification of the incoming air by means of a 'curtain of water' introduced at the inlet appears to have corrected the problem.

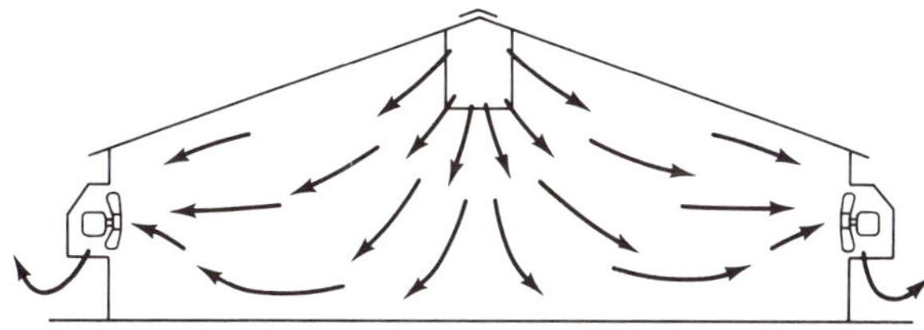

Fig. 5.30 Ventilating wide-span building by central ridge duct inlet and fan extraction through side walls.

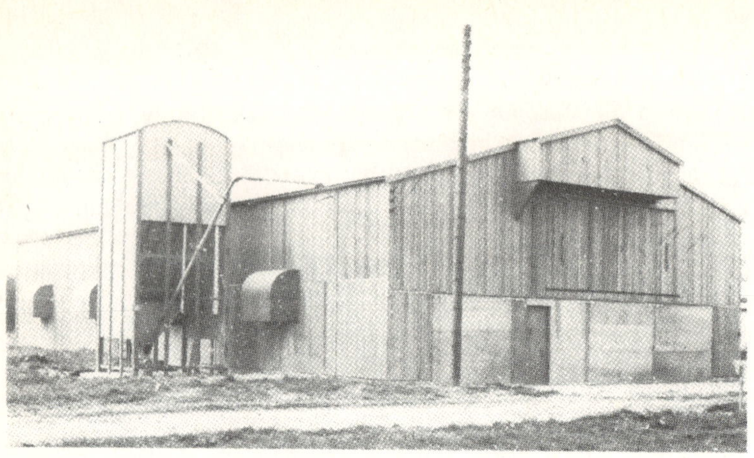

Fig. 5.31 Wide-span deep-pit poultry house with ridge intake and side wall extraction.

Recirculation systems

There is a simple system for small buildings which involves a minimum of equipment and gives a recirculation arrangement using only one fan and which runs at a fixed speed. The fan is mounted 0.9–1.2 m from the end of the duct running the length of the house, above or below the ceiling. The duct is of two-skinned insulated construction, with outlets at the base, and placed centrally over feed or service passages to avoid down-draughts on the livestock. At the base of the duct is a shutter (A in Fig. 5.32) hinged at the point marked P. When the shutter is fully closed the fan will pull all the air from outside to distribute entirely fresh air into the building. When, however, the weather becomes cold or there is less weight of stock in the building, the shutter A is moved back progressively. As this is done, less fresh air comes in but more of the warmed air is recirculated. Stale air passes out at the side of the building through small outlets 700–800 mm from the floor. The recirculating shutter can be mechanically and thermostatically operated if desired. If the building is more than about 15 m long, fans should be placed in the duct at both ends. This system is unsuitable for buildings divided into individual compartments unless the ducts draw in the air from the sides of the house, one duct serving one compartment.

An automatic and more sophisticated proprietary arrangement–the Fristamat–is now used in a number of controlled environment buildings (Fig. 5.33). With this arrangement there are no ventilating inlets or outlets in the house other than the Fristamat units, which are set in the roof and which serve as inlets and outlets. A special fan is provided with two sets of blades, an inner row for exhaust and an outer row for supply into the building. In addition there is an automatic damper assembly that controls the mixing of the incoming and exhaust air, depending on the climatic conditions. At high outside temperatures, the thermostat and servo-motor device that adjusts the damper arranges for the

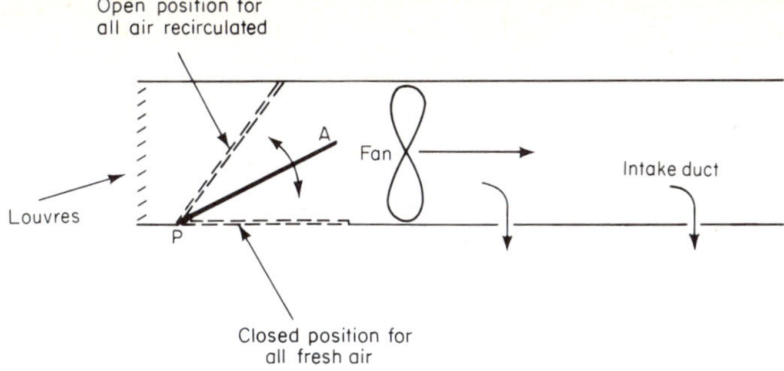

Fig. 5.32 Detail of duct construction for recirculation ventilation.

supply of 100 per cent outside air, but at decreasing outside temperatures the amount of fresh air is gradually reduced and a corresponding volume of internal air is recirculated, so the total air moved never varies.

Plenum or pressurized ventilation

There are a number of good reasons and special cases where it is much better for the ventilating air to be forced into a building with impeller fans. Such examples are the Danish-type piggery with fans placed in or near the ridge and above the centre passage, and those piggeries with outside yards where, by forcing the air into the building through the wall on the opposite side to the yard, the likelihood

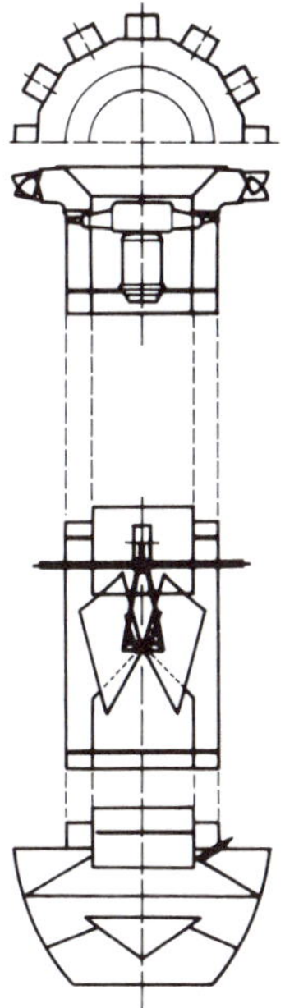

Fig. 5.33 Fristamat automatic system.

of draughts is reduced, since air should pass out of the pen into the yard. Strong winds may overcome the effect of the fans, so care with the construction of the baffle doors is still required.

The plenum system may be achieved quite simply by installing a fan in the type of ridge chimney described on p. 94. Alternatively, it may be done by placing fans in the gable ends and using an insulated duct running along under the ridge in the angle between the wall and the ceiling or above the false ceiling where this is present (Fig. 5.34). With such an arrangement great care must be taken to prevent down-draughts on the pigs by placing deflectors below the air exits, or directing air towards a wall or passage. The outlets from the duct must keep the air velocity low and be fully controllable.

The glass-fibre ceiling. One way of achieving a good reversed system and pressurized ventilation arrangement is to use the whole ceiling of up to 50 mm of glass-fibre through which the incoming air is diffused. It has the advantage that the incoming air passes into the house over a very wide area, so that the circulation is draught-free and uniform. The degree of pressurization helps to overcome the wind's adverse effects and the reverse flow affords a more dust-free atmosphere for the operator. The filtration may have useful health effects through partial purification of the air. Whenever the roof space is used as the pressure chamber, as in this case, it is important that it be well sealed from air leakage and it is desirable that it be both lined and insulated, otherwise there is a real danger that during warm and specially very sunny weather the roof space will become so hot the incoming air will be pre-heated.

Another special need is to ensure that there is an alarm system and/or an automatic standy generator, since otherwise in such a well-sealed house the animals will very quickly suffocate.

An alternative to this type of system is to fit an electro-magnetic failsafe system at the base of the fan inlet trunks and the top of the outlet boxes (see A, Fig. 5.35), so that if there is an electricity failure, the two arrangements pivot out of position and allow the whole system to go into reverse and act temporarily as a conventional system.

An economical way of achieving pressurized ventilation of livestock buildings is to use perforated polythene ducts which may be suitably served by ordinary propeller-type fans running usually at the higher speeds. The system has been

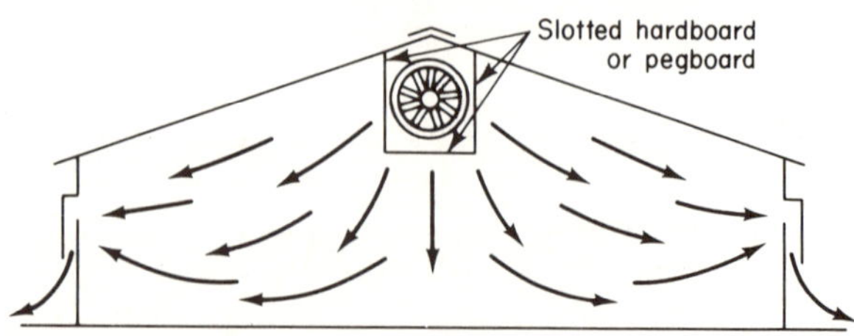

Fig. 5.34 'Pressurized' ventilation with fan blowing air through slotted hardboard ducting at ridge level, and air outlets in side walls.

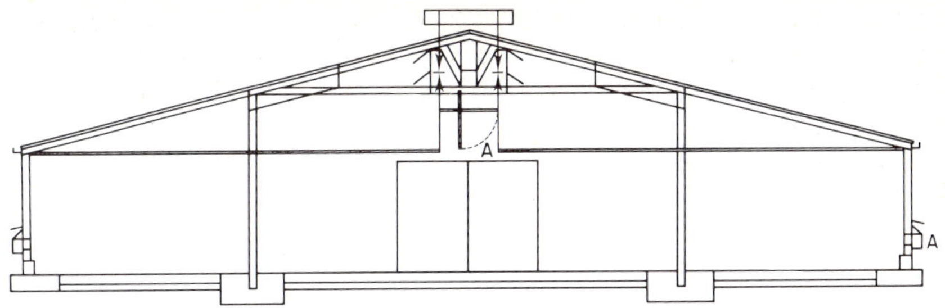

Fig. 5.35 The failsafe system. (A) Electromagnetic failsafe system to base of fan trunk and top of outlet box (pivot at base). (B) Weather sealing to joint between outlet box and wall. (C) Back-draught shutters of roof gauge reinforced polythene sheet. (D) Vermin-proof grid to airway from outlet box. (E) Airways to be not less than 0.1 m^2/1500 m^3/h except at fan. (F) Maximum airway to fan back-draught shutters: $1\frac{1}{2}\times$ fan area. (G) Fan mounting as manufacturer's specification of diaphragm ring and running mode for maximum volume output.

most widely used in piggeries and calf buildings and has been especially developed by Carpenter of the National Institute of Agricultural Engineering. It is important with such a system to study the literature referred to or take specialist advice.

Regulation of mechanical ventilation

Whichever system of mechanical ventilation is used, it requires an excellent control arrangement to cope with the variations between seasons and ages of the animals within the house. Fans should therefore have thermostatic devices, preferably electronic, which will vary the ventilation rates. Control panels are available which alter fan speeds gradually, preventing abrupt changes, while still leaving it in the hands of the stockman to fix a *minimum* rate below which the ventilation will not drop.

The use of a system of inlets with fan ventilation known as the 'high speed inlet' is often preferred. Using a limited area of high-level inlets a better mixing of the incoming air can be achieved and the adverse effects of the wind are eliminated. Care must be taken with this system to have: (a) totally smooth interior surfaces, (b) automatic motorized damper control on the inlets; and (c) a specialized design of fan and regulation by an expert so the whole system is totally balanced at all times.

THE DANGERS FROM GASES IN FARM BUILDINGS

Problems associated with gases in and around the livestock farm have been highlighted recently, particularly in association with gas effusion from slurry channels under perforated floors, but it would be wrong to regard these as the only dangers. Also, while there are now numerous fatalities recorded of livestock, and indeed in man, due to gas intoxication, there is also mounting evidence that there may be concentrations of gases in many livestock buildings that may adversely affect production by reducing feed consumption, lowering growth rates and increasing the animals' susceptibility to invasion by pathogenic micro-organisms.

Sources of harmful gas concentrations

The most serious incidence of gas intoxication arises from areas of manure storage in slurry pits or channels under the stock, usually but not always associated with forms of perforated floors. The greatest risk arises when the manure is agitated for any reason, usually when it is removed. There is also an ever-present danger if a mechanical system of ventilation fails and this is the only method of moving air in the house. Several cases of poisoning have been reported when sluice-gates are opened at the end of slurry channels and the movement of the liquid manure has forced gas up at one end of the building.

High concentrations of gases–chiefly ammonia–may also arise from built-up litter in animal housing. This is most likely in poultry housing since the deep litter system is the commonly used system with broiler chicken, poultry breeders and some commercial egg layers. The danger has undoubtedly been exacerbated in recent years, owing to the necessity of maintaining relatively high house temperatures in order to reduce food costs while at the same time there has been good scientific evidence that higher temperatures than hitherto should be maintained in the poultry house for optimal egg production. The farmer has often attempted to achieve such temperatues by restricting ventilation and in the absence of good thermal insulation of the house surfaces, so that the result may often be generally harmful if not actually dangerous.

The most popular form of heating poultry buildings has long been by gas radiant heaters which are suspended from the ceiling. Well over half of all poultry housing is heated in this way and because the cost of gas appears to be improving in relation to that of electricity, this system is being used more for pig housing and especially for piglets in the early weaning system. There is a risk that with inexpert use such heaters may be improperly serviced and the house insufficiently ventilated to give complete combustion and toxic quantities of carbon monoxide can be produced.

The gases produced

The most important gases generated from stored manure are carbon dioxide, ammonia, hydrogen sulphide and methane; in addition there are a large number of trace organic compounds. In the following paragraphs limits of concentrations that are said to be acceptable are expressed as threshold limit values (TLV) and given in parts per million (ppm). A threshold limit value is the maximum concentration to which industrial workers may be repeatedly exposed in an eight-hour day during a working lifetime, without adverse effect. It is argued that the

TLV for animals may be lower than for man since they may be exposed continuously to the gases.

Carbon dioxide

Carbon dioxide is a colourless, odourless gas considerably heavier than air and highly soluble in water. Normal air contains about 300 ppm and more is released in respiration of animals and by manure decomposition. Most of the gas in bubbles coming from stored liquid manure or from lagoons or oxidation ditches is carbon dioxide. Concentrations of up to about 2000 ppm can be commonly measured in normal controlled environment houses.

There will, however, be considerably more than this where there is any interruption in ventilation or the ventilation is very poor. Carbon dioxide is not highly toxic to animals or man but the risk is that its formation contributes to an oxygen deficiency and so results in asphyxiation. The TLV for carbon dioxide is said to be 5000 ppm. Concentrations of 100 000 ppm (10 per cent) cause violent panting and higher concentrations have a narcotic effect. Death will occur after a few hours of concentration of 250 000 ppm (25 per cent) or more.

No significant distress has been recorded when pigs inhale air containing 20 000 ppm (2 per cent) carbon dioxide if normal quantities of oxygen are present. Air containing 40 000 ppm causes deeper and faster breathing. More than 100 000 ppm may produce dizziness and even unconsciousness. Even concentrations of 200 000 ppm are not necessarily dangerous to animals for a limited period.

Ammonia

Ammonia is a colourless gas with a very characteristic pungent odour. It is lighter than air and very soluble in water. It does not burn readily but air mixtures of over 16 per cent ammonia are considered explosive. It is a gas that is released from fresh manure and during anaerobic decomposition of organic matter. The problem is less with slatted floors than with solid flooring, because of the high solubility of ammonia in water. Concentrations are measured as high as 170 ppm in piggeries and poultry houses which are badly ventilated. A TLV for man of 50 ppm has been set to protect against irritation to the eyes and mucous membranes of the respiratory tract. Air containing 50–100 ppm, however, can be inhaled for some hours by man without apparent effect. A concentration as high as 5000 ppm may cause suffocation. Since it is an irritant, ammonia does produce discomfort in animals but only in quite high concentrations does it cause permanent damage. At 100–200 ppm it induces sneezing, salivation and loss of appetite.

It is known that in the chicken lower levels of 50–100 ppm act by slowing growth rate, inducing kerato-conjunctivitis and reducing appetite, so a practical limit that should be aimed for is suggested as 50 ppm. In any case it seems reasonably unlikely that concentrations higher than 50 ppm would be found except in the worst ventilated of poultry or other livestock houses.

Hydrogen sulphide

Hydrogen sulphide is a colourless gas and has the unmistakeable smell of 'rotten eggs'. It is soluble in water and is produced from the decomposition of organic wastes under anaerobic conditions. A concentration of 0.09 ppm in a normal ventilated house may rise to about 0.30 ppm if ventilation is poor. Dangerous concentrations can be released into a house if there is any form of agitation of stored slurry. Concentrations reaching 200–300 ppm have been found a few moments after pumping out a storage pit and as much as 800 ppm during vigorous agitation. The presence of hydrogen sulphide can be noted by black accumulations of copper sulphide that form on copper thermostats and electrical wiring, the white deposits of zinc sulphate on galvanized metals and black discoloration where lead pigmented paints are used.

Hydrogen sulphide is one of the most toxic gases associated with liquid manure storage, even at low concentrations. Even its characteristic odour does not give adequate warning because the sense of smell can be rapidly dulled by hydrogen sulphide and high concentrations do not give a proportionally higher odour. Its TLV has been set at 10 ppm. Concentrations of 20–150 ppm can affect the eyes after 6–8 minutes and cause severe irritation to the eyes and respiratory tract if inhaled for an hour. Exposure to 500 ppm for 30 min will cause severe headaches, dizziness and excitement.

High concentrations of 800–1000 ppm cause immediate unconsciousness and death through respiratory paralysis unless artificial respiration is immediately applied.

Animals (pigs and cattle) are made uncomfortable by prolonged exposure to low concentrations of hydrogen sulphide. If exposed continuously to at least 20 ppm they display loss of appetite and hyper-excitability: concentrations of 50–200 ppm cause vomiting, nausea and diarrhoea. In acute poisoning hydrogen sulphide acts so rapidly that there are few symptoms of an impending hazard. Sudden nausea and unconsciousness are followed by death at concentrations of 800 ppm and above. Pigs may recover from exposure but may be susceptible to pneumonia.

Methane

Methane is a colourless, odourless gas and is much lighter than air. It is not very soluble in water and is highly inflammable. Methane is generated from the anaerobic deceomposition of manure. Since it is lighter than air and insoluble in water, methane tends to accumulate near the ceiling in stagnant corners or in the top corners of tightly enclosed manure pits. When the air moisture reaches 50 000 ppm any small spark can cause a dangerous explosion. Methane is not considered a toxic gas but characteristics can develop that produce an asphyxiatory atmosphere. Animals suffer no known harmful effects from inhaling methane and since it is considerably lighter than air it will be dissipated rapidly if there is adequate ventilation. Concentrations in controlled environment houses are normally well below the hazardous 5 per cent level, but explosions attributed to methane have occurred around manure storage pits.

Carbon monoxide

It seems to be unlikely that carbon monoxide will appear in a livestock building other than due to the effect of incomplete combustion of gas burners. There are, however, many circumstances under which this may occur. At certain periods, as in brooding chickens or turkeys, the demands for heat are high but the need for ventilation is minimal. If management is careless, the ventilators will be so closed that there is insufficient oxygen for the burners and substantial quantities of carbon monoxide rather than carbon dioxide are produced. Also, if the maintenance of the burners is neglected deposits of dust build up around the air inlets to the burners and starve the oxygen supply. Normal levels of carbon monoxide range up to 5 ppm but harmful effects may arise in livestock from levels of 50 ppm or more.

Fumigation

An increasingly used method of disinfection of animal buildings is to use formaldehyde gas. Clearly, there are potential dangers with this process if care is not taken but fortunately it is so pungent a gas that there is early warning of risk and it is usual nowadays to use remote controlled generation of the gas from solid paraformaldehyde rather than the much more dangerous production of the gas from the interaction of liquid formalin and potassium permanganate.

CONCLUSIONS

There is adequate evidence that gases cause intoxication in and around livestock buildings but there is little information on the precise magnitude of the problem. Reports in recent years have been sufficient to show up the extreme and spectacular dangers when, for example, ventilation fails, slurry is agitated or the combustion of burners is incomplete. They emphasize the inherent dangers in some systems of housing and the measures that can be taken to reduce them by careful planning of ventilation systems and their control. Very much less is known about the effects of sub-lethal concentrations of gas on livestock given a prolonged or even lifetime's exposure to them. One of the authors (D.W.B.S.) is especially aware of the dangers, as on two occasions when it has been necessary to investigate problems of ill-health in livestock, he has inhaled sufficient concentrations of gas to cause fainting – in one case high concentrations of hydrogen sulphide were found and in the other carbon monoxide.

It is of much concern that in many controlled environment buildings the odours and gases arising from manure are offensive and indicate that considerable amounts of gas are passing back into the building. There seems no doubt that since systems that are capable of generating gas are increasing, more investigations of these problems are indicated.

6

Disinfection of Animal Houses

It is generally agreed, and indeed was especially emphasized by the Swann Report[1] on the use of antibiotics in animal husbandry, that there is a much greater need under intensive systems of animal management to have improving standards of hygiene rather than rely on the use of drugs to control disease. One of the most important ways of achieving this is by the regular and thorough implementation of planned disinfection programmes in all livestock units. The disinfection of a building should eliminate from the house all microorganisms that are capable of causing disease thus converting the place from a potentially infective state into one that is largely free from infection. A disinfectant is the agent that is capable of achieving this and in livestock farming it is usually a chemical agent.

DEFINITIONS

In the general context of disinfection terms are used that need precise definition. A *disinfectant* is an agent that is by custom applied to buildings and land. In contrast, an *antiseptic* is an agent that attempts to eliminate infection on living tissues, but it may also sometimes be used to signify a disinfecting agent used in a weaker concentration than a disinfectant that will render harmful microorganisms innocuous either by killing them or by preventing their growth. Another term frequently used is *sanitizer*; this is an agent that reduces the number of bacterial contaminants to a safe level as may be judged by public health requirements. In the 'disinfection' of animal houses an absolute elimination of microorganisms is the general aim so that sanitizers play little part. They do have a part to play, however, in the partial aerosol cleansing of the atmosphere in populated buildings which is resorted to increasingly nowadays.

Other terms that are used include *sterilization* which means nothing less than the complete destruction of all forms of life. It can rarely, if ever, be achieved in the cleansing of animal accommodation though it remains the aim. A *germicide* is an agent that kills all microorganisms and may therefore be considered synonymous with disinfectant, although it is sometimes taken to exclude the destruction of bacterial spores. A germicide may therefore be a less potent agent than a disinfectant. Likewise, a *bactericide* kills bacteria; a *viricide*, viruses; and a *fungicide*, fungi. In general, the suffix -cide applies to any agent that kills microorganisms, while -stat means that the agent merely prevents growth; thus *bacteriostat* is a term that is occasionally used, but has little application in the critical needs of animal housing.

The processes of disinfection of a building can take place by the action of nature (natural disinfection) and by artificial means (artificial disinfection). Before discussing these processes in some detail, it should be emphasized at the outset that 'cleansing' is an essential preliminary to disinfection (Fig. 6.1). Organic matter has the power to reduce considerably the power of disinfectants, so that without good cleansing, the action of the disinfectants is often readily nullified.

NATURAL DISINFECTANT AGENTS

Most pathogenic microorganisms do not survive long outside the animal body, but unfortunately sufficient may always remain to cause renewed infection. While vegetative bacteria and viruses can live several months if protected with organic matter, the spores of bacteria can live almost indefinitely in the soil or protected in cracks and crevices of the building. For example, *Clostridium tetani* and *Bacillus anthracis* can live many years. Even the coccidial oocyst may survive for years in infected quarters.[2,3]

The factors contributing to natural destruction of microbes are nevertheless important, as they do reduce the numbers and this in itself is a worthwhile aid

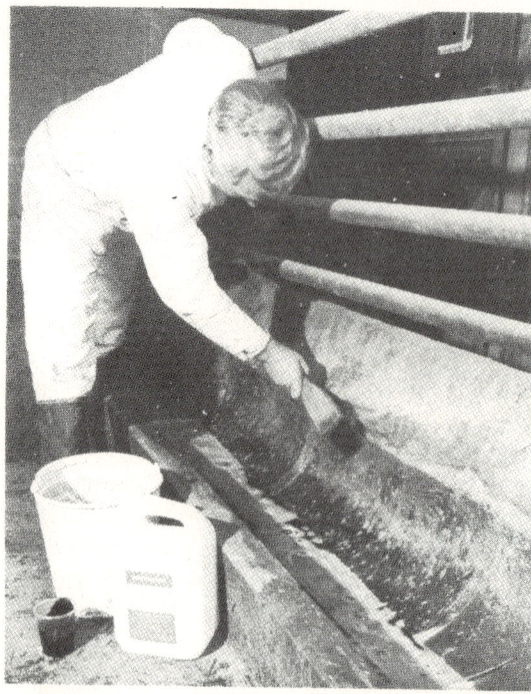

Fig. 6.1 Scrubbing off caked muck may be the only way of cleaning and disinfecting feed troughs.

to the artificial processes. Sunlight, heat, cold, desiccation and agitation all contribute. Sunlight is the most potent and its powers of destruction are enormous. Its efficiency is entirely due to the ultra-violet range of wavelengths and its most effective range is between 2800 and 2400 Å.[3] Unfortunately, these ultra-violet rays have little penetrating power and cannot pass through glass or translucent roofing sheets or through clouds of industrial haze; the value of sunlight in animal buildings is therefore wholly unreliable. Desiccation from fresh air and wind will also contribute to the destruction, particularly when the microorganisms are exposed to this by prior cleansing of the building. In Chapter 3 the reader will also have learned of the effect of temperature and humidity in assisting in the destruction of pathogens. Another process is antibiosis; many bacteria and fungi produce substances which are antagonistic to other organisms. Penicillin and streptomycin are agents of this nature whose antibacterial action is well known. In the soil, in floors and buildings generally, pathogenic organisms will be acted upon by antibiotics produced by non-pathogenic organisms which are normal inhabitants of the soil. Warm, moist conditions will assist the action of such saprophytic agents.

The action of heat

For many years heat has been used for disinfection, dry heat being used with the 'flame-gun' and moist heat in the form of the 'steam-jenny', but both tend to be inexact and uncontrolled methods of applying the agents.

Many bacterial spores can easily survive the transitory attention of the heat source and pathogenic organisms may readily be protected from the heat in cracks and crevices of the building.

CHEMICAL DISINFECTANTS

Disinfection on the farm is generally carried out by using chemical agents (Fig. 6.2). The lethal action of disinfectants (Figs. 6.1 and 6.2) is due in the main to their ability to react with the protein and, in particular, the essential enzymes of microorganisms. Therefore any agents that will coagulate, precipitate or otherwise denature proteins will act as general disinfectants. Among these agents are phenols, alcohols, acids, alkalis, aldehydes, halogens, chloramines and quaternary ammonium compounds, as well as heat and certain radiations. The manner in which chemical disinfectants exert their germicidal activities varies with the type of compound. The halogens generally depend on their reactivity with proteins. Because of this they are highly sensitive to organic matter, which has the effect of reducing considerably their germicidal power. Other oxidizing agents, hydrogen peroxide and the permanganates, also react vigorously with cell proteins. Formaldehyde is almost equally reactive in this case with the amino group of the cell proteins with the same destructive effects.

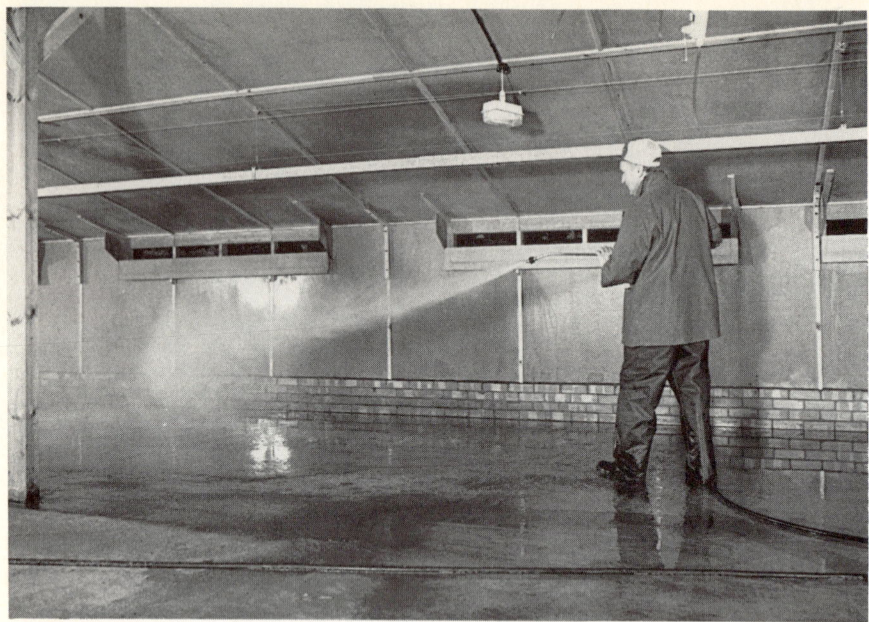

Fig. 6.2 Pressure cleaning a poultry house with a detergent disinfectant — the most effective method of cleaning animal housing.

Acids and alkalis are active mainly through their hydrogen and hydroxyl ions, respectively. Their disinfecting action is related to the concentration of the ions concerned, and acids are more effective than alkalis because at equal concentrations the hydrogen ion is more effective than the hydroxyl ion.

Phenols also act as protein denaturants. The action in this case is by absorption of the phenol by reason of its greater solubility into the protein phase, yielding a complex which may ultimately be coagulated. The quaternary ammonium compounds constitute the large group of substances, some of which are germicides, possessing high surface activity which are cationic by nature. With its surface absorption the material is brought into more effective contact with the bacterial cell and consequently there is an increase in local concentration around the cell. The evidence for the germicidal action of the quaternaries, as they may be termed, is that they induce cytolytic damage, resulting in leakage of cell constituents into the suspending fluid. They may be germicidal to both vegetative microorganisms and their spores at quite high dilutions and are also active against viruses.

SELECTIVE ACTION

Many disinfectants have a selective action on different types of microbes. For example, Gram-positive and Gram-negative bacteria differ in the structure of their membranes, the latter being of a more complex nature. Microorganisms also respond to changes in pH value, and as every protein has its own characteristic isoelectric point, each responds individually and will be influenced by the acidity or alkalinity of the disinfectant; for example, fungi are extremely acid-resistant, whereas viruses tend to be more susceptible to acid disinfectants such as the iodophors. Another factor affecting the behaviour of disinfectants is the lipoid content of the cells; in some the content is high, as in acid-fast organisms, and it will thus attract a lipophilic moiety in a disinfectant substance and dissolve it more readily, increasing its germicidal activity thereby. Some disinfectants which are called 'broad spectrum' are almost equally active against most species of microorganisms, while others show specificity and are only active against a restricted number of species.

DISINFECTION OF VIRUSES[4,5,6]

For disinfection purposes viruses can be classified into two groups: lipophilic and hydrophilic. Lipophilic viruses have lipid envelopes which make them sensitive to the majority of disinfectants. The majority of animal pathogenic viruses are in this group including fowl pest, Aujezsky's disease, Marek's disease, inclusion body rhinitis of pigs, infectious laryngo-tracheitis, pox viruses, bovine rhinotracheitis and duck plague. However, hydrophilic viruses are enveloped and are less sensitive to disinfectants in general and some very important viruses are in this group and which have a tendency to a dangerous persistency on farms and in animal buildings. Examples are porcine enteroviruses, and reoviruses, including Gumboro (IBD), blue comb and viral arthritis of poultry. Against this latter group quaternary ammonium compounds have a poor effect but are very good if associated with formaldehyde, glutaraldehyde and chloramines.

Dynamics of disinfection

Disinfection is not an instantaneous matter; it takes place gradually. However, many more microbes are killed at the beginning of the process than at the end, although there is an initial lag period before activity commences. An examination of the number of organisms surviving at different stages during disinfection shows that the number of bacteria killed in unit time bears a constant relationship to the number of surviving organisms. Thus, after the lag phase, destruction of the bacteria is very rapid at first but tends to slow up, so that eventually destruction of all the organisms takes a considerably longer time. The usual time/survivor curve is of the sigmoid type.

The concentration of disinfectant and temperature of disinfection influence the rate of death and also alter the shape of the time/survivor curves. As the death rate is increased by using higher concentration of disinfectant, the initial lag phase is eliminated or, in fact, is so quick that it goes undetected.

Temperature and dilution

The activities of most disinfectants increase as the temperature is increased, although there are a few exceptions. The so-called 'temperature coefficient' is the measure of the change in velocity of disinfection per degree rise in temperature:

$$\text{temperature coefficient (per } 10^\circ \text{ rise)} = \frac{\text{time to kill at } x^\circ}{\text{time to kill at } (x+10)^\circ}$$

The coefficient is an exponential factor, as is the dilution coefficient. The effect of dilution, however, varies widely between disinfectants. For example, phenol is considerably affected by dilution and hence the coefficient is high.

The accepted formula for calculating the concentration exponent or dilution coefficient is:

$$\frac{\text{log initial number of organisms}}{\text{log survivors}} = \mathrm{K}tc^n \text{ (Sykes)}^2$$

where K = the reaction velocity constant;
t = time of disinfection;
c = concentration of disinfectant;
n = the concentration exponent.

The effect of organic matter

Almost invariably when disinfection is carried out on the farm, organic matter will be present. It can be said that organic matter always interferes with the action of the disinfectant and may do so in the following ways:

1 The organic matter may protect the cell by forming a coating on it and preventing the ready access of the disinfectant.
2 The disinfectant may form an insoluble compound with the organic matter to remove it from potential activity.
3 The disinfectant may react chemically with the organic matter, giving rise to a non-germicidal reaction product.
4 Particulate and colloidal matter in suspension may absorb the anti-bacterial agent, so that it is substantially removed from solution.
5 Fats, etc. in serum and milk may inactivate the disinfectant.

APPROVAL OF DISINFECTANTS

There is no completely satisfactory method of assessing or standardizing disinfectants and an enormous number of different techniques have been used in the past. There is also no universally effective disinfectant, so that different disinfectants are required for different purposes.

In the UK Approvals are under four headings, as follows:

Group 1A are for disinfectants active against foot-and-mouth disease.
Group 1B disinfectants against swine vesicular disease.
Group II covers those against fowl pest.
Group III against tuberculosis.
Group IV for general farm use, the test organism being *Salmonella chlorae-suis*.

The official test lays down a rigid procedure for specified reduction of the organisms in the presence of organic matter. The most recent order, The Diseases of Animals (Approved Disinfectants) (Amendment) Order 1975, specifies some 300 disinfectants in the various groups.

MALODOURS

Many intensive livestock farming operations are liable to cause pungent and objectionable odours. For example, malodours can result from the storage areas or the spread of slurry, from deep-pit cage layer units and from large numbers of pigs and cattle kept housed together. While more careful consideration of the dangers would often enable the risk to be reduced by good planning, sometimes the only practical solution is to use an odour controller such as Antec Maskomal. This is a complex forumulation of aldehydes, ketones, terpenes, acetates, butyrates, esters, perfume compounds and emulsifiers. The material is miscible with water and may be mixed in with the material causing the odour or can be washed over or sprayed on to the offending material or surface. Farmers should, however, look upon all such measures as temporary whilst they recognize procedures to prevent the smells. The odour of agents masking smells is sometimes considered offensive and by its nature must be powerful.

DISINFECTANTS

Phenols and related compounds

The phenols and related compounds are a very important group of disinfectants which were once the most popular of all.

All phenols can act bactericidally or fungicidally but generally are neither sporicidal nor particularly virucidal. They have high dilution coefficients – that is, small concentration changes give rise to large differences in their killing rates. They are always more effective as the temperature rises, and are more active as acid solutions. Organic matter can severely interfere with their efficiency and small quantities of faeces can reduce their effectiveness to 10 per cent. However, the higher the phenol coefficient the greater the influence of organic matter; for this reason the cresols, which are related compounds and have a low coefficient, are only slightly affected by organic matter.

Cresols

The three isomeric forms of cresol – ortho-, meta- and paracresol – form the basis of a large number of proprietary disinfectants. The cresols are only slightly soluble in water and are usually emulsified in soap. Cresols are effective against spores. The presence of soap renders solutions of the cresols suitable for cleaning purposes and this increases their effectiveness, although excess quantities of soap are harmful. Liquid Cresolis Saponatum BP or Lysol D contains 50 per cent by volume of the cresols, the solvent being prepared by the action of an aqueous solution of KOH or NaOH on linseed or other vegetable oil. Lysol is some three times more powerful a disinfectant than phenol, although different preparations vary considerably in their germidical action. There are also many proprietary 'coal tar disinfectants', also phenolic in nature.

In view of the inevitable low solubility in water, they are either solubilized or emulsified. The solubilized types, known as 'black fluids' are those in which the phenol fraction is dissolved in a soap base, and the emulsified types, known as the 'white fluids', are those in which the phenol is emulsified into a permanent suspension with the aid of gelatin or dextrin.

In more recent years a number of synthetic phenols have been marketed. These may be chloroxylenol, o-phenylphenol or one of the other diphenyl derivatives. Such preparations, in contrast to the cresols or coal tar disinfectants, are non-toxic, non-irritant and a more pleasant colour.

Examples of the synthetic disinfectants are Dettol, Ibcol and Antec Aerial disinfectant.

ALCOHOLS

Alcohols tend to be bactericidal rather than bacteriostatic against vegetative organisms, but have no real action against the spores. For example, anthrax spores have lived in alcohol for 20 years. Nevertheless, they can be rendered sporicidal by adding 1 per cent of a mineral acid or caustic alkali, or even by adding 10 per cent of amyl-m-cresol, so that even the most resistant spores are killed in four hours. The only alcohols having practical application are ethyl alcohol, benzyl alcohol and ethylene and propylene glycols. The glycols are mainly active in the aerosol form and as virucidal agents, and indeed it is these which are widely used in animal disinfection and are frequently added to complex mixtures to enhance the overall properties of the disinfectant.

FORMALDEHYDE AND GLUTARALDEHYDE

Formaldehyde is an excellent disinfectant in both the gaseous and the aqueous forms, being bactericidal, virucidal and fungicidal. Its gaseous and aerosol applications are discussed later. In aqueous solutions, formalin, which is an aqueous solution of formaldehyde gas containing 40 g of formaldehyde in 100 ml of the solution, is widely used at 5 per cent strength as a general disinfectant, but it does need to be in contact with the surface for some time to be effective. Its action is greatly affected by temperature (i.e. it has a high temperature coefficient) and the warmer it is the better, blood heat being most satisfactory. It also acts more efficiently when the surface is wet. In agricultural use formalin is largely used as a gas or an aerosol spray.

A very active complex disinfectant which is useful against the most persistent viruses is one containing formaldehyde, glutaraldehyde and a quaternary ammonium compound. This is active at much lower temperatures than formaldehyde (Tegedor, T. Goldschmidt, Ltd.). Glutaraldehyde alone is widely used as a hatching egg cleaner and for hatchery hygiene, e.g. Ovation (Antec International, Ltd.).

PHENYL MERCURIAL COMPOUNDS

Certain mercurial disinfectants are available and a 2 per cent phenylmercury dinaphthylmethane (disulphonate), known as Zeetagen (Antec), is a useful terminal spray in animal houses and also at dilutions of up to 1/640 for the control of egg-transmitted aspergillosis as a dip solution. There is also a satisfactory effect as a bacteriocide.

QUATERNARY AMMONIUM COMPOUNDS

These are cationic neutral detergents available as aqueous solutions, powders or pastes. They are effective against a wide range of bacteria, viruses and moulds and have a high surface activity. Generally, when dissolved in water, they have a high wetting power and the ions adhere to the surfaces, giving a long-lasting residual effect. They also have low toxicity and lack odour or taste. Such products are popular in hatcheries, for aerial disinfection, egg dipping and general disinfection around incubators and equipment. They are often combined with other disinfectants to give a very wide spectrum of activity.

The halogens

Chlorine

In agriculture, chlorine is widely used for disinfecting water and in the cleansing of dairy and other farm equipment. Also, it is common practice for poultry processing plants to introduce between 10 and 20 ppm in their water supply. Chlorine-releasing compounds containing up to 90 per cent available chlorine are available and have an important use in the formulation of bactericidal detergent powders of the alkaline variety. Products of this type are suitable for use in the washing down of an animal house. The inorganic chloramines, being a concentration of chlorine and ammonia, are used in water and sewage treatment and also organic chloramines, such as Halazone, which is an excellent water sanitizer.

The normal use of chlorine in cleaning milk and other utensils is to have a detergent wash with a solution containing 250–300 ppm of available chlorine followed by a rinse with a weaker chlorine solution. Failure of chlorine disinfectant is most likely due to the presence of organic matter, which does seriously interfere with its action, so that it is not normally used where much dirt is present. In favourable circumstances it is best used warm and it will act quickly. Chloramines, such as Halamid (Duphar Veterinary), are much more active in the presence of organic matter and have found a secure place as general disinfectants.

Iodine and iodophors

Iodine is an effective germicide, although like chlorine it is much depressed by organic matter. It is effective against vegetative organisms and spores. The most widely used iodine preparations are the iodophors in which iodine is mixed with surface-active agents, which act as carriers or solubilizers for the iodine. They lack any real odour and are not irritant.

They have been used at dilutions of around 25 parts of available iodine per million for utensils. They have built-in indicators which reveal quickly the approximate concentration of the use-dilution; a yellow tinge or pale amber colour is imparted by an iodophor even when only a few ppm of free iodine are present in the solution. Higher concentrations give deeper shades of amber or brown to the solution. The use-dilution of 25 ppm is equivalent to available chlorine concentrations up to 200 ppm. Iodophors are an ideal germicide to use in water utensils.

The commercially available products, iodophors, contain up to 3 per cent available iodine. For the iodine to exert the maximum bactericidal action it is necessary for the pH to be acid, and phosphoric acid is often added. The iodophors are unaffected by hardness, but organic matter and contact with alkaline detergents are detrimental; they have a wide spectrum of activity and are widely used in the livestock industry as aerosol disinfectants, being safe and pleasant to use.

Sodium carbonate (washing soda)

About 4 per cent solution (that is, 0.5 kg or two handfuls) in 10 litres of water is a traditional general cleaning and detergent agent. Its powers in hot solution make it a useful material, more as a preparation for the site before applying an approved disinfectant. In fact, sodium hydroxide (caustic soda) is a more effective agent, combining good detergent properties with powerful disinfectant action. It is most effective against viruses and Gram-negative bacteria. A 1 per cent solution is more advisable on very dirty surfaces, while a 5 per cent solution is required when there are likely to be numerous spores present. Warning must be given of the caustic nature of this material, which makes it unpopular. When using, it is necessary to wear rubber gloves, protective clothing and an eye-shelter or goggles. This product, incidentally, is the exception that proves the rule in that it becomes *less* active when warmed.

Ammonia

A 10 per cent aqueous solution of ammonia is an effective agent for the destruction of coccidial oocysts. This is the only use for ammonia as a disinfectant. Antec Tryad combines an ammonium compound for this purpose with a general disinfectant.

Quicklime

Quicklime (calcium oxide) is occasionally used as a disinfecting agent; infested land is sometimes treated at the rate of 2 tonnes of quicklime to the acre: also, when disease carcases are disposed of by burial, it is a normal procedure to cover them with quickline. There seems no evidence that either process is particularly effective.

RADIATION STERILIZATION

This is a comparatively new field and it has been only very rarely applied to the field of animal housing, where it admittedly has only slight possible application at present. The two forms which are of importance are (1) the ionizing radiation comprising X-rays, gamma-rays, cathode rays, beta-rays, neutrons, protons, etc., and (2) the ultra-violet radiation. Of the former we can say that they have the greatest application in food and pharmaceutical fields. The radiations have powerful penetrating powers and produce no thermal effect, but the equipment required for generating these radiations is at present quite outside the scope of the agricultural industry and there are also the inherent dangers to personnel.

Ultra-violet radiation has been used on a number of occasions for the aerial disinfection of animal buildings, but the results have not been successful. The problem is that the radiation has negligible properties for penetrating solids or even liquids. It is not a sterilizing agent; it is only capable of reducing the number of organisms, but in any case equipment is too expensive and the radiating tubes have too short a life for economic justification in animal buildings, particularly in view of the dust pollution of the atmosphere which is inevitable.

FILTRATION

Interest has centred on the use of air filters for the supply of air into animal buildings since the advent of large intensive houses in which cross-infection can easily take place between units. Air filtration can be carried out with many types of physical filter or by electrostatic precipitation; the latter is not at present economically justified, as the equipment is expensive and the removal of microorganisms only partial.

Many forms of materials are used for filter media, including cotton-wool, slagwool, glasswool, asbestos and polythene. Particles down to 0.1 μm size can be removed but in fact virus and bacterial particles will travel through the air in dust and organic matter and it is considered satisfactory to filter out particles above 3 μm in diameter and it is reasonable to look for something approaching 100 per cent efficiency at this size. Filters are either the disposable type, which are used for a defined period and then thrown away, or the washable type, which can be regenerated by cleaning in a disinfectant detergent mixture. There is little doubt that the former is more satisfactory for animal buildings. Perhaps the most satisfactory type are the filters which are impregnated with a disinfectant: for example, the Fram filter consists of filter fibres impregnated with a disinfectant.

It has been found that such filters can be used successfully for filtering air into broiler houses for up to the full 7–9 week-cycle. Broiler houses are the dirtiest buildings on the farm, so these will represent extreme conditions. It is always desirable for the filters to be placed on the inlet side of the system, as they will stay viable for longer periods in this way; fans must be used with this arrangement to impel air into the house and maintain a moderate pressure, so that the air will pass out of the unfiltered outlets and the cracks and crevices in the construction of the building. Necessarily, no filtered arrangement is absolute and whether it is worthwhile in practice remains to be proved. An advantage of the filtered system, which is not without importance, is that the air will pass into the house well diffused and draughts are less likely to occur. Certain recent investigations by the author (D.S.) with the use of germicidal filters on broiler sites have shown their value in limiting cross-infection when placed on the inlet side of the ventilation system with mechanical extraction arrangement. The filters apparently lowered the introduction of *Escherichia coli* organisms below the threshold in two selected houses on grossly contaminated site and also helped the control of environmental conditions by diffusing the entering air and acting as a partial light-trap. A full description on the potential use of filters is given by King, Charles and Walker.[7] These workers have also been responsible for the development of a whole-ceiling glass-fibre filter that diffuses the air and reduces the bacterial contamination of the air. Although such a procedure cannot be absolute, the aim in the practical field is to reduce the challenge, and this is a procedure which is likely to do this. Certainly results have been most encouraging. Great care must be taken to see filters are never choked with dust, nor frozen with ice in cold weather.

GASEOUS AND AEROSOL FUMIGATION

The use of gases and vapours for disinfection purposes has recently come into great prominence. There are a number of reasons for this. It is cheap and usually does no harm to the materials used in the construction of the house. It is also comparatively simple for any disinfecting gas to be removed from the house after use. A further advantage, which applies generally to gases, is that they may be applied at normal or only slightly above normal temperatures. Gases tend to be toxic to humans, so care must always be taken in their use.

Formaldehyde

Formaldehyde has been used for many years as a comprehensive germicide and fumigant. All bacteria, including spores, are susceptible to formaldehyde gas, even in the presence of organic matter, so it is clearly the type of material to use for general purposes. It may be used in a number of ways. A popular way is by the interaction of formalin and potassium permanganate: 80 ml of formalin per 10 m^3 for buildings up to 1000 m^3; and for larger buildings up to 2000 m^3, 40 ml per 10 m^3. The ratio of permanganate to formalin required for optimal generation of formaldehyde is two parts of permanganate to three parts of formalin. Great care must be taken in this operation as the compounds react with violence. No more than 1 litre of formalin should be put into each container, which should have deep sides to prevent the mixture bubbling over. As there is a risk of fire, litter and wood members of the house should be kept out of range. The operator should wear a respirator while carrying out the procedure.

Formaldehyde gas may also be released from the solid paraformaldehyde which is obtained in a number of proprietary forms. For example, Alphagen Prills or Microgen are used by placing them on remote-controlled electric hot plates at a rate of 1 kg per 300 m^3 of building. For optimum results the building should be warmed to 20°C or above; many failures are recorded when reliance has been placed on formaldehyde at cold winter temperatures in the order of 0–10°C. If the building cannot be so warmed and virus infections are serious, an additional cleaning with a known active disinfectant must be used.

Formalin vapour

A rather more satisfactory method of carrying out fumigation with formaldehyde is to disperse a mixture of formalin and water as an aerosol of small particle size.[8] For complete sterilization, it should be dispersed at the rate of 30–60 ml to each 6–10 m^3 of air space. For general disinfection rather less is recommended, viz. 30 ml per 15 m^3 for buildings up to 1200 m^3 capacity and 30 ml per 30 m^3 for larger buildings. In relation to the use of formaldehyde, humidity is an important factor in influencing its efficiency. The higher the humidity the better it works, 60–80 per cent being considered the optimum.[9] It also has a high temperature coefficient, so the warmer the better, and a temperature of 20°C is advisable. It is not well diffused into porous materials; it should be considered as primarily a surface disinfectant. If the humidity is below 60 per cent, it is as well to release water vapour to increase it, or mix the formalin with water. The space to be fumigated should be kept closed for at least 12 hours, particularly if a high concentration of bacterial spores is present.

Formaldehyde undoubtedly ranks as the best terminal fumigant. The only problem may be that the compound is difficult to remove after use, owing to the fact that the formaldehyde does not remain in gaseous form during sterilization but becomes absorbed on exposed surfaces as a film of polymerized formaldehyde. Although this appears rarely to be a worry in practice after a good aeration, it may be dealt with by sprinkling a dilute solution of ammonia in the house. The dangers of using formaldehyde alone in cold weather are very real and the material is relatively ineffective at freezing temperatures.

Liquid aerosols

Aerosol particles consist of suspensions of solid or liquid particles in the atmosphere which are of a size less than 200 μm diameter and in this form they remain in suspension a considerable time. Their lightness enables them to flow over and around any solid objects and they can penetrate behind equipment and divisions and so on. High velocity motor or electrically driven aerosol generators can be used to distribute disinfectants within a few minutes, in buildings as large as 1000 m^3 capacity even from a single point (Fig. 6.3). This dispersability of aerosols can be used to provide either an even distribution of vapour in the atmosphere or an even deposition of a film of disinfectant on horizontal and vertical surfaces. They may be used either for disinfection of the air when the animals are in occupation or for terminal disinfection when the building is empty.

Large particles of infected material are resistant to disinfectant, so that air containing large amounts of dust in suspension cannot be effectively disinfected by concentrations of chemical vapour that are not harmful to animals. Before attempting air disinfection in such situations the dust content of the air should be lowered and it is advisable to carry out air disinfection in conjunction with the deposition of dust-adhesive film on the surfaces. A film composed of triethylene glycol retains its dust-adhesiveness for long periods and if a disinfectant is included with it, gradual disinfection of the adherent dust occurs. The following procedure has been recommended on sound evidence for terminal disinfection of farm buildings after prior cleaning and formaldehyde fumigation.

An aerosol of large particle size composed of six parts of a 3–4 per cent

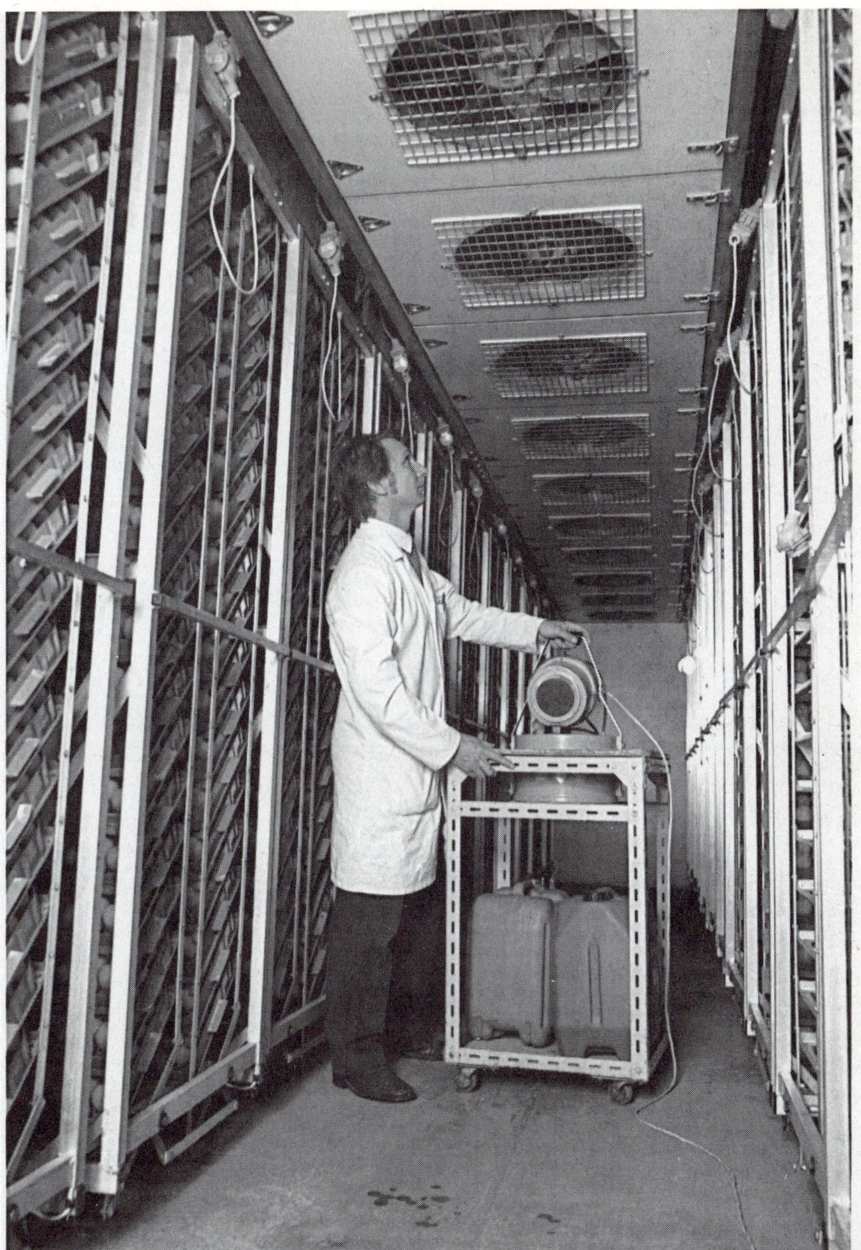

Fig. 6.3 Setting up a spraying machine for the sanitizing of eggs in a mammoth walk-in poultry incubator.

solution of a chloroxylenol mixture and four parts of triethylene glycol is generated in a concentration of 160 ml per 10 m^2 of floor space.. This deposits a film which has been shown to be effective in retaining its adhesive properties for at least one month on non-absorbent surfaces, and its disinfecting activity was only slightly reduced after 17 days. Thus, in this procedure, we are enabled to institute a useful residual activity.

Further work has shown the value of atmospheric disinfection of occupied stock buildings by the following procedures: chloroxylenol, one part; triethylene glycol, two parts; water, two parts. This is generated at the rate of 40 ml per 100 m^2 of air space. A mixture of three parts of chloroxylenol and two parts triethylene glycol provides a suitable formulation for a dust-adhesive and disinfecting surface film in farm buildings which are occupied. This is dispersed in larger-sized particles which settle out of suspension relatively quickly.

ECTOPARASITES

It is of great importance to control ectoparasites in and around the farm buildings (Fig. 6.4): they are a nuisance both to the attendants and the animals; they may be the cause of direct irritation and disease; and they may indirectly spread disease – indeed, any infectious agent can be carried by ectoparasitic vectors.

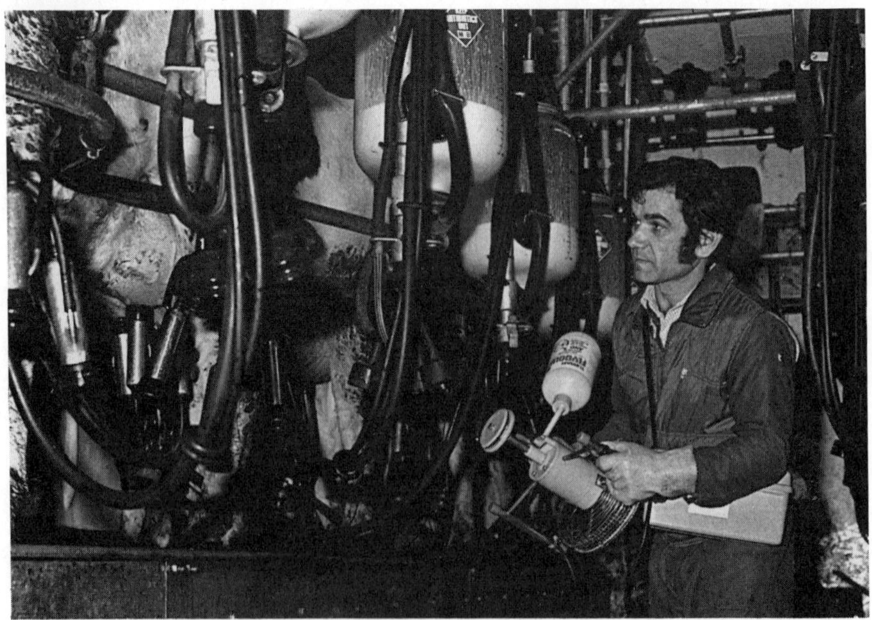

Fig. 6.4 A 'Turbair Flydowner' battery powered sprayer used in the pit of a herring bone parlour. Elimination of flies can be a considerable help in reducing infections such as mastitis.

These ectoparasites include flies (including the ordinary housefly, the lesser housefly and the stable fly), mites (including red mites and northern fowl mites), ticks, lice, fleas, bugs, beetles and cockroaches. For the control of external parasites of animals a variety of compounds are available, such as gamma benzene hexachloride (Lindane), piper-oxyl-butoxide pyrethrum (Pybuthrin) or *0,0*-dimethyldithiophosphate of diethylmercaptosuccinate (Malathion) and *0,0*-dimethyl 0.245 trichlorophenyl phosphorathroate (Fenchlorphos 12 per cent). These are marketed in forms to be used either for the treatment of individual animals or as aerosols, or for mixing in the litter, i.e. 1 per cent Lindane applied as a single application to the litter at the rate of 1.4 kg per 100 m^2.

Piperoxyl-butoxide pyrethrum can be successfully employed in a low-pressure aerosol dispenser, or Malathion at a level of 0.5 kg per 2 m^2 sprinkled on the litter. Compounds are also available in the form of paints for application on the perches or other fittings of poultry houses.

Commercial examples are as follows:

Antec 'Limite' consisting of 50% 1 naphthyl N-methyl carbonate is effective against mites, beetles, lice and fleas on a long-term basis.

Turbair 'Flydown' which is an oil-based formulation of pyrethrum, kills rapidly all flying insects; and Turbair 'Kilsect' is a blend of resmethrin and bromophos to kill all flying and crawling insects with a residual activity up to two months.

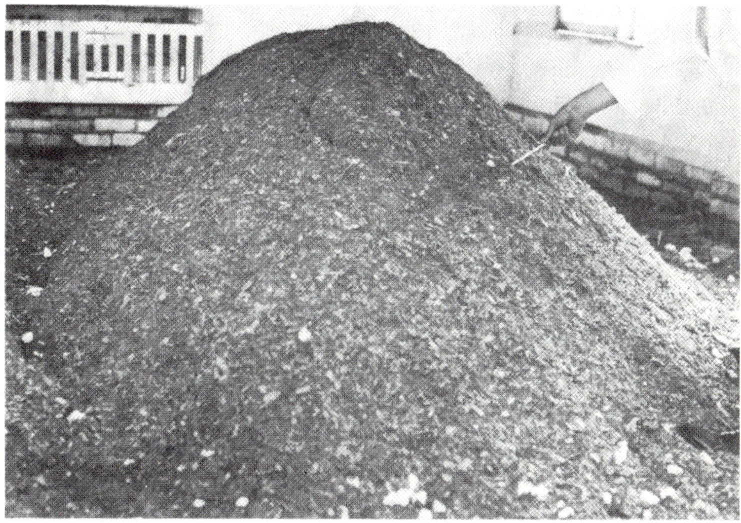

Fig. 6.5 Many organisms may be destroyed in deep litter from poultry houses if it is stacked and allowed to heat.

RECOMMENDED PROCEDURE IN DISINFECTION AND DISINFESTATION OF ANIMAL BUILDINGS AND EQUIPMENT

Basically two procedures should be adopted, the first being that used between batches of livestock within a building, in the absence of disease, and the second after an outbreak of disease.

Procedure of disinfection with no disease present

1 All equipment and fittings that are removable should be demounted and taken out of the building. It is advisable for them to be soaked in a bath of disinfectant where the materials are able to stand up to this treatment. Alternatively, they may be power-sprayed or steam-sterilized. Equipment such as poultry brooders will require fumigation after cleaning.

2 The roof and structural elements of the house should be dusted and cleaned, preferably with an industrial vacuum cleaner.

3 In a poultry house, any litter may either be removed (which is generally preferable) or stacked into heaps for at least 24 hours and preferably three days at least (Fig. 6.5). The temperature within this heap should reach 50°C and thereafter the heaps should be rearranged so that the external layers are in the centre and it must again be verified that it reaches a temperature

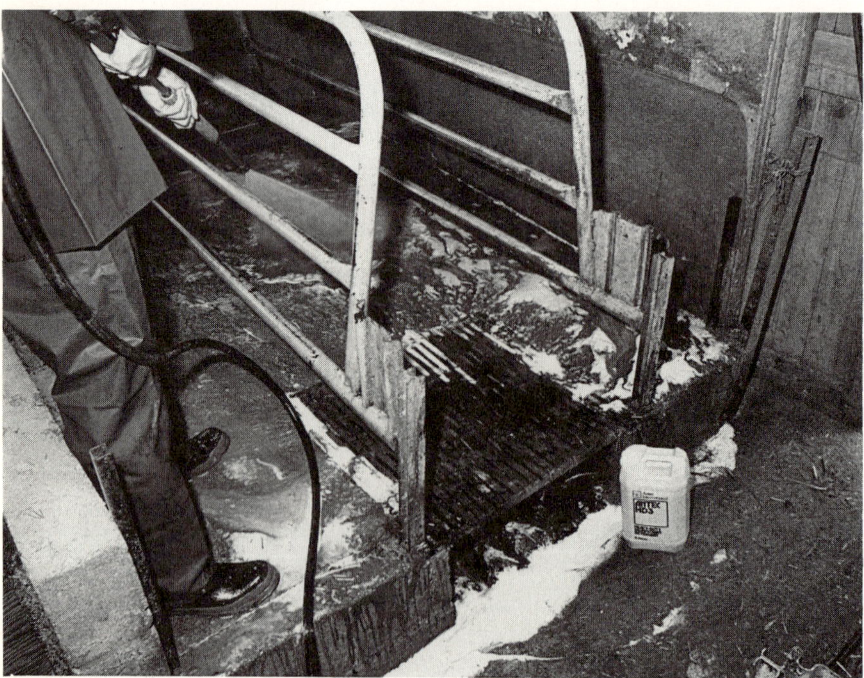

Fig. 6.6 A farrowing pen being cleared with a detergent disinfectant used via a pressure washer.

of 40°C. This temperature will greatly reduce the incidence of parasitic infection.

4 The lower part of the walls and floors should be soaked and cleaned – preferably with a pressure washer – with a heavy duty, wide-spectrum detergent disinfectant.

5 In the case of earth floors, these should be soaked in a solution of 0.5 litres formalin to 50 litres of water, or a suitable proprietary preparation.

6 After the house and equipment have been cleaned, this should be soaked with an approved disinfectant at the correct strength, and/or fumigated with formalin, or sprayed with an aerosol of formalin.

Procedure after contagious and infectious disease

1 The building should be closed and isolated from all visitors (Fig. 6.7).

2 The bedding and litter should be sprayed with a strong disinfectant, such as a phenolic type, and likewise similar treatment should be given to all areas in intimate contact with the stock.

3 The litter should subsequently be removed from the building and may be burnt or buried so there is no possible contact with livestock.

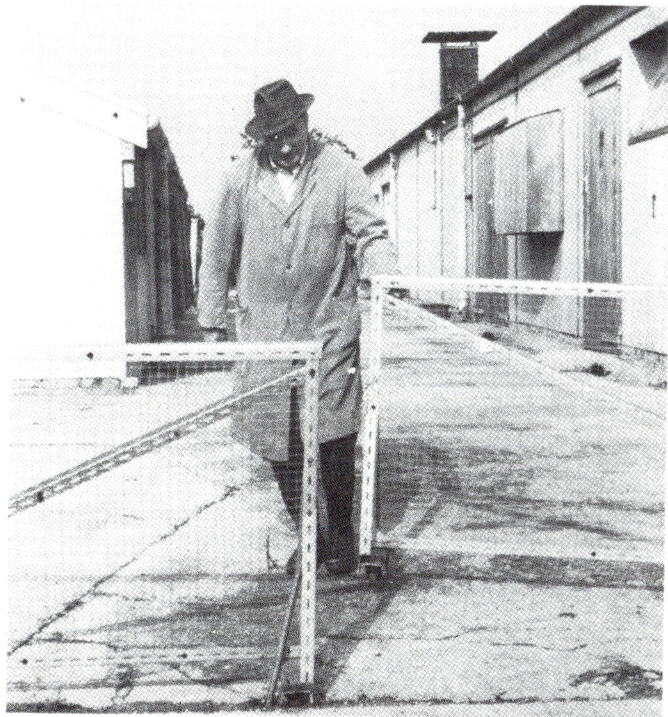

Fig. 6.7 Provide good fences and a gate or gates around the site. The cheap home-made gates here are made from Dexion angle iron, which is serviceable, light and cheap. Concrete surrounds and concrete floors are almost essential to achieve good hygiene.

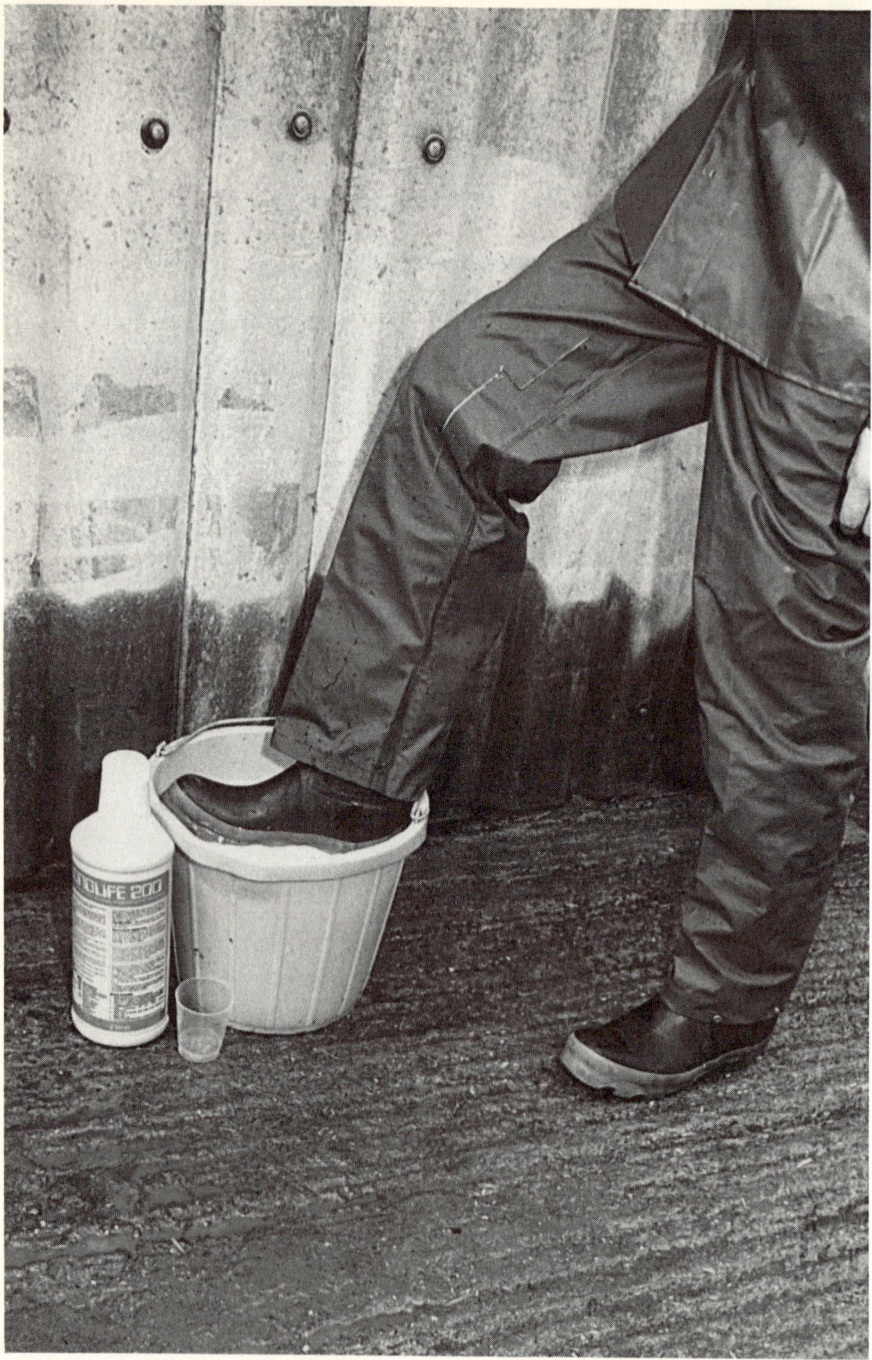

Fig. 6.8 A disinfectant foot drop is essential outside every animal house, and the visitors must wear protective clothing.

4 Portable equipment and fittings should be given the same treatment as previously suggested and preferably in the house, later to be taken out and aerated.
5 Clean the floors and lower part of the walls with detergent disinfectant.
6 The house should be treated in the same way as suggested in the previous section. Where the floor is of earth, it is wise to spread polythene or tarred paper over it before the new litter is put down, thus isolating the possibly still infected floor from the next batch.
7 It may sometimes be advisable to skim off the top few inches of the soil around a heavily infected area.
8 The approaches to the building should be treated with disinfectant and foot-dips provided (Fig. 6.8).

REFERENCES

1 *Report of the Joint Committee on the Use of Antibiotics in Animal Husbandry and Veterinary Medicine.* Chairman: M. M. Swann (1969). London: H.M.S.O.
2 Sykes, G. (1958) *Disinfection and Sterilization.* London.
3 Reddish, G. F. (1957) *Antiseptics, Disinfectants, Fungicides and Chemical and Physical Sterilization.* London: Kimpton.
4 Meulemans, G. and Halen, P. (1982) Efficacy of some disinfectants against infectious bursal disease virus and avian reovirus. *Vet. Rec.*, **111**, 412–413.
5 Gorman, S. P., Scott, E. M. and Russell, A. D. (1980) Antimicrobial activity, use and mechanism of action of glutaraldehyde. *J. App. Bact.*, **48**, 161–190.
6 Armstrong, J. A. and Froelich, E. J. (1964) Inactivation of viruses by benzalkonium chloride. *App. Microbiology*, **12**, 132–137.
7 King, A. W. M., Charles, D. R. and Walker, G. (1966) *Air Hygiene Studies: I. Disposable Filters.* W.P.S.A., U.K. Branch Meeting. UK 66/10.
8 Houghton Poultry Research Station (1962) Mimeograph: *The Disinfection and Disinfestation of Broiler Houses.*
9 Nordgren, G. (1939) *Acta Path. Microbiol. Skand.* Suppl. 40.

7

Dairy Hygiene

The production of milk over the last half-century has assumed a position of considerable economic importance. Recent changes in demand have curbed production and emphasized the necessity for the retention of the well-established systems of organized marketing in the United Kingdom.

Milk provides suitable conditions for the growth of bacteria which may contaminate it at some stage of its production, handling or processing. While some contaminants have little or no significance, the majority of organisms can spoil milk, whether it is destined for the liquid market or for processing into dairy products. Of greater importance is the fact that some of these organisms may be pathogenic. For many years there was an ever-present danger of contracting disease through drinking raw milk but this risk has been reduced to negligible proportions now that most milk for the liquid market is heat-treated.

In view of its public health significance, successive governments have made the production and handling of milk the subject of legislation designed to safeguard the consumer against disease and adulteration. Minimum compositional standards have also been laid down.

CLEAN MILK PRODUCTION

The concept of clean milk production has been changed considerably over the last 20–30 years, and by a variety of factors. The increase in population and in the consumption of liquid milk, together with the gradual depopulation of rural areas, has made it necessary to move milk in bulk over long distances from the dairying areas to satisfy the demand in the thickly populated centres. Apart from the public health considerations, it is commercially essential in these circumstances to heat-treat milk. Thus heat-resistant organisms have assumed greater significance than when raw milk was consumed within a few hours of production and there was insufficient time for contaminants to develop.

The economics of milk production must influence any system of dairying for, among other factors, labour is expensive and often difficult to obtain, so that the farmer has to make do with less than he formerly regarded as the essential minimum. Whatever the system of housing and dairy management, it must be designed to keep cows healthy and clean, and to milk them quickly with clean equipment and the least expenditure of time and labour.

The production of safe, clean milk begins with a healthy cow; in certain cases the sale of milk from an unhealthy cow may contravene public health regulations. Section 35(3) Schedule 3 of the Food Act 1984 prohibits the sale for human consumption of the milk of any cow suffering from tuberculosis, and certain other conditions listed in Schedule 3 of the Act. These are:

Acute mastitis.
Suppuration of the udder.
Actinomycosis of the udder.
Any comatose condition.
Any infection of the udder or teats which is likely to convey disease.
Any septic conditions of the uterus.
Anthrax.
Foot-and-mouth disease.

There are two primary sources of infection in milk which can have an important public health significance. The cow may be the natural host of an infective organism which is screted with the milk, as in brucellosis, for example. Alternatively, a human can infect a cow which acts as host, and ultimately the causal organisms or toxins find their way back to humans from infected milk. More frequently, however, infected workers or 'carriers' contaminate milk either by direct handling or indirectly from a polluted water supply. Therefore the health of the workers who are engaged in the production or handling of milk must also receive careful consideration.

PRODUCTION IN THE MILKING HOUSE

There are many points in the production and handling of milk where contamination can occur, and careful attention to detail with a properly planned routine is essential if results are to be consistently satisfactory. While it is possible to produce clean milk with poor facilities, the provision of equipment and premises designed for easy working and cleanliness assists in obtaining satisfactory results without unnecessary waste of labour.

There are well-tested and proven requirements which can be used as general guides, are likely to meet most regulatory requirements and are here summarized. Milking should be carried out in a building which is adequately lit and ventilated, provided with an impervious floor and walls where liable to soiling, the floor constructed so that liquids are conveyed to a suitable drain outside the building, the effluent being piped to a suitable point for disposal as required by the local public health authority. The milking house must be provided with clean approaches and away from any manure pit or cesspool liable to cause contamination of milk through flies, airborne contamination or odours. A milk room, having the same basic requirements for cleanliness, is necessary for the handling and storage of milk and for the cleaning and storage of the dairy utensils. The size of the room should be adequate for the amount of milk to be handled and situated in a cool place shaded from the evening sun. A supply of pure water, sufficient for washing the utensils, water cooling where applicable, and cleaning the premises, is absolutely essential. Dung should be removed from the milking house daily and floors and walls washed clean. Although the condition of the buildings is important, methods of production, handling and storage of milk require particular attention and will be discussed in the following sections.

The cleanliness of cows' udders and flanks is an important factor in clean and efficient milk production. The introduction of cow cubicles and kennels provides a system of loose housing in which most cows will keep clean with a minimum of attention. It is recognized that dirty cows will disrupt the milking and generally reduce the efficiency of clean milk production.

The milking routine will be one that will not only milk cows cleanly and efficiently but also be an important factor in the successful control of mastitis. This routine will incorporate the following functions:

1 There are aids to early detection of mastitic clots in milk. Whilst the use of the fore-milk cup before the udder is washed has been the accepted method and has various advantages, many milk producers now rely upon plastic in-line filter indicators which will retain clots and in severe cases cause the teat cup cluster to fall off. Their use has the advantage of reducing the necessity for handling the udder and teats.

2 Use individual (sterile) udder cloths or disposable paper towels for udder washing and drying.

3 Wear smooth rubber gloves which may readily be disinfected between cows and will thereby reduce the transfer of infection on the hands of the milker.

4 Treat the udder washing water with a suitable disinfectant at the recommended strength. The water should preferably be warm and changed frequently to prevent recontamination of the udder. In most milking parlours it will be more convenient, labour-saving and effective in controlling udder disease to use a purpose-made electrically operated udder washing water heater. This will be used in conjunction with a spray or pad, and about 1–2 litres of warm water at a temperature of approximately 43°C will be required to wash each cow. It is advisable to treat this water with a suitable disinfectant at the rate of 250 mg/litre available chlorine or 25–50 mg/litre available iodine.

Some types of warm water udder washing units where water is held at suitable temperatures for bacterial growth have been shown to be the predisposing source of mastitic infections caused by *Pseudomonas aeruginosa*. To avoid the water becoming contaminated and bacteria proliferating during storage, tanks should be connected directly to a rising main, properly covered and sited where dust and vermin cannot gain access. Additionally, the water should be treated with a disinfectant at the rate suggested above.

Providing that the udder and teats are clean there are many producers and veterinary advisers who have obtained better hygiene results with reduced mastitis problems by dry wiping the udder and teats with disposable paper towels.[1] It must be stressed, however, that where there is any doubt about the cleanliness of the teats or where regulations require, washing as previously described should be carried out.

5 Remove the teat cups as soon as milk flow ceases and avoid over-milking. Experience shows that where automatic cluster removers are used cell counts are lowered.

6 Teat disinfection after each milking by dipping or spraying is an important part of the mastitis control programme. The main groups of chemicals used are the iodophors, hypochlorite and those incorporating chlorhexidine as the active ingredient. These have good bactericidal efficiency over a wide range of organisms but expense and safety aspects in health and handling must be considered. Emollients to promote soft and pliable teat skin and the healing of teat sores can readily be added to disinfectants but they may decrease their bactericidal action.

Although teat dipping takes relatively little time in the milking routine various methods of teat spraying have been developed, from hand-operated sprays to fully automated systems. Spraying presents problems of ensuring complete coverage of all teats and could also present a health hazard but as yet this is not proven.

Automatic systems have been developed consisting of a floor-mounted spray which is activated, as the cow passes through a 'race' outside the parlour, by a light-sensitive electronic control.

7 Use antibiotic therapy, in consultation with a veterinary surgeon, on all cows with clinical mastitis or at drying-off.

It is most important to eliminate those predisposing causes of mastitis that are within the control of the producer, principally through the provision of dry, well-ventilated and draught-free housing, good hygiene and milking techniques and the correct operation and maintenance of the milking machine.

The indiscriminate use of antibiotics for the treatment of mastitis and the inclusion of milk from cows so treated in consignments for sale may be the subject of legislation and price and other penalties. For many years it has been recognized as a problem in the manufacture of cheese and fermented milks such as yoghurt. It is also possible that such milk could create a public health hazard in a few individuals either by sensitizing them and subjecting them to severe reaction if they are treated medically with these antibiotics or by causing an allergic reaction, particularly skin rashes. There is also the possibility that resistant organisms may develop in the alimentary tract from food containing antibiotics.

The important factors in avoiding the inclusion of milk containing antibiotic residues in the bulk milk are:

1 Strict observance of the manufacturers' recommendations for the correct use and milk withholding time.

2 Ensuring that treated cows can be identified, for example, by colour sprays or tail tapes, and that there is good communication between all the workers involved, particularly relief milkers.
3 Provision of bucket units or separate 'dump lines' for contaminated milk. Milk jar contamination with antibiotic residues can often be responsible for test failures.
4 Antibiotics used in dry cow therapy can persist in the udder for 5–6 weeks and careful and accurate records are essential. Care is required where cows or heifers have been purchased and may have been treated prior to sale.

Facilities for the personal hygiene of operators which are essential include:

a Hot water, soap, towel and nail-brush to enable hands to be washed before and kept clean during milking.
b A first aid kit with waterproof dressings and antiseptic for treating cuts and abrasions on the hands.
c Washable coats or overalls and hats.

The cleanliness of cows' udders and flanks together with good udder washing has already been stressed. Nevertheless, because of the pressures on the milkers in many systems, particularly during wet weather and where cows are walking through muddy gateways or fields, there is a possibility that some sediment could get into milk which could lead to a prosecution or rejection by the buyer.[2] Sediment is the extraneous insoluble matter which gains access to milk from soil, dung, feedingstuffs, dust, bedding and hair, and obviously every care must be taken to prevent it getting into milk in the first place.[3,4]

In practice it is impossible to ensure that every particle of foreign matter whatsoever can be excluded, so that some method of filtration is essential. For pipeline plants there are two types of filter available: disposable and non-disposable. Initially disposable sock-type filters held in tubular containers were the only type on the market. The milk flow in these is usually outward and should the flow be impeded, the sock is likely to break or be blown off the line in some cases. The quality of the filter is very important. A variation on this design is to support the sock over a wire frame with the milk flow from the outside into the centre of the container, which gives satisfactory results with fewer filters splitting. More recent developments are multi-service in-line filters constructed for performance and efficiency to the requirements of BS 5190: 1975, 'Pipeline filters for milking installations'.[5] The filter consists of a plastic body and cap and filter cones which are inserted into the body of the unit (Fig. 7.1) There are two filter cones, one fine and one coarse. After milking, the cone screens are removed, entrapped sediment rinsed away and then left soaking in a cleaning solution until required for the next milking. It is claimed that they provide more efficient filtration at substantially reduced filtration costs.

In the past the importance of fly control was often neglected but with larger units and increased publicity there is an increased awareness of the problem. If flies are allowed to breed unchecked, they carry dirt and disease, worry cows and reduce yields. Flies normally breed on dung heaps, slurry pits and on decaying vegetation. Where possible it helps to site natural breeding grounds as far as possible away from farm buildings. An effective fly control programme is required to provide both long- and short-term protection.[6,7]

Long-term protection aims to tackle the problem at source using residual insecticides. The organophosphorus insecticides can be used for spraying in places where flies can breed. They are particularly effective in controlling fly larvae and may be persistent for up to two months. They should be applied with a knap-sack or other sprayer at the commencement of the fly season.

Insecticides must be approved under the Medicines Act 1968 to ensure that there is no risk of the contamination of milk with insecticidal residues through indiscriminate use on lactating cows in the milking parlour. Safety for farm staff is also vital, particularly when operating in enclosed areas. Within the last few years synthetic pyrethroid insecticides have been developed which combine high insecticidal ability with low toxicity to man and animals.

Methods of control include:

1 Control at source to which reference has already been made.
2 Exclusion from the parlours by mechanical means using 'spray arches' or 'misters' of water either at the parlour entrance or in the collecting yard.

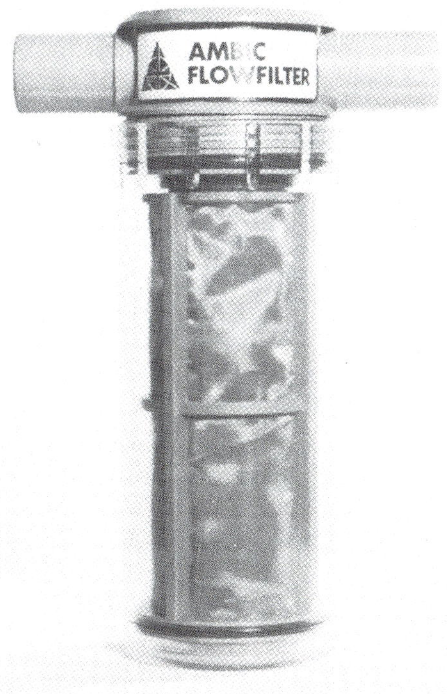

Fig. 7.1 The Ambic flowfilter.

The spray arch can be used with a plastic curtain to brush flies from the cows' backs.

3 Electrocutors which attract and kill flies can be used in the parlour. Approved knockdown sprays are quick and safe and help to keep cows quiet during milking.

4 Treatment with insecticides through a 'spray arch' at the end of milking.

5 Insecticidal PVC ear tags[8] containing cypermethrin have been used successfully and provide control for up to three months. The insecticide from the ear tag is transferred to the animal's coat by ear flapping, movement of the tail, grooming and contact between tagged cattle. The insecticide, which is rainfast, is slowly released over a period of about three months.

COOLING AND BULK COLLECTION OF MILK

All farms in the U.K. selling milk by wholesale contract now have their milk collected in bulk. It is contractual upon the producer that milk is cooled to and held at a temperature not exceeding 4.5°C before collection.

Some method of refrigeration is used for cooling the milk in all bulk tanks: this may be by direct expansion or indirectly through the use of chilled water. In tanks where the milk is cooled by direct expansion, the extraction of heat from the evaporator is used to cool milk directly, being an integral part of the wall of the tank. Where indirect methods are used the evaporator coil is immersed in a tank of water or water/alcohol mixture. This builds up an ice bank between

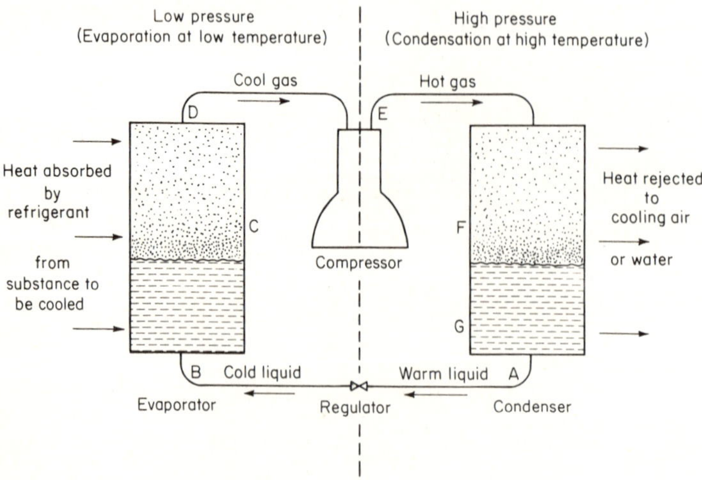

Fig. 7.2 Diagram of vapour compression refrigeration cycle.

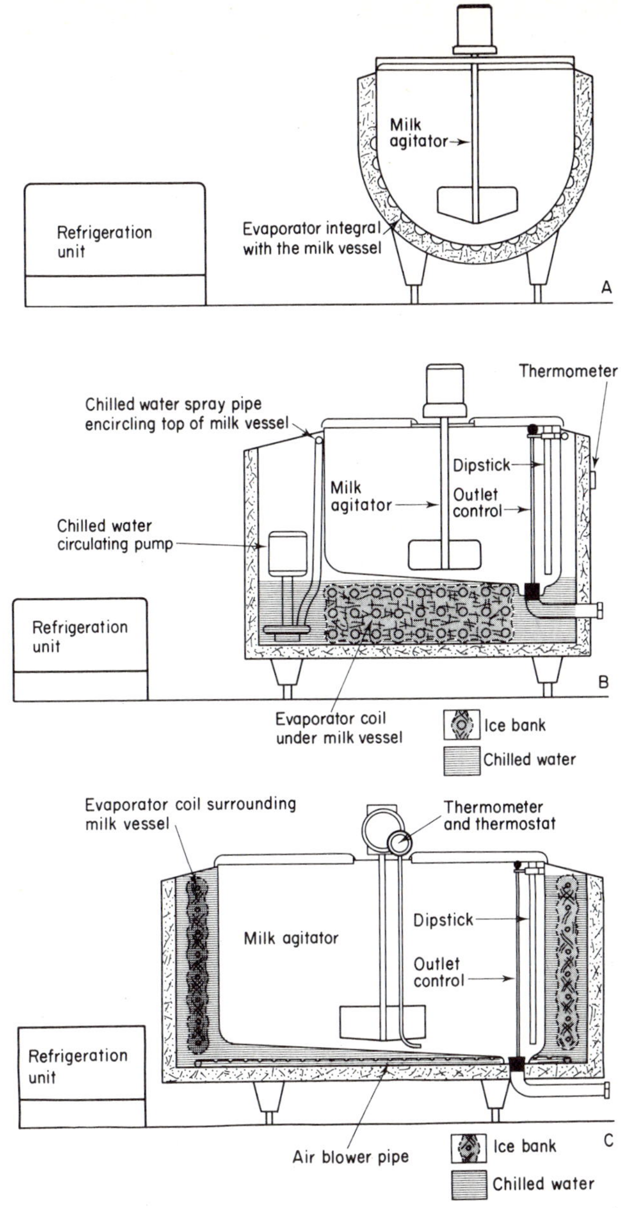

Fig. 7.3 Three types of refrigerated bulk tanks: (A) directly refrigerated bulk tank with refrigerant circulated against the milk vessel; (B) bulk milk tank with chilled water distributed by sump and spray method; (C) jacketed chilled water bulk tank with ice-bank round the milk vessel.

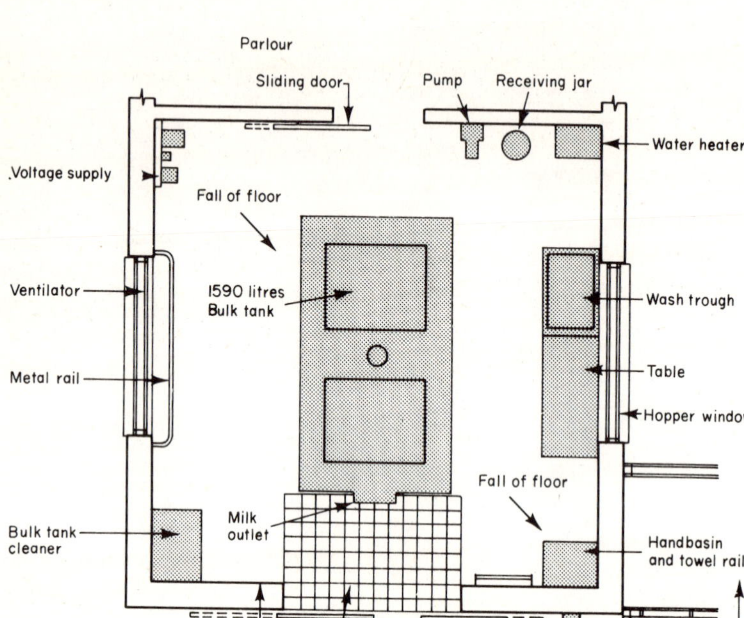

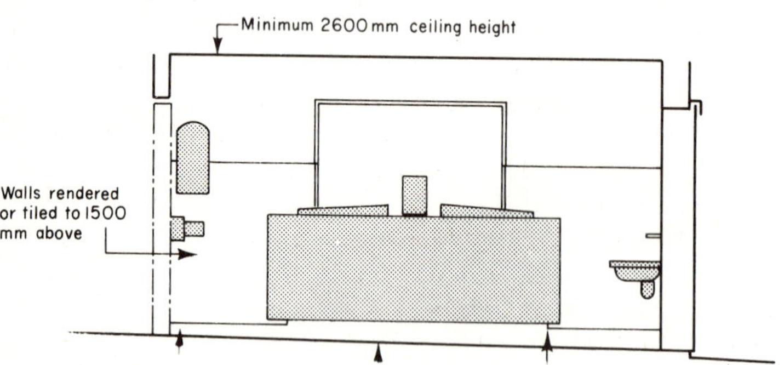

Fig. 7.4a Milkroom with tank for bulk milk collection.

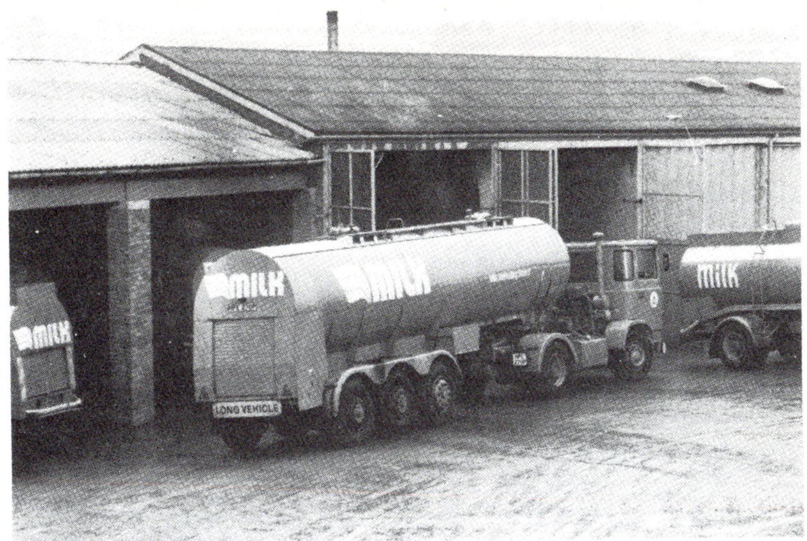

Fig. 7.4b Milk Marketing Board bulk tank collecting vehicles.

milkings which can be melted for cooling the milk when required (Figs. 7.2–7.4).

Since the introduction of bulk tanks there have been improvements designed to reduce costs, cool the milk more rapidly and hold it at a low temperature more effectively. A plate or tube heat exchanger is used initially with either water on its own or in conjunction with chilled water to reduce the temperature of the milk before discharging it to the bulk tank.

The standards required for the construction and performance of bulk tanks are laid down by the U.K. Federation of Milk Marketing Boards. Each type of tank offered for sale has had its performance tested and accepted officially. Briefly the specification requirement for cooling is based on the initial cooled evening milk, which is already in the tank, having morning milk added and the tests being taken under these conditions.

Most bulk tanks are of jacketed construction with a stainless steel inner compartment and an outer skin of stainless steel or glass fibre. With indirect refrigeration the space between the inner and outer skins is either filled with chilled water or has a sump containing chilled water for circulation through a spray rail. In tanks using direct expansion refrigeration the space will house the evaporator coils attached directly to the lower part of the milk tank so that no intermediate coolant is required (Fig. 7.3a).

Where chilled water is used as the cooling medium the refrigeration system builds up an ice bank between milkings. To avoid this being excessive a thermostat is set to cut out at about −2.2°C and to cut in at about 0°C as required. When milking commences, the refrigeration unit, of whatever type, starts up as soon as the temperature of the milk in the tank operates the thermostat. Fairly rapid cooling is encouraged by the operation of the agitator, which stops when the milk reaches the predetermined temperatures. As any rise in temperature of the milk occurs, the refrigeration unit and agitator will cut in and operate until the milk is returned to the correct temperature. Other fittings on the bulk tank will be a thermometer, an outlet plug with a rubber bung and there may be a calibrated dipstick and spinners for automatic cleaning (Figs. 7.3b,c).

These arrangements have worked satisfactorily for tanks of up to 4000 litres of milk per day. Quantities in excess of this have created difficulties; first, the size and handling of the tank and the size of the dairy to house it; and secondly, because of the area of the cooling surface in relation to the bulk of milk to be cooled.

With the larger tanks a different approach has been taken by using a heat exchanger to cool the milk before storage in a partially refrigerated tank until collection by the tanker (Fig. 7.4a). Pre-cooling through a plate heat exchanger can enable advantage to be taken of off-peak electrical current. The heat exchanger can be simple or two-stage, using either water or refrigerant separately or combined, to reduce the temperature of the milk before it enters the bulk tank.

Pre-cooling

With all bulk tanks, milk can be initially pre-cooled with mains or an approved water supply to within 2–3°C of the cooling water temperature; with a plate cooler a 2:1 ratio of water will be required to milk cooled. Tube pre-coolers are also available but are likely to use more water. In order to maintain a constant flow of milk a balance tank of about 2000 litre capacity may be required.

To obtain full value from pre-cooling it is essential that all the cooling water is re-used. This can have several advantages because the temperature of the water is likely to be raised by 6–8°C and can be used for supplying udder washing units, water heaters for plant cleaning, cattle drinking and washing down the parlour and surrounding areas. This can represent considerable savings in the use of electricity depending on the source and initial temperature of the cooling water and that the warmed water which is discharged can be used effectively.

The dimensions of the milkroom

Floor space

The floor area required will depend on the size and number of bulk tanks which have to be accommodated. Bulk tanks vary in size from 1 to 2.5 m in width and from 1.5 to 4.5 m in length.

Some of the more common tank sizes for normal capacities are:

Capacity	Width	Length
455 litres	1.00–1.20 m	1.10–1.50 m
900 litres	1.25–1.80 m	1.63–1.93 m
1590 litres	1.40–1.60 m	2.40–2.95 m
2270 litres	1.50–1.66 m	2.80–3.80 m
3410 litres	1.95–2.25 m	3.00–4.20 m

Additionally, a clear working space of at least 0.75 m around each side of the tank should be allowed.

Ancillary equipment will also require both wall and floor space, i.e. releaser jar, milk pump assemblies, wash trough, hand basin, water heater and automatic cleaner. To cater for these, a further 2.32 m^2 of floor space should be allowed.

Example. The minimum size dairy to accommodate the smallest tank size with 0.75 m clearance and space for ancillary equipment should be 3.70 m long by 3.00 m wide.

Height

Sufficient headrom is advisable and may be essential to obtain access for cleaning some of the largest capacity tanks. A minimum height to eaves level of 2.4 m will be adequate for all tanks up to 3640 litres.

Wall space

Clear wall areas should also be provided particularly on the adjoining parlour wall for mounting the releaser jar milk pump assembly.

Floor fall

Floor should have a fall of 1:40 toward the external trapped gulley and away from the exit door to avoid flooding when cleaning out the bulk tank.

Access to the milkroom

Access to the milkroom must be such that a large heavy tanker can drive up, turn easily, and get within 5 m of the tank.

Condenser unit

This must be large enough to accommodate the motor and condenser unit. As this unit gives rise to considerable heat it is best placed in a separate building as close as possible to the bulk tank. This building must be amply ventilated with vermin proof ventilators and preferably sited on a north-facing wall.

Mobile tanks have been developed for use on small inaccessible farms, there being two sizes: 270 and 500 litres. The one currently on the market is really a conventional spray rail tank on wheels with a remote ice-bank which is attached by flexible hoses to the tank when required for cooling. It has the disadvantage on many farms which are situated at the end of long lanes that four journeys a day must be made unless the tanker can be met. This may not be possible because of variable collection times, or practical where collection times occur within an ordinary day's outside work.

For larger farms milk porters are available in which to transport milk from farm to roadside. These are insulated tanks and milk is cooled and held for overnight storage in a conventional bulk tank.

Various methods are available for taking milk to the roadside or common collecting points during inclement weather and when tankers would be unable to get to the farm. These consist of glass-fibre tanks which may be trailed types or some for fitting to the tractor link box or a farm trailer. There are also MMB flexible emergency containers, which are for use once only and must be transported on a farm trailer.[9]

With bulk tankers travelling into farm yards and in close proximity to buildings associated with cattle (Fig. 7.4b), it is possible that in some circumstances they could become a disease hazard. If possible the tanker should be kept out of areas which are also used by cattle, from the point of view of both disease and also general hygiene and cleanliness. During the last major outbreak of foot-and-mouth disease the damage which could be caused by the collection of milk by bulk tanker was not fully understood in the initial stages of the outbreak. After the tanker has picked up milk from a farm it has to build up vacuum to transfer milk at the next farm. Operation of the vacuum pump extracts air from the upper part of the tanker and blows it to exhaust. If this air is already contaminated with virus from cows which are infected with foot-and-mouth virus but showing no clinical symptoms, the infection could be spread along roadside hedges and to the next farms visited by the tanker. A virus air filter has been developed which can be fitted by the exhaust outlet of the vacuum pump on the tanker and which could help to minimize the spread of infection from this source. It has been suggested that it is possible for the infective virus to be present in a cow's milk 36 hours before the disease is diagnosed.[10]

The cleaning of bulk tanks and other aspects of bulk milk collection will be discussed later in the chapter.

DAIRY EQUIPMENT

The most important single factor in clean milk production is the attention given to the cleanliness and sterilization of utensils and the milking plant. For several years the methods employed in cleaning and sterilizing dairy utensils have been subjected to modifications owing to the variety of surfaces which have to be cleaned, some of which are liable to damage from mechanical causes, high temperatures or corrosion by chemicals. It is also necessary, when planning a system, to consider the cost of materials and availability of labour. Provision of the right equipment and a well planned routine can reduce much of the monotony associated with dairy work.

In addition to the milking machine and cooling equipment, there are other basic essentials which must be provided whatever system is followed. Many of these offer a certain amount of choice according to the producers' requirements. They include:

1 Facilities for personal hygiene of milkers.
2 Udder washing facilites and strip cup.
3 Water heating and washing equipment (wash troughs, brushes, etc.).
4 A detergent.
5 Some method of sterilizing the utensils.

Personal hygiene

Requirements for this have already been dealt with. In addition a hand basin, cupboards, shelves and hooks for hygiene equipment should be provided.

Udder washing

The aims of udder washing are to stimulate milk let-down, to produce milk with little sediment and low bacterial counts and finally to avoid so far as possible the spread of mastitis by transfer from cow to cow.[11] Washing with water from buckets and udder cloths possibly caused more problems than it solved. The most effective method of achieving these aims is to use warm water delivered by spray nozzle, the teats being thoroughly dried with disposable paper towels (Fig. 7.5).

Small capacity water heaters specifically designed for udder washing are most suitable. About 1.14 litres of water at a temperature of approximately 43°C will be required for each cow. This can be provided by a 3 kW water heater, which can be used to wash up to 60 cows an hour if required. Chemical entraining devices can be fitted to most warm water wash systems to meter a controlled amount of disinfectant into the wash water. Recommended rates are 250–600 mg/litre chlorine or 25–50 mg/litre iodine. Where storage-type udder washing water heaters are used cases have been recorded of the contamination of water tanks with organisms which can cause mastititis and it is therefore essential to properly cover any tanks to exclude rodents, insects, dust and dirt.

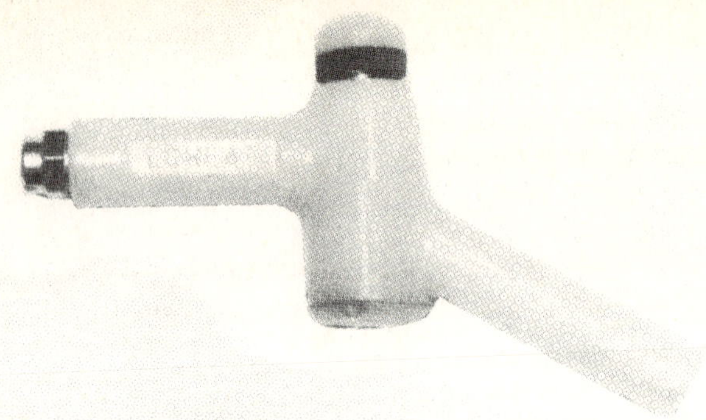

Fig. 7.5 Loheat-type 300 plastic udder wash spray gun.

Water heating and washing equipment

A hot water supply may have to provide sufficient hot water for washing dairy utensils, hands and udders, and it may be required for calf feeding (Table 7.1). It is also advantageous to incorporate some method for boiling water to use in conjunction with chemical sterilization. For small dairies, hand cleaning utensils, a 45 litre wash boiler is quite suitable and can be used with electricity, mains or bottled gas. The boiler can be fixed so that it gravity feeds into the wash-up trough.

For larger dairies hot water may be required on tap or for circulation or acid boiling water cleaning, in which case specially designed heaters are available (Fig. 7.6). In addition to those operated by electricity, there are also oil-fired water-heating systems, and although they are more expensive in first cost, it is claimed that they are relatively inexpensive to run.

Where electricity is not available, a geyser using bottle gas is satisfactory, particularly when used in conjunction with a wash boiler for providing boiling water.

There are opportunities for conserving energy in the form of heat which would otherwise be dissipated to the atmosphere. Milk is taken from the cow at about 35°C and cooled to less than 4°C. Some of the heat generated by the vacuum pump in extracting the milk or by the refrigeration unit in cooling the milk can be recovered to reduce electricity costs.

In the refrigeration cycle the highest temperature heat is available after the refrigerant has been compressed and this is normally lost. The hot refrigerant gas can be passed through water which it warms. A standard heat recovery unit (HRU) can be expected to provide warm water at a temperature of about 50°C depending on the amount of milk produced. The size of the HRU for the most economic savings has to be related to the size of the bulk tank and the anticipated amount of milk. The unit comprises an insulated heat exchanger located around a copper cylinder. The hot gas discharged through the compressor heats the

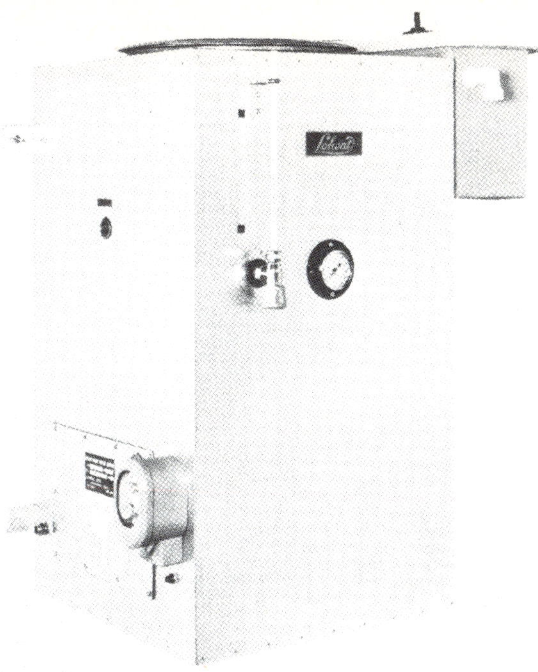

Fig. 7.6 Model BW AC 15 Loheat plant for high-temperature acidified cleaning suitable for a parlour of up to four units.

water which can be used to supply heaters for udder or utensil washing. If used for utensil washing the temperature can be boosted by immersion heaters and there are a range of dairy water heaters manufactured for this purpose.[12]

Electricity costs can also be reduced by converting the heat from the exhaust air of the vacuum pump, which normally goes to waste, to heat water for udder and utensil washing.

Wash-up troughs can be obtained in galvanized iron, rubber or polyurethane. Rubber and polythene troughs have the advantage that they cannot be attacked by chemicals or cause mechanical damage to utensils, but they are more costly.

Brushes, suitable for various types of equipment and hung on a rack accessible to the wash trough, should also be provided, although with circulation cleaning much less brushing is required than was hitherto essential. It is, however, important not to neglect the parts of the equipment which circulation of chemicals will not thoroughly clean and also external surfaces, which are important in the overall cleanliness of the plant.

Detergents[13]

The detergents required will consist of one or more chemical agents added to water to assist in the removal of milk or other residues from dairy equipment.

Table 7.1 *Summary of types of water heater and their uses on diary farms for utensil cleaning purposes*

Type	Range of sizes (litres)	Range of heater heater loaders (kW)	Method of controlling temperature	Mounting	Purpose on diary farm	Milking installation	Remarks
1. Wash boiler	20–50	2–3	Hand	Freestanding	Washing water (49 °C); occasional heat treatment of clusters (96 °C)	Up to 3-bucket	Frequent element replacement likely if used daily
2. Dairy boiler	90	3	2 Thermostats	Freestanding	Circulation cleaning (71 °C); heat disinfection (96 °C)	Up to 3-bucket and pipeline	
3. Open outlet water heater	6–22	0.8–3	Thermostat	Wall mounting	(a) Hand washing only; (b) immersion cleaning; (c) udder washing	(a) All types; (b) in-churn; (c) all types	(b) For washing off caustic soda before milking

4. Cistern-type water heaters							
(a) Domestic	20–50	1.5–3	Thermostat	Wall mounting	Washing water (49°C)	3-bucket	
(b) Farm	90–110	1.5–3	Thermostat	Freestanding	Washing water (49°C)	4-bucket and above	
(c) Farm (for circulation cleaning)	110	3	2 Thermostats	Wall mounting	Circulation water (71°C); heat disinfection (96°C)	Pipeline	Designed for circulation cleaning systems
5. Cistern-fed water heater	90–450	3–9	Thermostat	Freestanding	Washing water (49–60°C)	4 or more bucket and pipeline	For detergent washing; circulation cleaning; larger sizes for off-peak heating
6. Cistern-fed open-top heater with controlled inlet	65–220	3–6	Thermostat	Wall mounting	Boiling water (96°C)	4 to 10 pipeline systems	For acidified boiling (ABW) cleaning

The properties which the detergent should possess will be influenced by the chemical composition and nature of the residues and by the type of surface from which they have to be removed.

In hard water areas the water softening properties of the detergent will also require consideration. The residues can be one or more of the following kinds:

1 Liquid or air-dried milk residues on the surfaces to be cleaned.

2 Residues of either milk or calcium and/or magnesium salts from hard water supplies dried on by heat.

3 Various kinds of foreign matter, e.g. dirt and dung adhering to the outside of the utensils.

Milk consists of water together with fat, protein and lactose, and other mineral and organic matter in small quantities. The lactose and some of the milk ash are present in true solution. The proteins are present in the emulsoid state together with an emulsion of liquid fat particles. Because of these physical characteristics of milk the following points have to be borne in mind when selecting a detergent.

1 *Increase of the wetting power of water.* The reduction of the interfacial tension between the solution and the surface to be cleaned assists in the removal of dirt particles.

2 *Solution of protein and emulsification.* The reduction of residues to fine particles which are held in suspension in the cleaning solution – liquids are emulsified and solids deflocculated.

3 *Free-rinsing and non-foaming properties.* Where the solution is not completely rinsed from the surface, scale or slime will build up which will eventually reduce the penetration of a chemical sterilizer to the surfaces. It is also an advantage if the detergent does not foam excessively, especially for mechanical systems of cleaning relying on agitation.

4 *Water softening and scale prevention.* In a very few areas, up to 40° of hardness will be encountered and specially blended detergents will be required. With some of the more recently introduced methods of cleaning, water hardness requires special consideration. Sodium hexametaphosphate prevents the formation of a precipitate when alkaline detergents are used in hard water.

5 *Corrosion of metals.* This problem has been reduced by the increased use of stainless steel. On the farm there are really only two metals with which any difficulty is likely to be encountered – the aluminium milking pail, and equipment constructed of tinned copper tubing. Aluminium is soluble in alkalis, corrosion being caused by caustic soda, soda ash and trisodium phosphate. Corrosion by soda ash will be reduced by the addition of sodium metasilicate; corrosion by trisodium phosphate by adding a mixture of sodium silicate and sodium perborate. Attacks on tin appear to be dependent on the amount of dissolved oxygen present in the solution, and the addition of sodium sulphite, a reducing agent, will prevent corrosion.

6 *Other properties.* Detergents should not be toxic, affect the flavour of milk,

be catalytic to oxidation in milk fat, or be injurious to the skin when used for hand-washing utensils.

The composition of detergents

Because of the complexity of these requirements the provision of an all-purpose detergent may not be easy. Most detergents consist of mixtures of chemicals designed to meet as many as possible of the conditions required for a particular purpose. For example, the normal cleansing technique for hand-washing a bucket-milking plant will require a different blend of substances from a detergent designed for circulation-cleaning a large milking plant piping milk to the dairy.

The main groups of detergents are as follows:

Alkalis

Sodium hydroxide (caustic soda)
Sodium carbonate (soda ash, washing soda)
Trisodium phosphate
Sodium metasilicate

Polyphosphates (for water softening)

Sodium hexametaphosphate
Tetra-sodium pyrophosphate

Synthetics

Anionic e.g. sulphated primary alcohols
Cationic e.g. quaternary ammonium compounds
Non-ionic, various ethers and esters.

In addition, other ingredients may be added, such as sodium sulphite, sodium aluminates, sodium silicate and sodium perborate.

The main constitutents of a mixture of inorganic compounds should possess an alkaline reaction, which is necessary for dissolving casein and for the solution and emulsification of fat. Table 7.2 lists the chief characteristics of some of these chemicals.

The organic and synthetic detergents generally possess very good wetting properties and have many advantages, the chief of which are that they are harmless to most skins and are suitable for use in hard water areas. They are liable to excessive foaming and rinsability is poor.

Milkstone

Milkstone can also be considered a problem of detergence, and most utensils will require periodical treatment with a milkstone remover. The principal constituents of milkstone are protein, milk ash, traces of detergent, and calcium

Table 7.2 *Properties of chemicals used in or with detergents*

Characteristics	Caustic soda	Sodium silicate	Sodium carbonate	Sodium hexametaphosphate
Wetting power	good	good	poor	fair
Emulsification	poor	good	good	poor
Rinsability	poor	fair	fair	very good
Water softening	good	fair	good	very good
Action on metals	very corrosive	fairly corrosive	not corrosive	not corrosive

and magnesium salts, precipitated from hard water supplies. Build-up of milkstone may occur through air-dried films and, particularly where steam is used for sterilization, traces may be baked onto surfaces. Places where troubles are most likely to occur are on rough metals, particularly those which are difficult to brush owing to shape or inaccessibility. Milkstone is removed by using either a mineral or an organic acid. Phosphoric acid is often used and there are several proprietary brands of organic acid which are quite suitable. Whatever method is used, care has to be taken to avoid corrosion of metals. The presence of milkstone on utensils is masked when they are wet, and a periodic inspection when they are dry will make detection more certain.

In some plants using an acid boiling water (ABW, described later) cleaning routine, even where the correct procedure is followed, a build-up of scale or film on the plant surfaces takes place. The film is probably protein in nature and could cause disappointing results with milk quality tests. This type of film can generally be removed with a strong hot solution of approved hypochlorite. Precautions in the use of hypochlorite for this purpose are essential because of the reactivity between traces of acid remaining in the equipment and the strong solution of hypochlorite. It is therefore essential to ensure that every trace of acid is rinsed away before introducing the hypochlorite. After the acid container has been rinsed throroughly, 1.14 litres of approved hypochlorite is added. Then the normal ABW technique is followed and, if necessary, another 1.14 litres of hypochlorite added. Finally, the plant is flushed with cold water and the stock acid solution added again to the acid container. It may be necessary with stubborn deposits to repeat the treatment.

STERILIZATION OF UTENSILS[14]

The term 'sterilization' in the context of farm dairy utensils is not taken to mean the destruction of all forms of life, as it would, for example, in relation to instruments in a hospital operating theatre. 'Disinfection' is a more accurate term, implying the elimination of a majority of undesirable organisms from utensil surfaces.

There are three methods of sterilizing farm dairy utensils:

1 Boiling water
2 Steam
3 An approved chemical agent, which can be used as an alternative to 1 or 2, above.

Correct application of the plant and materials is essential to obtain satisfactory results.

Chemical sterilization

Chemical agents approved to meet the requirements of the Milk and Dairies (General) Regulations 1959, are listed in circulars issued by the Ministry of Agriculture, Fisheries and Food. The groups listed are:

1 Sodium hypochlorite solutions.
2 Detergent sterilizers based on available chlorine.
3 Sterilizers based on available chlorine.
4 Detergent sterilizers containing quaternary ammonium compounds.
5 Solutions of quaternary ammonium compounds.
6 Iodophors.
7 Ampholytic surface-active compound sterilizers.

Chlorine compounds

Two sources of chlorine for sterilizing dairy utensils are available:

1 Sodium hypochlorite (NaOCl) in liquid form.
2 Organic chlorine compounds, e.g. chloramine T, dichlorodimethyl hydantoin and the potassium or sodium salts of dichloro- or trichloroisocyanuric acid. The organic compounds may be blended with a detergent to produce a stable powder combining detergent and sterilizer, and many of these products are approved by the Ministry.

The requirements for approved hypochlorite are that at the time of dispatch it must contain 9–12 per cent available chlorine (w/w), not less than 0.7 per cent sodium chlorate and not more than 2 per cent free caustic alkali. The label attached to the container must give the date of dispatch and a guarantee that within a specified time thereafter it will not fall below 8 per cent available chlorine provided that it is stored in the dark at a temperature of 16.0 ± 0.6°C. Care should be taken in the storage of the stock solution, and the small quantities required for daily use should be stored in dark glass bottles and kept out of direct sunlight. The presence of any foreign matter in the stock solution will reduce its strength very rapidly. It is illegal to add hypochlorite to milk; its presence is revealed by the chlorate ion in the sodium chlorate.

Table 7.3 *Strength of hypochlorite*

Purpose	Parts per million	Stock solution (ml per 40 litres water)
Hot detergent chlorine wash	250	100
Chlorinated rinse	75	25
Double strength chlor. rinse	150	50
Udder washing	175	25 ml–10 litres
Water sterilization	10–20	1–2 teaspoonfuls

The efficiency and effectiveness of cleaning dairy utensils with chlorine compounds depends on factors which affect their bactericidal action: (1) concentration; (2) temperature; (3) contact time; (4) pH value; (5) condition of surfaces and the presence or absence of organic matter.

Concentrations of hypochlorite for various purposes are shown in Table 7.3. An approved detergent/sterilizer should be used at the strength at which it was approved. When the water supply is open to suspicion, the final rinse water should always be treated with approved hypochlorite.

Quaternary ammonium compounds

Other materials available are the quaternary ammonium compounds (QACs) and the iodophors. The iodophors have been in use for some time both in this country and the USA and they have advantages which recommend their use. Iodine is employed as the sterilizing agent and it is chemically combined with a detergent. This is a safe, convenient way of using iodine which is a powerful germicide. Since iodine is most effective as a bactericide in an acid solution, the iodophors usually contain phosphoric acid for dairy use. Loss of effectiveness in sterilization in the presence of organic matter is not so marked with the iodophors as with the QACs and chlorine compounds. They help to prevent the deposition of milkstone and alkaline salts on the surfaces of milking equipment.

Containers of approved chemical agents are required to include the following information:

1 A statement that the product has been approved by the Ministry of Agriculture, Fisheries & Food and the Ministry of Health to meet the requirements of Regulation 27 of the Milk and Dairies (General) Regulations 1959.

2 The concentration at which the product has been approved as being satisfactory in use.

3 The date by which the material must be used.

THE CLEANING AND STERILIZING ROUTINE IN THE DAIRY

The most recent figures indicate that over 87 per cent of producers in England and Wales are using circulation or acid boiling water (ABW) cleaning of pipeline plants whether in milking parlours or cowsheds. Over the last few years milking machine pipelines have been designed and modified where necessary to give satisfactory results with circulation cleaning. Providing that the installation is technically sound, the surfaces in good mechanical condition and that a satisfactory cleaning routine is followed methodically, it is possible to produce milk having an acceptable total bacterial count. There are two well-established methods of cleaning pipeline plants:

1 circulation cleaning
2 acid boiling water cleaning (ABW).

There are also other well-tried systems – VP – which give satisfactory results (Figs 7.7–7.10).

Circulation cleaning

The routine for this is in four stages which should be carried out twice daily:

1 Preparation of the plant
2 Cold or tepid water rinse
3 Hot circulation wash
4 Final rinse.

Preparation of the plant. As soon as milking is finished, the milk line is drained of all milk and the filter and pipe removed from the bulk tank. External surfaces of the clusters are brushed to remove all traces of milk and dirt. This is more

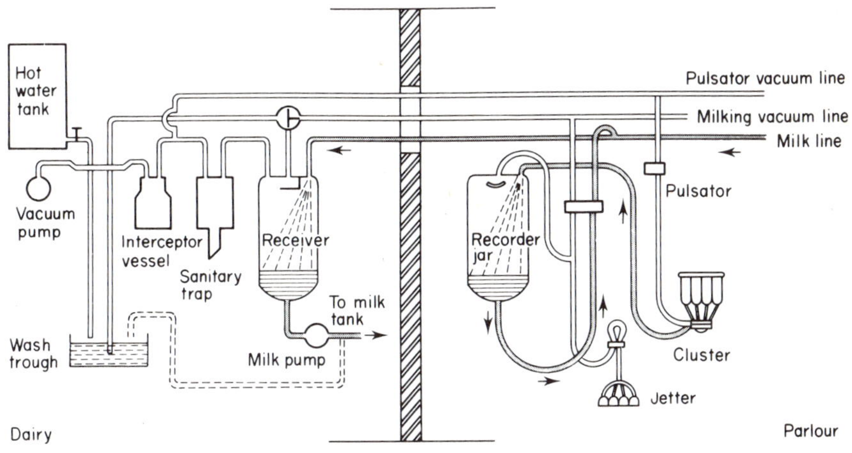

Fig. 7.7 Acidified boiling water (ABW) sterilization: parlour set for milking.

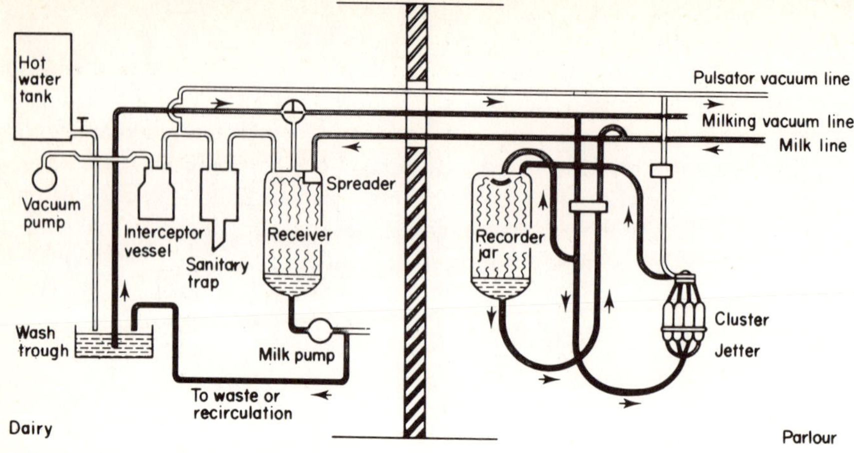

Fig. 7.8 ABW sterilization: parlour set for cleaning.

effective if warm water is used and some detergent sterilizer added to the water. The plant is then set to the 'wash' position, attaching the clusters to the jetters or, where applicable, taking the clusters into the dairy to attach to the wash-line manifold.

Cold or preferably tepid water is drawn through the plant and run to waste until the water is clear of residues.

Hot circulation wash. The solution for cleaning and sterilizing is then prepared. This may be a single product combining detergent and sterilizer or can be a separate dairy detergent used in conjunction with hypochlorite. For parlour

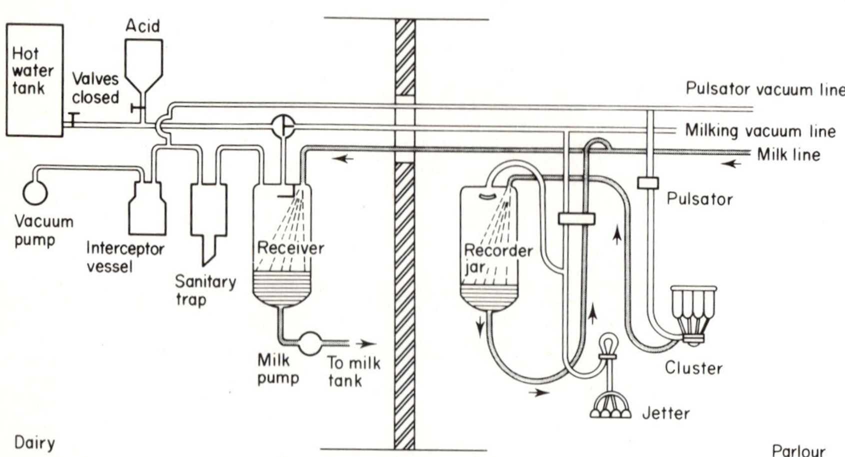

Fig. 7.9 Chemical sterilization: parlour set for milking.

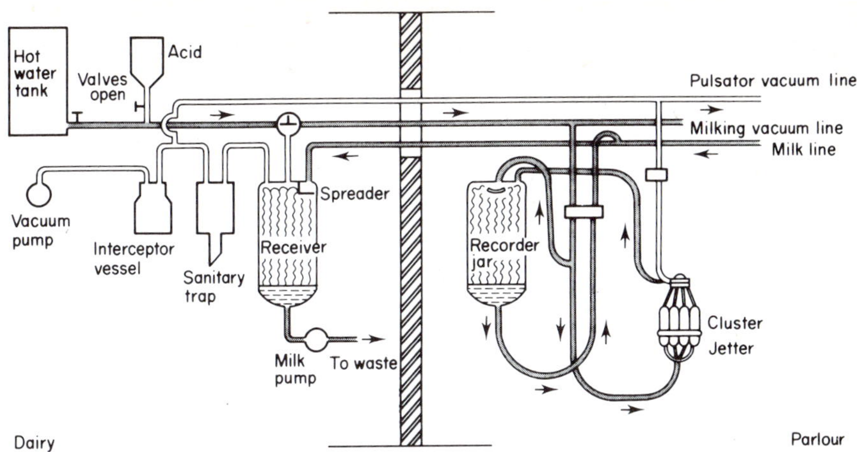

Fig. 7.10 Chemical sterilization: parlour set for cleaning.

plants with jars the recommended amount of water recirculating is 15 litres per unit at a temperature of 85°C. The hot solution is drawn into the plant and circulated for up to 10 minutes. The time depends very much on the amount of cooling of the solution and the aim should be that at the finish of circulating the temperature of the solution should not be less than 45°C. Heat loss can be reduced by running the first 10 litres or so of solution to waste. If tepid water is used for the initial rinse it will help to warm up the pipeline.

Final rinse. The plant should be rinsed in clean cold water to which has been added approved hypochlorite at the rate of 25 ml of hypochlorite/40 litres of water. It should be ensured that the plant is properly drained.

Non-foaming detergents should be used and there are many specially formulated proprietary detergent/sterilizers on the market.

In hard water areas it will probably be necessary to circulate a descaling solution of acid periodically to avoid the formation of milkstone.

Recent studies[15] have drawn attention to those factors which can adversely affect the efficiency of circulation cleaning. These are:

1 Poor flow distribution.
2 Incorrect flow rate.
3 Uneven distribution to all jar assemblies.
4 Incorrect distribution of the solution to the recorder jar and cluster.
5 Insufficient water – this should be 12–15 litres per unit.
6 Temperature of the hot water too low: this accounts for many of the unsatisfactory results.

As plants have become more complex these problems are more likely to occur and observation of the solution during circulation can give some indication of likely trouble spots.

Acid boiling water (ABW) cleaning[16]

A single operation system of cleaning was developed at the National institute for Research in Dairying using boiling water. The routine consists of drawing boiling (scalding) water (96°C) into the plant at the rate of 14 litres per unit during approximately 5 minutes and letting it run to waste. To prevent deposition of calcium salts in the plant, a solution of acid is drawn into the plant during the first 2–3 minutes of the cleaning process. All components of the plant must attain a temperature of 77°C within three minutes of the start of cleaning and this temperature must be maintained during the process. Initially the plant must be heat-balanced to ensure that correct temperature can be maintained. Great care must be taken in handling and dispersing strong acids as they are highly corrosive. After use the solution should be discharged direct into the drainage system to avoid damage to the dairy floor.

Among the problems which can arise in this routine are:

1 Partial blockage of the acid bleed with dust and dirt, which could cause the acid solution to be below strength.
2 Deposition of protein on the jars and pipeline. This can be removed using hot, strong, approved hypochlorite solution. Great care should be taken to wash the acid bleed container thoroughly to remove all traces of acid, as acid and hypochlorite can be highly reactive and therefore dangerous if mixed. 1.2. litres of approved hypochloride is added to the hot water. Ensure that all hypochlorite is rinsed away and if film is persistent repeat as nccessary.
3 In hard water areas the high temperatures required can lead to the deposition of calcium salts on the elements and thermostat of the water heater which may prevent the water reaching the minimum temperature of 96°C. The elements can be descaled with commercial formic acid and in some cases it is possible to remove the scale by wiping it off. Where scale formation is persistent it may be necessary to reduce build-up by using a scale dispenser or water softener.

Manual cleaning routines

These routines will apply to bucket plants and will consist of an initial rise, a hot detergent sterilizing wash with a thorough brushing of all surfaces and finally a cold or hot rinse. The temperature of the hot wash should be about 50°C which will be just about as hot as the hands can bear. To ensure that satisfactory results are obtained, the routine must be carried out methodically after morning and evening milking and all surfaces, both metal and rubber, should be in good mechanical condition.

CARE OF THE MILKING PLANT RUBBERS AND THE VACUUM SYSTEM

To obtain satisfactory results for hygiene and to reduce the risk of udder disease, the rubber components of the milking plant must be maintained in a mechanically sound condition. With circulation and ABW cleaning systems using synthetic rubbers these will have a longer life than manually cleaned natural rubberware. They should, however, be renewed when necessary and because of the cost of replacing them throughout a milking plant, a rotational system is recommended to deal with each component in turn.

The cleanliness of the vacuum system is often neglected because it is not considered to be an obvious source of contamination. It can, however, become contaminated with milk residues, dust and moisture and as there is a movement of air between the milk and vacuum lines of the plant there can be a risk of the cross-flow of air. Periodic cleaning should be carried out using a warm non-foaming detergent/disinfectant solution followed by a warm rinse using clean water. Care should be given to avoiding moisture entering the pulsation system or any electrical equipment.

CLEANING BULK TANKS

Bulk collection of milk from most farms is by tankers equipped with flowmeters to measure the milk and a totalizer and print out unit to record it.

The tanker driver having visually inspected, sampled when appropriate, transferred and recorded the litres of milk, either rinses the interior of the tank with cold water or sets in motion the washing sequence of an automatic bulk tank washer.

Bulk tank cleaning can be carried out manually, automatically or semi-automatically.

For hand cleaning after the preliminary rinse a detergent/sterilizer powder may be sprinkled on, either by hand or by a purpose-made dispenser which is worked up into a paste by brush and the tank hose rinsed. Alternatively, an iodophor solution can be sprayed over the interior surfaces, brushing carried out as necessary and after suitable contact time the tank hose rinsed with cold water. All cleaning with bulk tanks is carried out with cold water and cold solutions of cleaners; otherwise damage to various components and possibly the tank itself could result.

Automatic cleaners for bulk milk tanks were introduced into the U.K. in 1965. Equipment for cleaning consists of a water container with a measure on one side for containing an approved cleaning agent. Water from the container is pumped by a centrifugal pump through piping to two spinners attached to each of the tank's two covers. When the pump is set in motion, water is drawn from the container entraining a cleaning and sterilizing solution which is fed to the spinners, and distributes it all over the tank. A plastic trough is placed under the tank outlet into which the dipstick, plug and outlet cap can be placed. A final rinse is given and this can have hypochlorite entrained if the water supply is not bacteriologically acceptable.

In the fully automatic systems the driver has only to place the plug, dispstick and outlet plug in the trough and initiate the cleaning sequence, control with each step being by a process timer. With the semi-automatic cleaner the final rinse of the tank has to be initiated separately.

Whatever system of cleaning is used, there are places on the tank on which milk tends to accumulate and contamination to build up. These areas are on the underside of the bridge, on the stirring paddle and the thermometer, on the dipstick, on the rubber outlet bung and on the outlet itself. Special attention is required to ensure that these parts of the tank are kept in a satisfactory condition.

When deciding upon the system of cleaning, points which must be considered are:

1 The accessibility and shape of the tank for hand cleaning.
2 Milk collection at times which conflict with labour being available for hand cleaning the tank.
3 Capital cost.

MILK

Sampling

Milk samples may be required for either chemical or bacteriological examination, and if the analysis is to be of any value, it is essential to ensure that they are representative of the bulk. For chemical tests the sampler must be provided with a dipper, preferably of not less than 85 ml capacity and a plunger to agitate and mix the milk. The equipment must be thoroughly clean and dry to avoid adulteration and preferably sterilized to avoid contamination. For some chemical examinations a suitable preservative can be added; the nature of any such additive should be noted on the bottle.

For bacteriological purposes equipment, including plungers, sample bottles and stoppers, must be sterile. Glass sample bottles are provided and may have a nominal capacity of 85, 120, 170 or 230 ml. Closures can be either screw cap or rubber bungs. The bottles may be sand-blasted on a suitable area for recording details of the sample.

Samples should be transported to the laboratory as quickly as possible and precautions taken to prevent deterioration and exposure to fluctuations in temperature. If samples are required from individual cows for bacteriological examination, the cow's udder should be thoroughly washed and rough-dried and the udder washing water should be treated with 30 ml of hypochlorite to every 10 litres of water. After discarding the fore-milk, a few squirts of milk from each quarter should be directed into the sample bottle. The milk can be cooled by immersion in a bowl of water or held under a running tap for a few minutes.

Abnormal milk

When milk was collected in churns abnormal flavours or colours could be detected more readily than with bulk milk because it was often held at a higher temperature allowing taints to develop or the milk to absorb odours from strong smelling substances. There was usually a lower dilution factor making it easier to detect any abnormality. There are, however, some faults which have become more important and could be responsible for the spoilage of large quantities of milk.

Abnormal milk can be caused by or derived from a variety of factors:

1 External influences on milk already produced, e.g. absorbed odours from strong-smelling substances.
2 Ingested feedstuffs, weeds or medicines.
3 Physiological disturbance of the cow (mastitic milk, lipase and acetone taint).
4 Bacterial contaminants.
5 Chemical reactions.
6 Miscellaneous causes.

These conditions may give rise to milk which is abnormal in odour, colour, taste or consistency, and many taints are recognizable by more than one of these faults.[17] A survey[18] carried out by Thomas et al. on the flavour of raw milk lists 15 different flavours which could be described as abnormal; of the samples examined, roughly 22 per cent were described as having an abnormal flavour. Taints and abnormal conditions in milk are not always easy to locate and remedy, and in some cases a full-scale bacteriological investigation may be necessary. Although some attempt has been made to classify these conditions into broad groups, a specific taint can arise from one or more of the groups – for example, a fishy taint, which can be caused in more than one way.

Taints and tastes from external influences

Milk which is badly stored close to substances such as paint, paraffin, disinfectants, animal medicines, fishmeal, silage or fruit will tend to absorb the taint of them, particularly when the milk is warm.

Taints and tastes from ingested materials

These are mainly seasonal, and where the taint is from a food being fed to cows, it can be reduced by not feeding any of the material within at least two hours of milking and preferably longer. Bad or rotten feeds are more likely to produce off-flavours. There are at least three factors involved:

Weeds. Many weeds are known to be responsible for tainting milk. They will probably only be eaten in quantity when pastures are burned up, keep is scarce or an individual cow develops a liking for the weed; the most common and easily recognizable is garlic. Others are camomile, stinking mayweed, ivy, yarrow, buttercup and tansy; chicory (not always regarded as a weed) is said to impart a bitter flavour.

Feedstuffs. Silage, kale (particularly when old), turnips, lush clover, fishmeal, sugar-beet (giving a fishy taint due to the production of trimethylamine) are the most common offenders; some of these taints can be removed by aeration of the milk, e.g. with a surface cooler.

Animal medicines. Some medicines with which animals are drenched will cause taints; such milk should be excluded from the bulk for at least 48 hours.

Physiological disturbance of the cow

Mastitis. Large numbers of cows in a herd with mastitis will cause strong 'bad' taints and bitter flavours due to the rise in chloride content and the drop in lactose.

Acetonaemia. Cows suffering from this condition secrete milk described as having a 'sickly cowy' smell due to the presence of ketones. This condition usually occurs 3–6 weeks after calving and is associated with a disturbance of the carbohydrate metabolism.

Lipase taint. Lipase taint is generally due to an abnormal physiological condition of the cow. It mostly occurs in cows in late lactation and develops some hours after production, even if the milk is held at low temperatures. It is thought to be due to the production of certain of the lower fatty acids, of which butyric acid is the most important. Lipase taint is described as a rancid off-flavour.

Lipolytic or rancid taints may also be associated with pipeline milking systems, particularly where long lengths of pipe are used, as in 'round-the-shed' milking. It is due either to the mechanics of the milking installation or to a combination of this factor and the presence of milk from certain cows which is apparently more susceptible to this type of taint.

Mechanical factors which are thought to induce the taint are excessive agitation and foaming, partial churning of the milk at any stage, admittance of air to the pipeline and continuous operation of centrifugal pumps. Milk produced from cows during the grazing season appears to have more tolerance to agitation, whereas milk from cows in late lactation or with mastitis is more susceptible to the development of the taint.

Bacterial contaminants

Faults caused by bacteria and yeasts almost always arise from poor methods of milk production, dirty utensils, inadequate cooling or contaminated water supplies.

Souring. This is by far the most common fault in milk and is usually due to lactic streptococci, which produce lactic acid from lactose; almost invariably the root cause is dirty milking utensils.

Malty or caramel flavour. Variously described as malty, caramel or burnt flavour and a fairly common fault. The causal organism is *Streptococcus lactis* var. *maltigines* and the main source of infection is again dirty utensils. Eradication may be difficult and requires special attention to hygiene.

Frothiness. This is due to the production of gas by organisms of the coliform group, or more rarely by yeasts.

Ropy milk. The bacteria which cause ropiness usually come from a contaminated water supply, and the outbreak will be characterized by its persistence and the difficulty of complete eradication. The milk will pull out in long strings and be very viscous. Another source of infection is the teats and udders of cows which have become contaminated through wading in ponds. The main group of bacteria known to be responsible are strains of the coli-aerogenes group.

Other off-flavours and taints. These can be caused by bacteria or yeasts, and are fishy, earthy or fruity. They are rarely encountered.

Chemical reactions

Oxidized flavour. There are a variety of off-flavours included in this group – oily, tallowy, cardboardy and metallic. Changes in the milk arise from oxidation of the fat or fat globule membrane and of the constituents of the milk connected with the fat phase, i.e. lecithin, cephalin and oleic acid and its glycerides. Factors which induce the off-flavour are:

1 The presence of traces of dissolved metals, in particular copper, which acts as a catalyst to oxidative changes. It has been found that milk over a badly worn surface cooler with exposed copper will contain 1–2 ppm of copper, compared with an average of 0.2–0.5 ppm in normal milk.
2 Exposure of milk to strong sunlight will produce a tallowy flavour which can develop very rapidly. It is believed to be due to the oxidation of the unsaturated fatty acids of the milk fat and to be accelerated by the presence of riboflavin.
3 Individuality and feed. Some cows appear to secrete milk which is more

susceptible to this off-flavour. It is possibly associated with lack of green food and carotene in the diet.

The presence of dissolved oxygen is essential for the chemical action to proceed and therefore the taint is less likely to develop in milk contaminated with large numbers of bacteria, which will use up oxygen rapidly. When milk is refrigerated to extend its life, additional time is given for the chemical change to take place and the low temperature restricts the growth of organisms which would require oxygen.

Chlorophenol taint

Phenolic and chlorine compounds which come into contact with milk can react to produce an offensive taint which is not detectable by smell and only by taste. It will therefore not be apparent to the tanker driver and could lead to the spoilage of large quantities of milk. It can also be difficult to pin-point the source. Phenol is the main ingredient of many general purpose disinfectants and may be present in some udder salves. Chlorine compounds are almost invariably available on dairy farms and traces may be present on milking equipment or in chlorinated water supplies.

Miscellaneous causes

Stringy milk. This is a fault, usually very temporary, due to the physical condition of the protein giving stringy threads, particularly on surface coolers. Mastitis milk may also be stringy owing to high leucocyte content.

Blood in milk

The presence of blood in milk may be a frequent occurrence in some herds and such milk should, of course, be excluded from the bulk. It may also be responsible for defects in cheese manufacture. It is not always easy to detect and the strip cup in this respect may not help a great deal. There are several possible causes, the most common of which are:

1. Milk of freshly calved cows where heavy stocking of the udder has caused the rupturing of blood capillaries, due to pressure within the udder.
2. Internal injury to the udder, caused by horning or blows.
3. Warts, cowpox or abrasions on the teats, which bleed, particularly when the milking machine is applied, the operator possibly being unaware that blood has got into the milk.
4. Some types of mastitis.

Apart from visual examination, the method of detection at the creamery usually consists of centrifuging a quantity of milk in a boiling tube. Ramell[19] has suggested a technique for the accurate quantitative determination of the presence of blood.

REFERENCES

1 Dutton, J. (1983) Parlour processes to cut mastitis. *Farmers Weekly*, 26 August 1983.
2 Longstaff, G. W. (1977) Focus on quality – sediment. *Milk Producer 24*, 10 October 1977.
3 Hoyle, J. B. (1977) Sediment in milk and filtering for farm use. *J. Soc. Dairy Technol.*, **30**, 2, April.
4 Millard, D. and Cheeseman, G. C. (1974) Determination of extraneous matter in milk. *J. Soc. Dairy Technol.*, **27**, 2, April.
5 Dawkins, J. (1977) The reduction in sediment levels in milk through the use of commercial pre-production multi-service filters. *J. Soc. Dairy Technol.*, **30**, 4, October.
6 Bramley, A. J., Dodd, F. H. and Griffin, T. K. (1980) Mastitis control and herd management. *N.I.R.D. Technical Bulletin*, No. 4.
7 MAFF (1983) *Fly Control for the Dairy Herd.* Leaflet No. 656.
8 Liddell, J. S. and Clayton, R. (1982) Long duration fly control on cattle using cypermethrin-impregnated ear tags. *Vet. Rec.*, **110**, 502.
9 Anon. (1975) Emergency – snow, ice, floods. *Milk Producer*, November.
10 Anon. (1972) Virus trap for tankers. *Milk Producer*, **19**, 2 February.
11 Chammings, R. J. (1984) Effect of different methods of udder preparation on the somatic cell count and bacterial count of herd bulk milk. *J. Soc. Dairy Tecnol.*, **37**, 4, October
12 Minister, Patience (1979) Saving energy is cool. *Dairy Farmer*, September 1979.
13 Hipkin, D. W. (1976) The economic use of detergents and sanitizers in the diary industry. *J. Soc. Dairy Technol.*, **29**, 4, October.
14 British Standards Institution (1975) BS 5226. *Recommendations for Cleaning and Sterilization of Pipeline Milking Installation.*
15 Sinclair, George (1984) Problems of Circulatory Cleaning. *Dairy Farmer*, February 1984.
16 MAFF (1981) *Acidified Boiling Water Cleaning of Recorder Milking Machines.* Leaflet No. 718.
17 Orr, Margaret J. (1954) Some common faults in milk. *J. Soc. Dairy Technol.*, **7**, 2.
18 Thomas, S. B., Griffiths, D. G. and Morgan, K. J. (1959) The flavour of raw milk. *J. Soc. Dairy Technol.*, **12**, 3.
19 Rammell, C. G. (1963) The occurrence and significance of blood in bovine milk. *J. Dairy Res.*, **30**, 1.

8

Stock Water Requirements

SOURCES OF SUPPLY

Potential sources of supply of water for farm stock may be from public mains or a private source. Abstraction of water for farm use from a private underground source is controlled by law. The veterinarian and agriculturist will be principally concerned with an adequate quantity of water of satisfactory bacteriological standard free from any toxic substances which could affect its use for domestic, dairying or stock purposes. For domestic and dairy use the bacteriological standards will be most important, and very hard water will require treatment. A contaminated supply could be responsible for causing disease both amongst humans and stock.

Supplies obtained from public mains can generally be regarded as suitable for all purposes, the maintenance of quality being a statutory obligation of the water undertaking.

The suitability of streams and rivers for stock drinking depends on the nature of pollution which is liable to occur from the source to the point at which water is to be extracted.

Linton[1] classifies supplies according to their palatability and wholesomeness as follows:

Wholesomeness	Source	Palatability
Wholesome	Spring water	Very palatable
	Deep well water	
	Upland surface water	Moderately palatable
Suspicious	Stored rain water	
	Water from cultivated land	Palatable
Dangerous	River water	
	Shallow well water	

Palatability gives no indication of the purity of a supply or its suitability for stock drinking purposes over a prolonged period.

WATER REQUIREMENTS

On most farms water will be required for:

a Domestic and dairy use.
b Stock drinking and washing down.

It may also be required for irrigation.

The availability of a supply of pure water in sufficient quantity can often be the limiting factor in the farming policy. Lack of water can result in thriftlessness in stock generally and free access to water is essential for the maximum production of milk and eggs and efficient food conversion. For dairy farms an adequate supply is required for cleaning utensils and milking premises and, where applicable, for cooling milk. The Ministry of Agriculture, Fisheries and Food recognize the importance of farm water supplies by offering grant aid towards the cost of approved new water schemes from private sources or of connection to public mains.

The requirements for individual farms will vary according to the number and type of stock, the type of enterprise and the time of the year. Peak demands are likely to coincide with times when water is scarce, and so adequate storage is essential. Where stock is concerned size, functional activity, dry matter content of feed and season will affect water consumption from day to day but some basis for the calculation of likely requirements is needed and Table 8.1 can be used as a general guide.

Ideally all stock should have free access to fresh clean drinking water at all times. Stock will not drink their fill of muddy or unpalatable water which, if contaminated, could cause an outbreak of disease and could also result in retarded growth, digestive troubles and where applicable reduced milk yields. Piping water to all fields used for stock will save labour and generally increase farming efficiency. Where private supplies are used it is essential that the source works, storage and distribution systems are soundly constructed and regularly maintained.[2]

The whole system should be inspected at least once a year to check on the soundness of fencing where needed and that collecting and storage tanks have not deteriorated structurally. Where necessary tanks and reservoirs should be cleaned out and chlorinated. If storage is required for mains supplies these tanks should be checked to ensure their cleanliness. Attention given to the effective lagging and insulation of exposed pipes will be well repaid in a severe winter.

For field supplies there must be sufficient troughs available, conveniently sited and with either a free-draining or built-up access. A concrete apron may be desirable on some soil types and where large numbers of stock are being catered for. In some situations one centrally placed trough can serve two fields which could be suitable for young stock or store cattle. For strip grazing movable troughs will be required together with a sufficient number of accessible hydrants

Table 8.1 *Water requirements of livestock*

Use or type of stock	Approx. requirement (litres)	
Milking cows (including cooling and cleaning)	135	per animal/day
Milking cows (drinking only)*	47–70	per animal/day
Other cattle	45	per animal/day
Horse	25–35	per animal/day
Pig	5–13	per animal/day
Sheep	7	per animal/day
Poultry (intensive)	0.6	per animal/day
Hosepipe for washing down	9–23 per minute	
Domestic	135–180 per head	

*Consumption of water by cows in milk can be calculated: 4.5 litres per 50 kg liveweight + 13.6 litres per 4.5 litres of milk yielded. In summer, on grazing only, grass will provide about 45.0 litres of water per day but will be influenced by weather conditions.

from which to connect a temporary pipeline. All troughs should have ball valves of the correct type for the pressure available and a service pipe large enough to carry a sufficient flow of water during peak draw-off periods. Protection of exposed pipes from frost damage has already been mentioned. Protection is also required to prevent mechanical damage and the trough should be provided with a plug for emptying and periodic scrubbing. This may be particularly necessary when there is a heavy growth of algae which can occur when troughs have not been in use for some time.

For the dairy herd adequate trough space and rapid refill rate are particularly important so that cows can drink in comfort without stress or bullying. The peak drinking periods are after evening milking until sundown or in mid- or late morning and it has been found that up to 10 per cent of the herd will drink at any one time during the peak drinking periods. It has also been shown that up to 40 per cent of the total daily consumption may be drunk during these periods.

Provision must be made for supplying some 20–70 litres of water per cow per day, the amount depending on weather, dry matter content of the ration, stage of lactation, milk yield and breed of cow. Between 450 and 600 mm of trough face will be required to enable the cow to drink in comfort and water intake can be from 16 to 25 litres of water per minute.

The total drinking space available will be determined by the size, shape and number of troughs together with their situation. Troughs are usually constructed of galvanized iron, pre-cast concrete or built *in situ* of brick or block work treated with a waterproof rendering. The usual size of a rectangular galvanized trough is 1830 mm long × 460 mm wide × 380 mm deep and holds 305 litres when full. Interest has recently been shown in large circular troughs similar to those used in New Zealand. These are available in pre-cast concrete or glass reinforced cement and have capacities of about 1600 litres. Advantages claimed are easier access because of a pronounced fanning-out effect whereby larger numbers of cows can drink together at any one time than would be possible with most rectangular troughs.

Minimum effective drinking perimeter spaces have been suggested which allow 10 per cent of the herd to drink at any one time:

Minimum effective drinking perimeter	
Herd size	mm
50	2250
100	4500
125	5650
150	6750
200	9000

Where water bowls are used it is suggested that with cows on a high dry matter ration one bowl should be provided for every six cows. Water bowls and troughs in yards should be situated so that they are clear of scraping routes and if in strawed yards built up on a concrete platform to minimize poaching.

When considering the total demand for water on dairy farms, in addition to young stock, allowance must be made for plant cleaning, for both milking equipment and bulk tanks, and also for cleaning of dairies, parlours and associated areas. Many milk producers are also economizing in electricity costs by pre-cooling the milk going into the bulk tank with water. As there are wide variations in plant size and methods of cleaning it is not possible to suggest exact amounts needed although general guidelines can be given.

The amount of water required for washing down parlours,[3] dairies and yards will be decided by the method of washing and the type of soiling to be removed; high-pressure washers are not necessarily suitable for all purposes. Indeed washing down with a bucket of water could in some cases be the most effective and economical method. Some types of soiling need to be flushed away whereas other types – for example, dried-on dung splashes on walls – need to be scoured or hosed away so that with pressure washers flow rate for a particular cleaning job has to be considered together with the most effective pressure. The correct balance between the flow rate and pressure will ensure the most economical use of labour, power and water and achieve the most satisfactory results. Plant is available to suit all these requirements and may also be satisfactory for other cleaning jobs on the farm – for example, machinery.

When cleaning floors of yards and parlours after removing the solid or semi-solid material with a scraper or squeegee, the use of a high-volume/low-pressure washer is in most cases the most effective. For wall cleaning where dry or semi-dry dung splashes stick a high-pressure/low-volume jet of water is required and this could also apply to yards where dung has dried on. Probable water requirements for this purpose are from 10–20 litres per cow per day and with properly planned cleaning methods the lower figure should be obtainable.

Table 8.2 *Amounts of water required for plant cleaning*

	Parlours			Bulk tanks		
				Automatically cleaned		
	with jars	without jars	Pipeline plant in cowshed	up to 1800 litre capacity	1800 litre + capacity	Hand- and spray-cleaned
Litres of water per unit (hot and cold)	35	45–65	45–65 (+65 per 30 m length of pipeline)	90–135	160–230	25–70

Table 8.2 gives an indication of the amounts of water used for plant cleaning.

For udder washing with clean cows 2 litres of water per cow per day should be sufficient but this will depend on the type of washer used and the cleanliness of the cows so that at some times during the year this figure could be much higher.

To assess the suitability of a supply for all purposes a full examination may be required which will consist of:

1 Inspection of the source of supply.
2 Physical examinaton of the water.
3 Application of chemical tests.
4 Application of bacteriological tests.

The bacteriological examination of a single sample of water is of little value and may give results which are completely misleading. To reach a firm opinion a series of samples must be examined, the results being interpreted in conjunction with the details of the source of supply and possible points of pollution. For details of bacteriological techniques reference should be made to *The Bacteriological Examination of Water Supplies*.[4,5]

REFERENCES AND FURTHER READING

1 Scorgie, N. J. and Willis, G. A. (1952) *Linton's Veterinary Hygiene*. Edinburgh: Green & Sons.

2 MAFF (1977) *Farm water supply leaflet* no.5. *Maintaining Water Supply Systems*. London: H.M.S.O.

3 MAFF (1976) *Planning for Parlour Milking*. Management Aids No. 16. Washing Down Parlours. Section I. Static Parlours. II. Rotary Parlours. London: HMSO.

4 Ministry of Health (1956) *The Bacteriological Examination of Water Supplies* Report No. 71 (3rd edn.). London: H.M.S.O.

5 MAFF (1968) Technical bulletin no. 17. *Bacteriological Techniques for Dairy Purposes*. London: H.M.S.O.

9

Manure Disposal from Livestock Farms

For many years farmyard manure was the main fertilizer used on farms. There was an age-old belief that the fertility of the land was best maintained through the animals and their dung, and in some areas, such as the fens of East Anglia, the principal reason for keeping animals was to provide this fertility. In more recent times inorganic artificial fertilizers have tended to replace farmyard manure as the main source of plant fertilizer. There have been a number of reasons for this: the high cost of handling farmyard manure; the use of housing systems without or with very little bedding; the emergence of intensive animal units without any relationship with farm land or crops; and the relatively lower cost of 'artificials'. All these factors have contributed to animal manure becoming something of an unwanted waste product, difficult to dispose of, and a liability instead of an asset. Instead of the solid farmyard manure many livestock units now produce a semi-liquid slurry, which is a mixture of faeces and urine suspended in water, occasionally with a little bedding and various other additions, such as disinfectants. The material will not compost. It must be stored in tanks above or below ground, or in lakes or 'lagoons' which are simply artificial depressions excavated out of the ground.

In recent years, in most countries of the world, there has been a continuous trend towards the imposition of legislation that prohibits the farmer from polluting rivers, streams, water courses and even farm ditches with effluent from livestock enterprises. This has raised many severe practical problems, especially since it has happened at a time when the nature of farm wastes has tended to alter to semi-liquids.

Some idea of the huge quantities of slurry from all farm livestock can be gained from the following figures in Table 9.1, which apply only to the United Kingdom.[1]

Since animal wastes per population equivalent are twice as difficult as human waste to treat as sewage, this is equivalent to the waste disposal of 272 million people – about five times the human population of the United Kingdom. Most livestock units handle waste in the traditional manner and it has been estimated that 80 per cent will continue to do so if better machinery is developed and better control of smell becomes possible. The remainder, especially those with little land, may have to use more sophisticated systems of handling waste, and

Table 9.1 *Slurry quantities*

	No. of animals (millions)	Tonnes of slurry (millions)	Population equivalents* (millions)
Cows	3	45	30
Other cattle	9	50	50
Pigs	7	10	14
Sheep	29	10	30
Poultry	126	6	12
Total	174	121	136

*Standard measure of pollution.

some idea of the amount involved is gained from the fact that this will involve the U.K. handling an amount equivalent to that from all the present human population. Using human waste techniques the cost of a sewage works for 1000 pigs would be about £80–90 per pig so that vastly cheaper methods must be developed.

The chemical composition of undiluted pig, cattle and poultry slurries are given in Table 9.2. As an example, in one day 100 pigs weighing 70 kg produce approximately 400 litres of slurry containing 85 per cent water.

About 25 m^3 of undiluted pig slurry could be placed annually on an arable acre, but on grassland it is not uncommon to apply as much as 100 m^3 by frequent application. Hence an acre of land can deal with the slurry output of 60 pigs or more. These figures are for undiluted slurries. In practice many slurries must be diluted where pipeline and gun systems are used, and then the application rates can be increased in proportion to the dilution rate.

DISEASE AND HEALTH PROBLEMS

Along with the problem of the physical disposal of muck is the vital question of human and animal health. Whilst the smell from composted solid muck is a little objectionable, it rarely creates a grave problem and there is also little if any disease risk to the human or animal population from this form of muck under temperate climatic conditions. Slurry, however, is quite a different problem. Slurry applied straight on the land from the animal house or after holding in a tank anaerobically has an extremely offensive smell. Whilst masking

Table 9.2 *Each 4.5 m^3 (1000 gallons) undiluted slurry supply as available nutrients*

	Units per 4.5 m^3 (1000 g) undiluted slurry		
	N	P_2O_5	K_2O
Pigs (faeces and urine)	40	40	35
Cows (faeces and urine)	45	12	40
Poultry (fresh droppings)	100	100	50

agents are possible they are too expensive at present to be considered economic. The worst smell comes from the pipeline and gun spreader, because the droplet size is small and light and may carry considerable distances. The least smell arises from a tanker spreader because the slurry is much thicker and not spread by aerially dispersed small droplets. The most satisfactory way to prevent the slurry causing offence is to treat it aerobically in some way before spreading, which will be dealt with later. Human and health problems may arise and we know already of dangers chiefly from the salmonella group of organisms and *E. coli*.

In a recent survey it was found that potentially pathogenic bacteria were able to survive up to nearly three months in slurry kept under anaerobic conditions.[2] While the particular bacteria studied were salmonella species and *E. coli*, there is no doubt that more resistant organisms, such as *Bacillus anthracis, Mycobacterium tuberculosis*, clostridial species and leptospira species, could survive at least as long and probably much longer. There are thus three possible hazards from the distribution of anaerobically stored slurry: (a) smells objectionable to the human population; (b) hazards to human health; and (c) hazards to animal health. If the slurry should enter a river or stream the pollution may have far-reaching and infinitely more serious effects. It is thus essential to all enterprises with slurry as the disposal system that either the slurry is placed on land where it cannot be a nuisance or a health risk, or it is so treated before hand that the risks are removed. It is essential that slurry derived from pig units where copper is used as a feed additive is not placed on land where sheep may graze since they are highly susceptible to copper toxicity.

SOLID MANURE

Solid manure – that is, faeces and urine combined with bedding such as straw or wood shavings – forms the most common method of handling the effluent from livestock buildings. The equipment needed is straightforward, the mixture is easily stored for long periods on the ground and also transported easily. With a minimum of care it need create little or no nuisance and it is the best product for the land. After a period of composting, health hazards are effectively eliminated. It is, therefore, the method of choice wherever possible.

Equipment

(a) *Scraping and loading equipment*

(i) *Mechanical scrapers in dung passages*. This is frequently done fully automatically either by using a scraper and chain, or reciprocating blades, or it may be done semi-automatically by fitting a blade attachment to a small horticultural tractor. For wider passages a tractor-mounted scraper can be used fitted either to the rear of a tractor or as an attachment to the front-end loader.

(ii) *Tractor-mounted hydraulic loaders.* Generally front-end loaders are used but rear loaders are designed that can work well in more confined areas.

(iii) *Tractor-mounted ditch diggers with manure grabs.* In this case the tractor remains largely stationary and a ditch digger is fitted with an hydraulic grab used for handling solid manure.

(iv) *Industrial loaders.* Where large quantities of dung are to be shifted individual earth moving equipment is ideal. Such machines can handle up to 2 tonnes in one bucketful.

(b) *Spreading equipment*

The spreading of the solid muck can be carried out in two ways. One is the conventional land-driven solid-dung spreader. A very wide assortment of robust construction is available and well known to the industry. Alternatively, a rotary flail spreader can be used and this has the advantage that it can handle materials of almost any consistency.

SLURRY

Storage must be provided as it is unlikely that the farmer can move it on to the land at all times of the year. This is the main factor affecting the storage required. Alternatively, an area of land without any potential value in it should be set aside where the slurry can be dumped. Or, often on the smaller farm, slurry can be added to solid muck in its composting heap which is able to absorb considerable amounts (See Fig. 9.1.).

Storage

Storage systems are as follows:

Under the slats

Usually a channel is used at least 1 m to 1–2 m deep. This may provide storage for some months. There is usually a sluice gate at one end which, when lifted periodically, allows the slurry to discharge into a collecting sump or storage tank from which the slurry can be pumped and spread. Alternatively, they can be emptied by lifting up some slats and pumping out or by inserting a pipe through the outside wall. Channels should always have some water put in them before use and are made to a fall of about 1 : 100 to the collecting end. A sluice gate is not essential and the slurry can be allowed to trickle over continuously into a collecting tank.

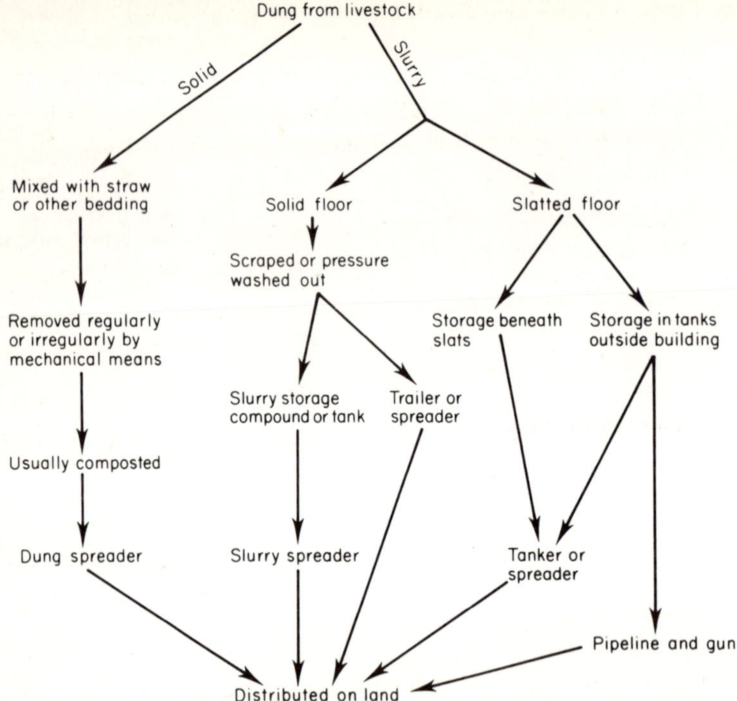

Fig. 9.1 Dung-handling systems.

Gases are produced anaerobically, including gases poisonous to man and animals. Great care is needed when emptying the slurry as gas may be driven up into the building. Ventilation systems with slats should always arrange to extract the stale air from above the slats. Under the slats the channel and tank must be completely sealed. The slats themselves should be maintained as cleanly as possible as they represent a serious health risk. Diseases such as haemorrhagic dysentery appear to be closely related to unhygienic slats either being of a poor design themselves or because they are placed in badly designed pens. Correctly built and disposed, slats are generally self-cleaning.

In tanks

Tanks are usual where large quantities of slurry must be stored. They are best in any case where pipeline and gun systems are used since water is usually added to a proportion of up to 2 : 1 water to slurry.

Three systems are used for storage:

Underground tanks. Usually up to 3–4 m deep and up to 4 m wide. They are mostly built of conventional lining materials such as concrete or brick and may be square or round. This arrangement is very suitable since it can be filled by gravity, but it is an expensive way of storing slurry.

Surface tanks. These may be cheaper to erect than underground tanks and are especially useful where the water-table is high. A large range is available and though a pump is needed to fill them they may be emptied by gravity.

'Lagoons'. These are artificial ponds excavated out of the soil for storing very large quantities. A depth of about 2 m is usual, but they should not be filled over about 1 m for aerobic working. Some further discussion on lagoons is given later.

Disposal of slurry in the field

Spreader

The slurry can be scraped along a ramp directly into a spreader, as used for solid muck. Normal slurry, however, has a dry matter content of 10–15 per cent and most of the urine must be drained off *en route* to the compound, or in the dunging passages, to raise the dry matter up to 20 per cent when the dung can be handled fairly well in this way. This is a reasonable system for a farmer to use where small quantities of slurry are to be disposed of. But it is not satisfactory otherwise.

Tanker

Using a tanker there is no dilution of the slurry and the capital cost is much less (Fig. 9.2). It is also more flexible since the tanker can go to several draw-off points. Though normally the tanker will have to go over the land, which can be a severe limitation on its use, some tankers can stand on the roadway and pump over the field by pipeline attachments.

Pipeline and guns

The advantages are that large quantities can be dispensed very quickly. It is a system which is satisfactory for most seasons (except freezing). Water must be available for dilution and cleaning the pipes after use. Very efficient agitators are essential in the storage tanks or a chopper should be used if bedding finds its way into the tank.

With all these systems a wide range of manufactured products is available but great care is needed by the farmer to choose the right one for the form of slurry to be disposed of.

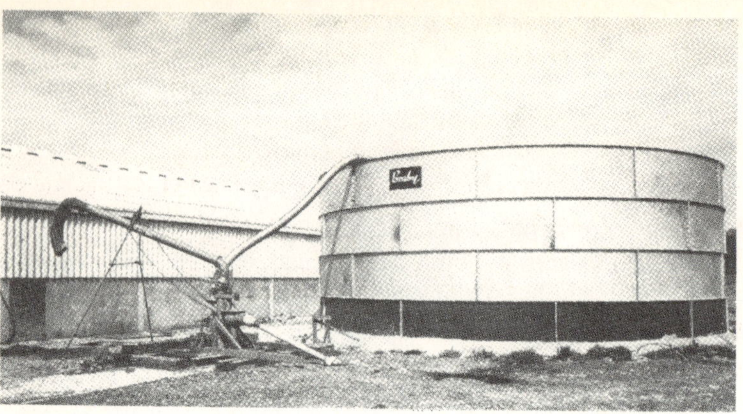

Fig. 9.2 Large surface slurry tank.

TREATMENT OF LIVESTOCK EFFLUENTS

Aerobic treatments

These rely on the action of microorganisms which use dissolved oxygen for their respiration. Organic material is broken down to mainly CO_2 and water with a residual sludge. There is no offensive smell from aerobic treatment.

If effluent is spread on land in thin layers this is the action that takes place. If the liquid is put into a shallow lagoon (or 'oxidation pond') this also may take place. It requires light to encourage the growth of algae which release oxygen for the bacteria to use. The light must reach the bottom of the pond and the mixture must be very dilute. With warm conditions, plenty of added water, and a shallow pond (say 1 m maximum) such arrangements can work in the right climate, but have not been particularly successful in Western Europe except where some solids have been removed beforehand. In warm climates lagoons can be loaded with very dilute waste to a total of about 20 kg biochemical oxygen demand (BOD) per acre per day: no more than the output of about 100 pigs.

Artificial means exist of mechanically introducing the oxygen. For example, oxidation ditches (e.g. Pasveer ditches), floating aerators, perforated pipes and proprietary fabricated floors and diffusers. These can all introduce oxygen into the water, reduce odour and provide good mixing. To date, however, these processes have not been successful for animal manure and much more work is required before they can be recommended with confidence. There is always a build-up of sludge in the bottom of the tanks which must be removed.

Anaerobic treatment

This relies on bacteria that break down manure in the absence of O_2 releasing mainly hydrogen sulphide, ammonia, methane and carbon dioxide. Water and sludge remain. This system is virtually impracticable for animal muck.

Drying

This is a possibility worth examining as there is a market for the end-product. At present, however, it appears too expensive using any of the currently available processing machinery.

Composting

This is aerobic decomposition of organic waste to a relatively stable humus. It usually requires the addition of straw, but there may be possibilities of adding pig slurry to municipal refuse and selling the product as a fertilizer.

Incineration

This is not used at present.

Vacuum filtration

This can be used to separate liquids and solids, but costs are too high for the system to be used at present.

Centrifugal separation of liquids

This is being used on several farms in the U.K. and elsewhere successfully, but there is too little information available to form a judgement on its effectiveness.

FUTURE PROSPECTS

Whilst it appears almost inevitable that livestock enterprises will grow in size, creating ever greater problems of effluent disposal, this is a good moment to pause and take stock of the position. From the point of view of animal health and effluent disposal, smaller units in the centre of sufficient land to take the muck and provide a barrier to the spread of disease are a much more satisfactory procedure. A number of such units controlled by a single efficient organization could provide the size the industry requires yet remove the hazards. Any extra capital cost, especially in the provision of automated machinery for moving food and muck, might well be more than compensated for by the improved health and productivity of the animals, the reduced costs in disposing of the muck, and the benefit to the land on which it is spread.

It is to be regretted that with so many processes of effluent disposal the benefit of this product to the land is so often squandered, and that the muck, instead of being an asset, becomes an expensive liability. There seems a considerable need to be more ruthlessly economic about the matter.

Large quantities of muck, especially if held anaerobically at relatively low temperatures, may cause disease to man and animals. They also may create a serious nuisance by their smell. Gases evolved from them under certain circumstances may debilitate or even kill animals and man. These risks must be reduced and traditional methods of effluent disposal after mixing with solid matter of some description mostly do this. Where, however, such disposal methods cannot be utilized, then techniques for the aerobic treatment of slurry appear to be the most promising ones, especially from the health and nuisance angles. Lagooning with some prior sedimentation or removal of solids where the climate demands it can be done relatively cheaply and can render the products safe. There are also a large number of processes for mechanical aeration of slurry to make it a safe product for disposal but their costs can be high and much more research needs to be done before they can be universally recommended. Two masterly surveys of the whole subject of muck disposal have been provided by Robertson[3] and Merkel[4].

REFERENCES

1 Slurry Disposal (1969) *Veterinary Record Members' Supplement No. 31.*

2 Rankin, J. D. and Taylor, R. J. (1969) A study of some disease hazards which could be associated with the system of applying cattle slurry to pasture. *Vet. Rec.*, **85**, 578–581.

3 Robertson, A. M. (1977) *Farm Wastes Handbook*. Aberdeen. Scottish Farm Buildings Investigation Unit.

4 Merkel, J. A. (1981) *Managing Livestock Wastes*. Westpoint, Connecticut: A.V.I. Publishing Co.

10

Housing the Dairy Herd

The essential requirements for housing dairy cows are animal health and comfort, hygiene, efficient and economical use of labour, proper handling facilities and compliance with the statutory regulations for hygienic production of milk.

Economic milk production is possible under a fairly wide range of temperatures and other conditions but there are many factors which must be considered when a new layout or the modification of an existing one is planned. There are many sets of farm buildings in use which were erected when labour was cheap and plentiful and which catered for systems of farming influenced by tradition and customs. As husbandry methods have changed over the years new buildings have been erected and old ones converted. Today the buildings on a dairy farm must be considered as an integral part of a complete system of dairy cow management.

Because recent advances in husbandry have made it possible to keep more stock and also because of the need for more specialization, the present-day trend in milk production is towards larger units planned with the latest technical and scientific advances to provide a system which is economically sound, has regard for healthy stock and makes the most effective use of a limited labour force.

A smaller number of milk producers are obtaining levels of milk yield from large and medium-sized herds which would hitherto have been thought impossible. During the last twenty years many improvements have been made in parlour design and performance and indeed some types, such as the tandem and chute parlour, are practically obsolete.

When new layouts for milk production are planned, general considerations arise regarding siting in relation to other farm buildings and the best possible access. Essentials include a suitably sheltered site with services, an ample supply of pure water and electricity and facilities for drainage and dung or slurry disposal. Proximity to fodder storage, both bulk and concentrates, calf accommodation, good access for wheeled traffic and cows with movement routes which can be kept clean and preferably separate are all desirable design factors.[1]

The type of layout and system will be guided by the following considerations:

1 *Farm size and system of husbandry.* The chief enterprise on the large, mainly arable, farm with plenty of bulk feeds and bedding will probably require a completely different system from the small all-grass farm, where skill in

stockmanship to encourage high yields could be more important than labour economy.

2 *Soil and climate*. Areas of high rainfall and humidity need special consideration particularly in the requirements for animal health and soil management.

3 Size related to the potential of the farm and the possibility of extension or adaptability to other systems of husbandry if the need arises.

4 Availability and skill of management and labour.

5 Economy in construction, use and maintenance.

6 Limitations imposed due to difficulties of waste disposal.

7 The position and appearance in relation to the surrounding landscape.

SYSTEMS OF MILKING AND HOUSING

The increase in the size of herds has required new systems of milking and housing to suit these requirements and which, with larger numbers, has needed a different approach to health and welfare considerations.

There are three principal systems for milking and housing:

1 The cowhouse.
2 The milking parlour with or without loose housing.
3 The milking bail, which may be a portable unit or fixed on a permanent site.

With the cowhouse system cows are milked throughout the year in the cowhouse (also called cow shed, shippon, byre or mistal) and housed by night or by day and night during the winter months, when ground may be wet and liable to poaching. This method of milking and housing cows has been well suited to the small and medium-sized herd where an increase in cow numbers is unlikely and where individual attention is a primary consideration. With a carefully planned routine efficient use of labour at milking time is possible. The most serious disadvantages are that the building is limited to a fixed number of cows and extension may be difficult. Adaptations for other classes of stock can be expensive and not always satisfactory. The use of pipeline milking and mechanized dung handling has helped to reduce the manual effort but nevertheless it is a fast-disappearing system which is mainly confined to the smaller herd.

With systems of loose housing cows are kept in straw yards, cubicles or kennels throughout the winter months and taken to the parlour for milking. An installation can be planned in which the limits of performance are known and which can be matched to a given set of requirements. The layout should be designed to minimize the disadvantages amongst which can be health considerations, disposal of slurry from cubicle passages or collecting yards and the cost of litter in the case of strawed yards.

Providing that the layout is well designed and properly managed, cows have more freedom of movement and less physical effort is required by the stockman, milking being carried out in a compact unit in which the cow comes to the milker. The system is flexible and it can be possible to leave room for extension should the need arise.

The design, construction and operation of dairy buildings are the subject of various statutory requirements. Those affecting hygiene and construction are:

The Milk and Dairies (General) Regulations 1959 (in England and Wales).
The Model Dairy Byelaws 1961 (in Scotland).
The Milk Acts (Northern Ireland) 1950 and 1963.

In addition, some buildings may require Town and Country Planning approval and will need approval for Building Regulations. The appropriate water authority should be consulted to ensure that there is no risk of polluting water courses with effluent. Other regulations concern the health and welfare of stock and staff, the provisions for which are to be found in the Health and Safety at Work Act and in the Codes of Recommendations for the Welfare of Livestock.

THE COWHOUSE

As it is unlikely that many new cowhouses will be erected in this country owing to cost and lack of flexibility, it is not proposed to discuss the design in detail. There are, however, certain basic design features which have been found desirable and which may be relevant when considering the comfort of stock in other housing systems (Figs. 10.1 and 10.2).

The double-range shed with tail-to-tail arrangement is the design which allows for most mechanization in cleaning out, milking and feeding. Where the site allows, advantage can be taken of the natural fall of the ground for gravity handling of dung and feedstuffs.

The usual requirements for hygiene are an impervious non-slip floor, impervious and easily cleaned walls and other surfaces, ample light and ventilation and disposal of effluent to an approved point.

The length and width of the standings should be decided by the size of the cow; typical averages are a length of 1600 mm for a Friesian and 1300 mm for a Jersey. The former figure may need to be more generous where there is Holstein blood. The width allowed for a double standing (per pair of cows) is usually 2100 mm. Where they are too wide they permit a cow to turn diagonally and foul the standing.

Other matters requiring consideration are the type of stall divisions which may have to be specially fabricated, provision of drinking bowls and the construction of easily cleanable approaches and traffic routes. For those milk producers who are still using cowsheds there is scope for reducing the labour requirement. Often it is inefficient work methods and a badly planned routine

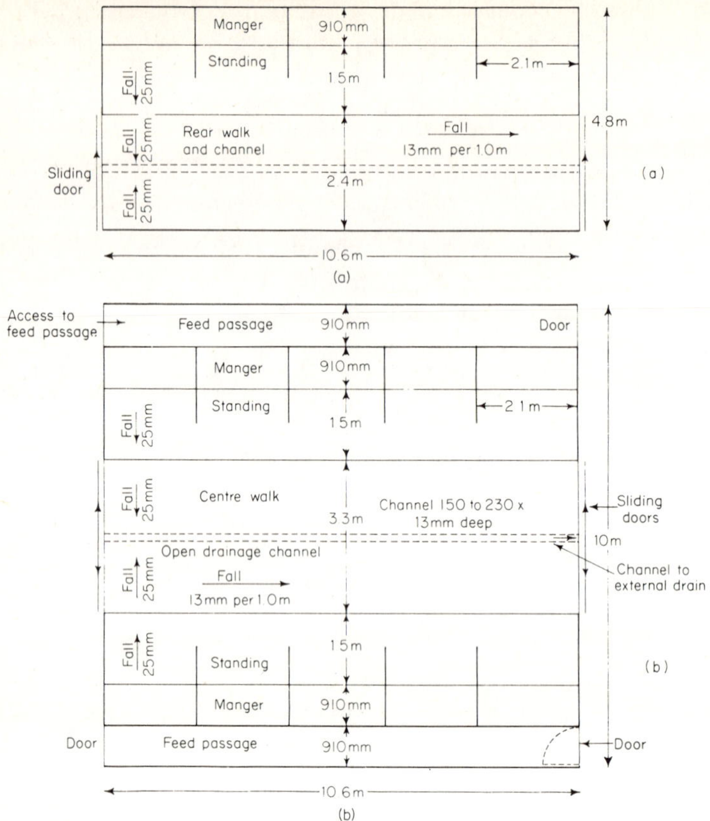

Fig. 10.1 (a) Typical dimensions for single-range cowshed without feed passage (10 ties). (b) Typical dimensions for double-range cowshed with central dung passage and channel with feed passages (20 ties).

that cause criticism of the cowshed system. The processes which have to be considered are:

1 Milking.
2 Cleaning out and washing down the shed.
3 Feeding.

Milking

Pipeline milking with milk conveyed direct to the dairy is the obvious choice. This system has become firmly established and fits in well with methods of economizing labour in milking, circulation cleaning of the plant and bulk collection of milk. Ideally, the pipeline should have a continuous fall from the point at which milk enters the pipeline to the milk room. Should the pipeline have an adverse fall or too many 'risers', the system may not milk cows efficiently and could cause taints in the milk.[3]

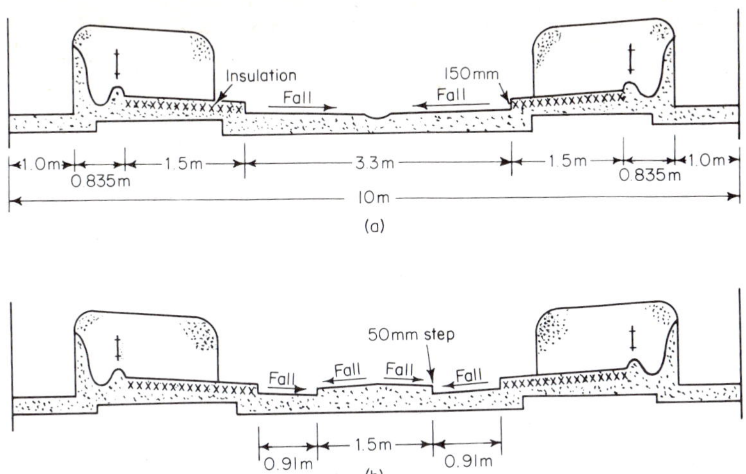

Fig. 10.2 Construction of floor section of double-range cowhouse showing alternative designs for the central passage: (a) central walk with central drainage channel suitable for cleaning with scraper blade; (b) 0.91 m gutters with 50 mm steps to 1.5 m wide centre walk.

Specially designed units are available which can be clamped to existing stalling so that a part of the cowshed can be used as a parlour during the summer months to avoid tying and untying cows and the movement of milking units and concentrate feed.

Cleaning out and washing down

With some types of floor section dung can be pushed out of the shed with a tractor-mounted scraper blade and then loaded into a spreader on a concrete area outside the shed with a fore-end loader or, where levels allow, pushed straight into a pit or onto a dung spreader.

Gutters can be cleaned out and trailers loaded with mechanical gutter scrapers.[4]

For washing down, pressure hoses are excellent but entail more expense. Bucketing from tanks is generally quicker and more effective than hoses on low pressure.

Feeding

Saving labour in feeding depends mainly on careful positioning of stored fodder, selecting the shortest possible transport routes to the cowhouse and using the most suitable type of transport.

THE MILKING PARLOUR

The milking parlour has developed over the last 50 years through various shapes and designs. Initially, hygienic requirements were considered more important than labour-saving. Little progress in developing the parlour as a completely integrated system of milking, housing and feeding was made until much more recently. Initially, many disappointing layouts were constructed. From this 'trial-and-error' approach, and as a result of investigational work and fundamental research, the essential data are now available for planning a complete system.

Units which will be required are:

1. The milking unit, which will consist of a milking parlour, a milk room, a power room, a holding box for cows which have to be segregated for individual attention, and a store or storage space for concentrated feedstuffs.
2. The cow housing unit, covered yards either strawed or with cubicle accommodation or purpose-built cubicle sheds, together with a feeding area and storage space for bulk feedstuffs.
3. Collecting and dispersal areas at the entrance to and exit from the parlour, which may be a part of the cow-housing unit provided that it is not connected in such a manner as to cause contamination to the approaches to the parlour.
4. Segregation and accommodation of cows for calving, veterinary attention and isolation. A crush and race incorporating a foot-bath are essential for most larger herds. Housing for calves and other young stock as well as facilities for handling and/or storage of slurry may also be required.

The parlour is a specialist milking shed in which the arrangement of the stalling, for milking batches of two or more cows at a time can be designed to suit various systems of herd management.

Parlour selection[5,6]

Stalling can be designed in various ways and several different shapes are available. Some of these – the tandem and chute – have become obsolete because of design limitations which slow down cow entry and exit, and cause more fatigue to the operator due to distances walked and the operation of gates. Other designs have failed because of frequent breakdown of working parts – e.g. some of the rotaries.

Parlours are equipped with a milking unit to each stall or two stalls may share a unit. Some designs – the rotary, trigon or polygon parlours – have one unit to each stall whereas the abreast or herringbone parlours offer a choice of one unit to each stall or one unit shared between two stalls. It is usual for the cows to be milked on a raised platform or the operator to work in a pit to eliminate stooping.

Within these basic designs a parlour can be selected suited to the number of cows to be milked, the labour available and the system of herd management adopted. Where possible room should be left for expansion and adaptation for automation if this is not installed initially. Capital cost in relation to herd management and labour requirements must also receive careful consideration to ensure value for money.

Some of the management factors which will affect parlour selection are:

1 Herd size and calving policy.
2 Yield produced per milking at peak yield.
3 Time allocated for milking.
4 Concentrate feeding policy.
5 Operations to be included in the work routine.
6 Number of operators.
7 The degree of automation in the installation.

The rate of removal of milk from the cow will depend on yield level, the size of the teat orifice and the correct stimulation of the milk ejection mechanisms. The design of the milking machine – vacuum level, pulsation rate and ratio and the type of lines – will also affect the rate of milk extraction.

The number of units required to milk a herd of a given size will depend on yield level, number of operators and the time allocated for milking. There are certain jobs which are an essential part of the milking routine and the time taken by the operator to carry out these tasks, some of which can be successfully automated, will determine how many units can be effectively handled. This time, known as the work routine time (WRT), is taken up by letting the cow (or cows) into the parlour, feeding, washing and drying the udder, fore-milking, applying and removing the units, disinfecting the teats and letting out the cow (or a batch of cows in some parlours), together with a notional time allowed for contingencies. The ideal WRT will be minimum time required for all the operations associated with the routine to be carried out effectively. Parts of this routine can be automated or mechanized which will result in a shorter WRT and allow the operator to milk more cows if the units are available. An example of a one-minute WRT is shown in Table 10.1.

Operations in the routine which can be automated or mechanized are cow entry and exit doors, gates or barriers, dispensing concentrates, removal of clusters (automatic cluster removers – ACRs) teat disinfection and milk recording.

In order to achieve the WRTs shown in Table 10.1 certain elements in the management of the herd are essential. Some of the component jobs which make up the WRT may be optional but others are considered essential on the grounds of hygiene and to satisfy milk regulations. If cows come into the parlour in a dirty condition udder washing will take longer and may be less effective; systems of housing designed to keep cows clean and to prevent them walking through excessive mud will reduce the time spent in udder washing. Collecting yards

Table 10.1

Operations in work routine	Mins/cow
Let in cow and feed	0.20
Fore milk	0.10
Wash and dry udder	0.23
Attach cluster	0.15
Remove cluster	0.10
Disinfect teats (dip or spray)	0.07
Let out cow	0.10
Miscellaneous (contingencies)	0.05
Total man minutes/cow	1.00
Cows milked/man hour	60

must be designed so that no time is wasted in waiting for cows to enter the parlour. Batch-handling of cows entering and leaving the parlour will also speed up the routine.

As a high throughput of cows requires close concentration it is desirable that the operator should aim to complete milking in $1\frac{1}{2}$–$1\frac{3}{4}$ hours, although with parlours where less physical effort is required through automation and working conditions are more congenial, this time can be exceeded.

Where concentrate feeds are fed in the parlour the amount which a cow can eat will be decided by the following considerations:

1. The time which the cow will have available for feeding.
2. The shape and height of the feed trough.
3. The type of material which is to be fed.

Although there are likely to be wide variations, probable rates of consumption of different types of feedstuff are likely to be:

Type of feed	*kg/min*
Meal	0.25–0.33
Cubes 10 mm diam.	0.34–0.50

More flexibility with concentrate rationing can be obtained where out-of-parlour dispensers are available. However, feeding some concentrates in the parlour will help to speed up cow entry.

The concentrate feeding policy and the anticipated average daily yield will determine, where there is a choice, whether the parlour chosen will be provided with one unit to each stall or one unit to two stalls. The latter will allow longer for a cow to eat her concentrate ration.

TYPES OF PARLOUR

Installations currently available are:

The abreast parlour
The herringbone parlour
The trigon and polygon parlour
Various rotary parlours.

Within these different types a design having various numbers of stalls and milking units can be found to suit most herd sizes and systems of management.

The abreast parlour

This is one of the earliest types of parlour and for the operator used to bucket milking it represented the least change in routine. (See Figs 10.3 and 10.4.) Cows are arranged in stalling in line abreast with a feed hopper between each pair of stalls. It consists of three areas: the work area behind the stalls which also forms the entrance to the stalls; the stalls; and the exit walk. The cows standing can be at the same level as the operator but it is more usual for it to be raised on a step 400–450 mm above the operator's floor level. Most abreast parlours consist of a single line of stalls, although there are variations. They can be arranged back-to-back with a central work area, in an L shape, or a circular design. Cows have to cross the work area to reach the stalls, and this may be considered an objection. It does however provide the operator with an opportunity to inspect the cows more closely.

The abreast parlour remains popular for the small and medium-sized herd. Advantages claimed are the ability to deal with cows individually, easy conversion of existing buildings, and in some cases extension if required. Furthermore, cost of installation is likely to be less than other two level parlours. However, because cows are not dealt with in batches, the operator is involved in more physical effort, thus extending the time of milking. More bending is required than a full two-level parlour.

Stalling varies in size according to make so that exact dimensions cannot be given. In practice there are standards which can be used for calculating the size of a parlour. The width is 4.88 m and the length will be adjusted to the number of stalls required (usually 2.13 m centres per pair of stalls, including feed hopper). If it is essential to install a parlour in a narrow building care must be taken to avoid cows turning at right angles. Sharp turns increase the risk of cows slipping and damaging themselves. The building should never be less than 4.57 m wide. Typical dimensions are:

Exit walk	910–990 mm
Stalls	2130 mm
Work area	2130 mm
Total	5180–5250 mm

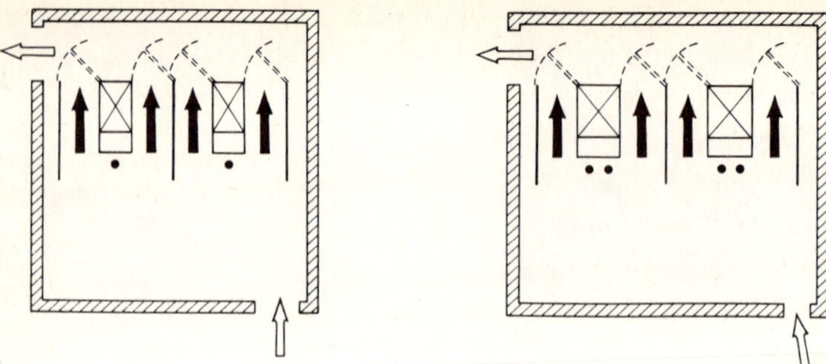

Fig. 10.3 Abreast parlour layouts. Left: four-stall abreast with two milking points. Right: four-stall abreast (wide centre sections) with four milking points.

Width. Each pair of stalls including feed hopper, 2130 mm per pair; one unit/one stall (two recorder jars), 2500 mm per pair; squeeze gap, 380 mm.

Where buildings are being adapted a side exit passage may be necessary; however if possible, this arrangement should be avoided.

Space must also be allowed where applicable for sliding doors and gear, and care given to the positioning of piers. The exit walk will have a width of 910–990 mm according to breed which will allow a cow room to walk without being able to turn around. The squeeze gap should be placed at the end furthest

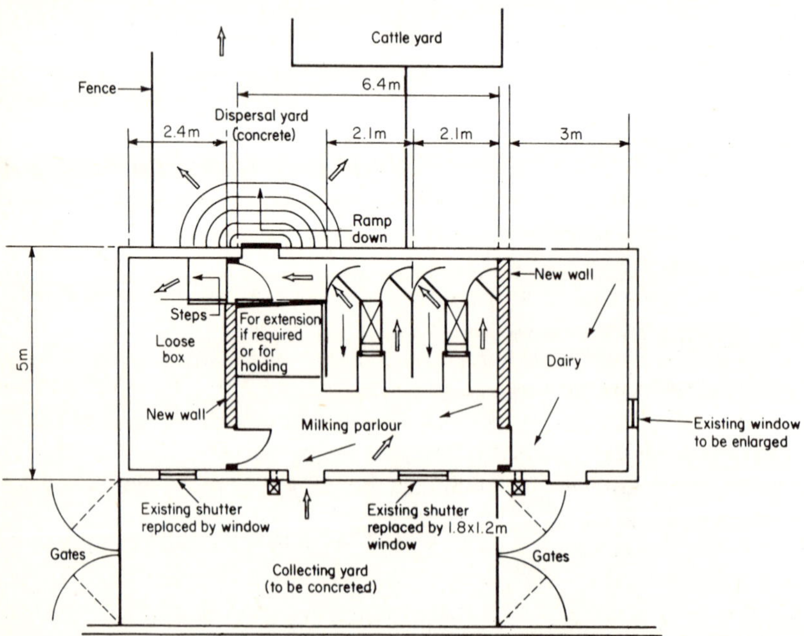

Fig. 10.4 Showing a two-level abreast parlour as it might be fitted to an existing cowshed.

from the exit door which will give the operator access to the exit walk when required to hustle a stubborn cow out of the building.

General points of construction, siting and ancillary buildings affecting all types of parlour will be discussed later. There are, however, some points peculiar to the abreast parlour in the construction of the floor section. As already indicated the whole floor may be at the same level as the operator, or the area of the standing and exit walk can be raised 400–450 mm above the level of the work area. A step of about 450 mm will be about the maximum that a cow with a pendulous udder can negotiate. This does not provide a full two-level parlour so that the operator will be in a semi-stooping position at times during milking. Provision of two steps to raise the cow higher is not satisfactory because the projecting step can be a hazard to the operator. A shallow pit in the work area is sometimes constructed but this can present drainage and cleaning problems. As it is impracticable to obtain full two-level working some degree of stooping with the raised standing will be unavoidable. A cutaway section is constructed between each pair of cows to provide working room alongside the cows which is facilitated by leaving toe-recesses under each standing.

An even fall of approximately 1 : 60 should be given to the whole floor and effluent discharged to a drain outside the building.

A loft or purpose-made bin in the roof space of the parlour can be used for the storage of concentrates, or separate storage can be provided outside the parlour and feed conveyed by auger to the hoppers in the parlour. Some degree of automation is possible with many abreast parlours to improve throughput. Most frequently the number of units is doubled up where space allows and automatic cluster removers installed. Where yields are high there may not be sufficient time to eat all concentrates in the parlour. Use of out-of-parlour feeders can overcome this problem. In some cases there may be room to extend the number of stalls.

It can often be difficult to justify mechanization and automation on economic grounds alone. Reducing stress on the operator, and indirectly on the cow, may however by fully rewarded.

The herringbone parlour[8,9,10]

The herringbone parlour is a high-performance, batch, full two-level parlour in which one man can handle five or more units successfully; it also lends itself to the installation of mechanical and automated devices. Design is such that cows are arranged for milking in echelon and the operator's work area is reduced to the minimum for the amount of units to be handled.

The use of herringbone parlours has been established in Australia and New Zealand for many years where it suits their systems of management using little or no concentrate. In the U.K. initially feeding concentrates presented problems. Once satisfactory mechanical systems were developed the potential advantages of this type of parlour could be realized.

Recently three (or more)-sided herringbones, the trigon and polygon have been introduced. The potential of this type of parlour for milking large numbers of cows with little labour was recognized by manufacturers and research and advisory organizations. The results of their research and investigational work have suggested optimum design factors, routines and limits of performance. It also provides a set sequence of operations which can be carried out in a compact area.

Where the batches of cows are placed in parallel lines the parlour can be provided with one unit to each stall or one unit to two stalls and recorder jars where used placed at high, eye or low level. Polygons and trigons will have one unit to each stall.

Internal design (herringbone with cows standing in parallel races)

The floor section of the parlour consists of two areas – the cows' standings and the operator's pit. The cows occupy a high-level area which can be constructed either as a solid concrete floor with a concrete or metal kerb, or it may be all metal or concrete with an overlapping metal chequer plate where the milking unit is low-line. Some floors incorporate a drainage channel covered with a removable metal grid constructed flush with the concrete section of the floor. This type of floor section is designed to reduce dung splashes and keep the floor cleaner at milking time, but it may complicate washing down.

Cows usually stand at an angle of 30–35° to the pit and approximate dimensions, depending on the angle of the cows, will be 1650 mm for the solid concrete floor with a concrete kerb, and 1600 mm for a concrete and chequer-plate floor using low-level jars.

In low-line parlours little or no fall is required for the pipeline. Longitudinal fall on the floor of the standings and pit will be made by constructing channels alongside the walls. The operator's pit can be excavated below ground level where disposal of effluent allows, or the high-level area can be built with the pit at ground level. Three factors will determine which will be the most convenient and least expensive: the situation of the milk room, drainage disposal arrangements, and site levels. Ramps should never be used. Where levels make it essential, steps may have to be used. Wherever possible though, it is desirable for the cows to enter the parlour at the same level as the collecting yard.

Stalling can be suspended from the roof or ceiling, supported from the floor, or it can be a free-standing unit independent of walls and ceiling and can be in round section or rectangular hollow steel tube.

The stalls and managers can be arranged so that the mangers and front rail are straight and the rump rail angled or zigzag, or straight rump rails are used with mangers either straight or angled. The dimensions and shape of the manger are important. It should be positioned so that cows are eating at about grazing height, roughly 150 mm above standing level. V- or U-shaped slots allow cows to place their heads at the right height of the manger. With correct design there is less poaching of feed and feed wastage and cows can eat more comfortably and quickly. Mangers can be built of brick or blockwork, suitably rendered but are usually fabricated from steel or glass fibre. Drainage holes make cleaning easier.

The pit will usually be 1370–1530 mm wide depending on the position of the recorder jars. If they are at eye level the width should be increased; a width of 1800 mm is desirable. Depth of the pit should be about 760–910 mm. Toe-in spaces of 75–150 mm should be allowed and recesses left in the pit walls make useful shelves. The Milk and Dairies Regulations (England and Wales) allow a trapped drain to be placed in the pit and the fall on the pit floor should match that of the floor or drainage channels of the high level area. Where levels present a problem it may be necessary to discharge drainage through a trapped gulley to an airtight sump provided with a float operated pump to discharge effluent to the high level drains. This arrangement, known as 'sump and pump', should be avoided unless there is no alternative. High level drains should be placed outside the parlour (Fig. 10.5).

Other requirements for the pit are access to the milk room and collecting yard and, where possible, windows in walls or doors giving on these areas are advisable.

Typical dimensions of the floor section are:

Width of high level area including manger)	1370–1850 mm
Width of pit	1370 mm (average)
Depth of pit	760–910 mm
Length of parlour (depending on cross passages)	910 mm/stall + 1060 mm

Entrance and exit passages may be added if required.

As it was often found that these dimensions allowed too much or too little room for some cows, a panel set up by MAFF suggested variations for different breeds of cows, i.e. Friesians, Ayrshires and Jerseys.[10]

Concentrates can be stored in a full-width loft, a purpose-made split loft or a free-standing bin outside the parlour. The two latter allow for a lighter and more pleasant parlour in which to work.

Carefully designed entry and exit arrangements will assist the smooth working of the parlour. Cows should preferably be channelled to come straight into the parlour without having to turn at right angles. Collecting should be at the same level as the high-level area of the parlour. It is usual to allow an area of 1.2–1.4 m^2 per cow for collection so that cows are packed tightly into the yard when milking starts. The shape of the collecting yard should be either circular or rectangular. Access to the yard should be at the end furthest from the parlour entrance and may be provided with backing gates. It is important to protect cows waiting to enter the parlour from draughts which can be a predisposing cause of chills and mastitic conditions. Cows can leave the parlour through doors directly ahead or, if turning to the left or right, a separate exit passage will be required. Circular collecting yards can also be used for dispersal.

Provision is necessary for segregating cows for A.I. or veterinary attention.

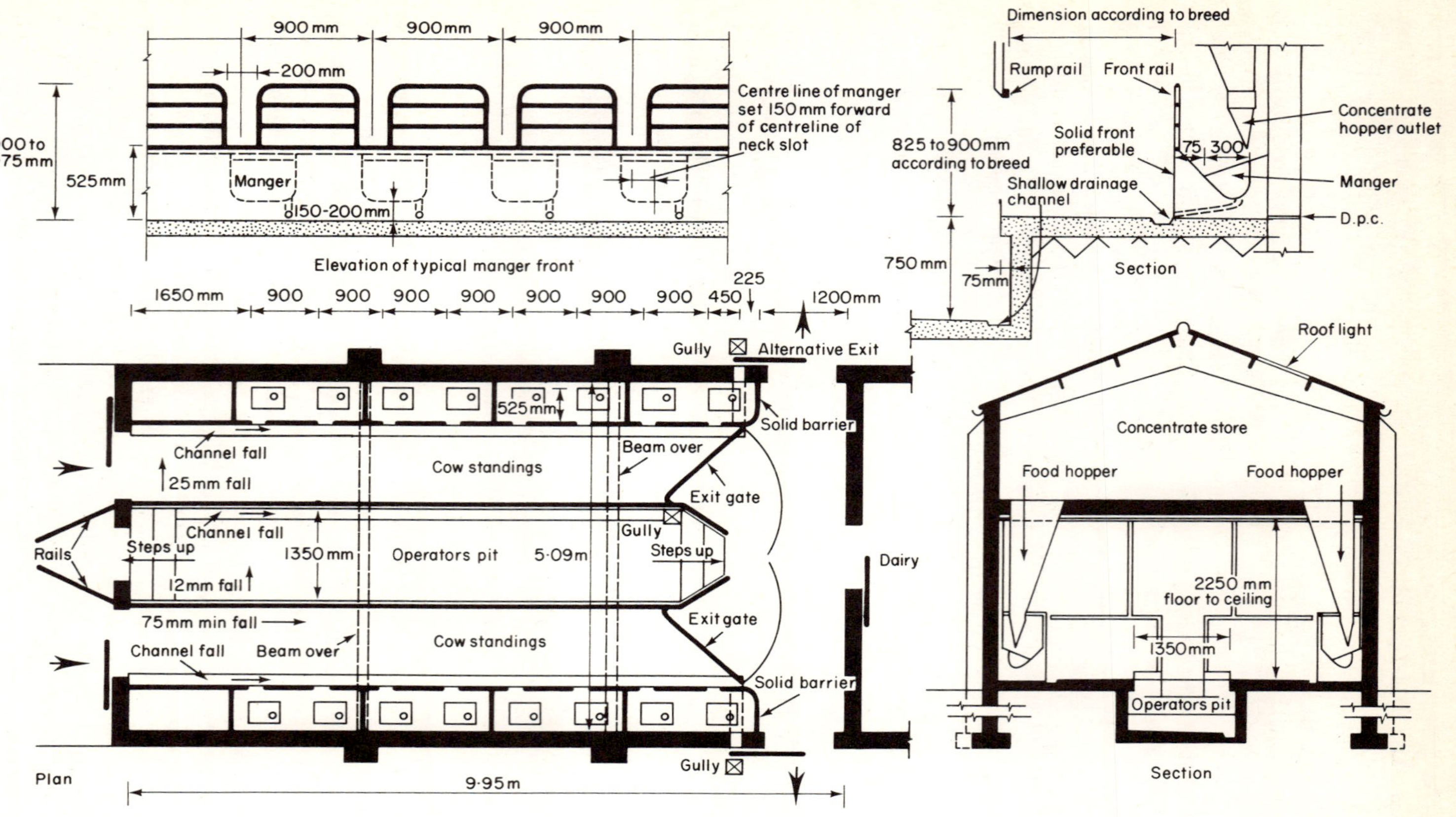

Fig. 10.5 Milking parlour, herringbone type, sixteen standings, eight points.

Trigon and polygon parlours

These are batch parlours developed from the herringbone, the trigon being suitable for herds of from 150–300 cows and the polygon designed for still larger herds. At present it has only a very limited application. Cows are positioned in three triangular races in the trigon around the pit, the size according to the number of stalls required. The polygon consists of four races arranged in a diamond shape. Both of these parlours are restricted to one unit to each stall.

The layout is shown in diagramatic form in Fig. 10.6 (a–c) together with entry and exit arrangements. Some side passages may be needed but these need not be required in the modified version. Side passages could hold up the smooth flow of cows into and out of the parlour and possibly disrupt the milking routine.

General design requirements and stallwork are similar to a conventional herringbone parlour. A larger building will be required and extension may not be possible unless provision is made for this at design stage. It is a parlour which can provide congenial working conditions for the operator in a well-lit and uncluttered work area.

The rotary parlour

Various layouts for rotary parlours were fully described in the previous edition of this book. This drew attention to the success of many layouts but emphasized that there were disappointments in the high cost of maintenance and the smooth operation of many parlours of this design. We suggested then that 'it would be difficult, if not impossible, to predict the future of this type of parlour'. Many of the initial problems of management have now been overcome but it would be impossible to speculate on whether there might be a revival of interest in this design of parlour (Figs. 10.7 and 10.8).

Details of parlour construction

Walls

The parlour may be constructed of traditional materials such as brick or blockwork or it may be prefabricated in either concrete panels, metal sheets, wood or a combination of these. Prefabricated types have the advantages of easy erection and greater flexibility. The internal finish of the walls with a smooth and impervious surface is not only a requirement of the regulations but will also be an important factor in labour economy in keeping the walls clean and help in the general cleanliness of the premises. Ledges and crevices encourage dust and dirt to accumulate so that, if possible, they should be avoided: wall-to-floor junctions should be coved to facilitate brushing and hosing down. Whatever wall finish is chosen, it will have to withstand really hard wear. An impervious finish can be given by cement rendering which can subsequently be treated with one of a range of paints which are suitable for providing a hard and longlasting surface which can be hosed down. Suitable paints are chlorinated

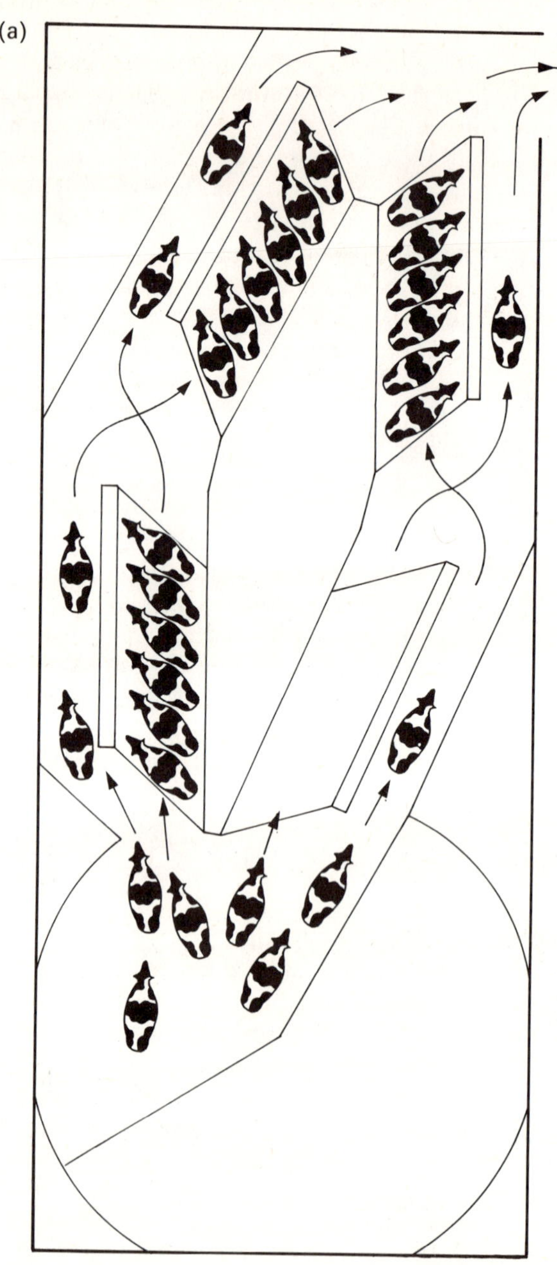

Fig. 10.6 (a) The polygon; (b) The trigon; (c) The modified trigon.

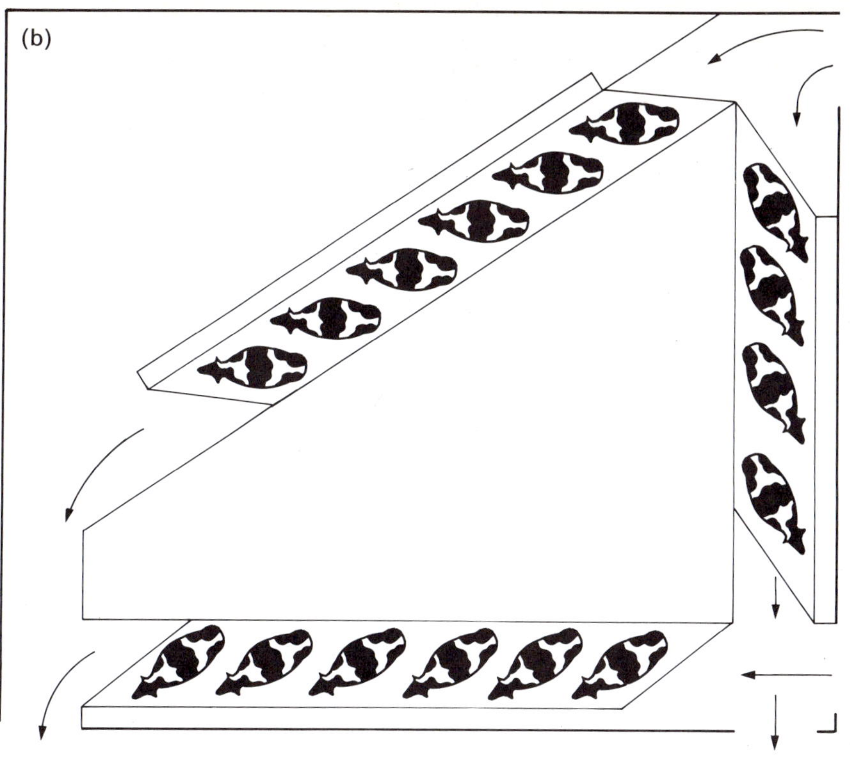
(b)

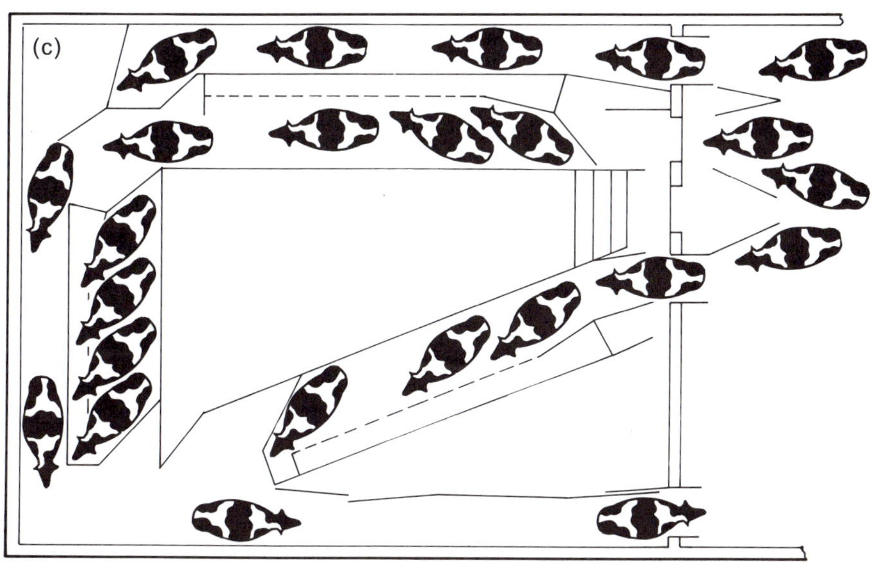
(c)

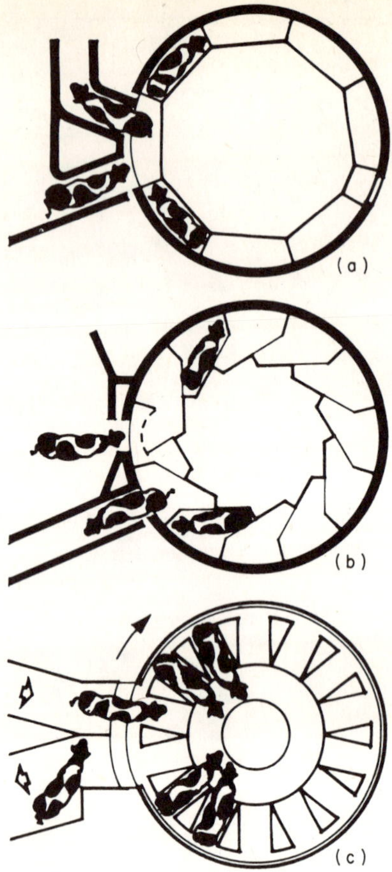

Fig. 10.7 Types of rotary parlour. (a) Tandem: cows stand nose to tail around the platform while the operator works inside the circle. (b) Herringbone: cows stand in echelon around the platform, heads towards the outside while the operator works inside the circle. (c) Abreast: cows face radially inwards, the operator working on the outside of the circle.

rubber, epoxy resin paints or light-coloured bitumastic. To avoid disappointing results the paint must be applied to properly prepared dry walls.

Glazed blocks which can be purchased in a variety of colours provide an attractive, easily cleaned and durable finish but will be higher in initial cost. Other materials available are tiles which must be well fixed and of good quality, Terrazo marble-chip rendering and plastic sheeting. Pit walls can be lined with stainless steel sheeting which is not unduly expensive and easily cleaned.[11,12]

Roofs

The roof will usually be clad with corrugated asbestos or metal sheeting. In order to keep the internal temperature more uniform throughout the year, the underside of the roof covering can be insulated. Where concentrates are stored in the loft, it should be sealed with damp-resistant (i.e. oil-tempered) hardboard, flat asbestos sheets and other suitable building boards available.

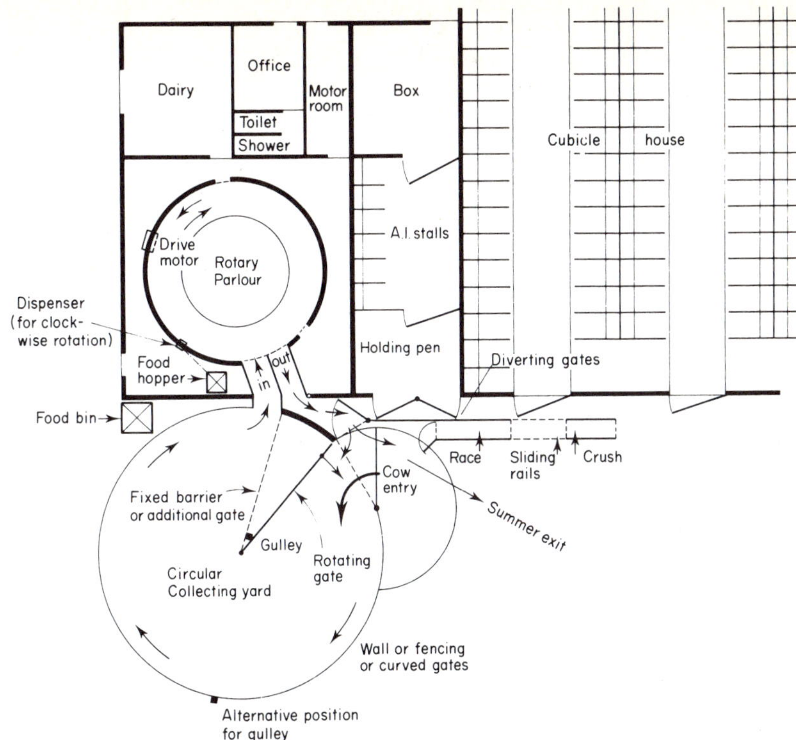

Fig. 10.8 Layout for rotary parlour.

Stallwork

This is usually constructed from tubular or box section steel rails with a galvanized or flat finish. Often too little attention is given to the cleanliness and maintenance of the stallwork and thus can lead to expansive replacements.

It is important to ensure that the earthing of the electrical installation is fully effective. Cases have been recorded where through faulty earthing cows have received electrical shocks through the stallwork which adversely affects behaviour and production. It has also been suggested that this could be linked to increased levels of mastitis.[13,14,15]

Light and ventilation[16]

This does not usually present much of a problem in an abreast parlour where it is usually possible to use windows for both, even where there is a full loft for the storage of concentrates. Windows are also desirable to enable the operator to see the cows waiting in the collecting yard. With many herringbone parlours the cake loft can be constructed in two sections, leaving an area between from which roof lighting can be obtained. It is desirable to provide an area of window or roof light at the rate of 10 per cent of the floor area of the building.

As much of the work will have to be carried out during the hours of darkness adequate artificial lighting will be needed. The aim will be to eliminate shadows as much as possible and to keep glare to a minimum to provide pleasant working conditions and as an aid to a generally high standard of hygiene. Fluorescent fittings are most suitable and in the herringbone parlour are usually concentrated over the pit. The recommended minimum illumination is 200 lux. Lights outside the parlour doors will help speed up entry of cows into the building.

All electrical fittings should be installed and maintained by a competent electrical contractor and should meet the requirements of the Regulations for Electrical Installations.

Floors

The floor should be: durable, impervious, resistant to chemicals and urine, non-slip, easily cleaned, and laid to falls for effective effluent disposal.

The most commonly used material for flooring is concrete although it has already been shown that some herringbone parlour floors are all or part metal; the pit floors are often finished with quarry tiles which give an attractive, hard-wearing and non-slip finish.

The surface given to the parlour floor is important because if it is too rough or slippery it can cause accidents to livestock or operators, foot problems with the cows and difficulties with cleaning. A non-slip finish can be provided by sprinkling carborundum onto the nearly completed floor at the rate of 1 kg/m^2.

Floors should be laid to falls, 1:50 being the usually accepted figure, to discharge effluent to drains outside the building. A properly trapped gulley is permitted in a herringbone pit floor. In general, the high level in a herringbone parlour should have a uniform fall with the pit but in the case of low jar parlours advice should be sought from the suppliers of the milking equipment.

Two factors which may need consideration are the repair or retexturing of concrete which is breaking up or has worn smooth through years of tractor scraping and other wear. Yards in this state can make cows nervous and form a hazard to operators and livestock, as well as causing foot problems. There is often only a short time in which to carry out the treatment or repair between milkings.

Information on methods of dealing with slippery floors is given in Chapter 2.

Repair of small areas of concrete is rarely successful because it is usually difficult to obtain a good key between the old and new work. Therefore re-laying is the most satisfactory method. However, in some cases the use of products based on fairly quick drying mortars or epoxy resins may be justified.[17]

Collecting and dispersal

This aspect needs careful planning as clumsy circulation arrangements can spoil a layout which is excellent in other respects.[18] Cows coming up quickly to the parlour entrance will help to maintain a good throughput of cows. Fundamentals of design which should be considered are:

1 Whatever the shape of the collecting yard, either rectangular or circular, allow 1.4 m^2 per cow collecting space.
2 Full protection from draughts is essential and overhead cover may be considered desirable despite extra expense.
3 The entrance gate to the collecting yard should be placed so that when cows are driven in, they are facing the parlour entrance. This means that usually the entrance gate will be at a point furthest from the parlour entrance.
4 Rectangular collecting yards should be long and narrow so that cows are funnelled to the parlour entrance.
5 Circular yards have the advantage that backing gates are easy to install and enable batches of cows to be dealt with separately if required. The backing gate, either manually or mechanically operated, can be moved up behind the cows to keep them up to the parlour entrance (Fig. 10.9).
6 Cleaning the yard is important. If not regularly cleaned slurry may be carried into the parlour on cows' feet. It may be scraped mechanically or by hand: hand-scraping is more usual for circular yards. Dirty yards and cubicle passages predispose cows to foot trouble.
7 It is desirable that cows enter the parlour at the correct level. If this is impossible then steps are preferable to a ramp. Steps having a length tread of 900–1500 mm with a rise of 150–225 mm are suitable; for ramps a width of 900 mm is suitable. Dirty ramps get slippery so that it is important to keep them clean.
8 Table 10.2 gives sizes for circular collecting yards. The radius of the circle will be as for the length of the backing gate, which can be obtained in lengths up to 9 m. In order to keep the cows moving up to the parlour door some form of backing device may be used. With a circular collecting yard a backing gate can be moved mechanically by a weight operating through a series of pulleys, by a motorized wheel, by winding a cable in the parlour or by water pressure which gradually moves the gate behind the cows. Some gates are fitted with a heel rail which will help to move them up steadily.

Table 10.2 *Size of Circular Yards*

Radius of circle (m)	No. of Cows in a $\frac{1}{2}$ circle	No. of Cows in a $\frac{3}{4}$ circle
4.9	30	47
5.5	40	60
6.0	50	75
6.7	60	90
7.3	70	110
7.9	85	130
8.5	100	155

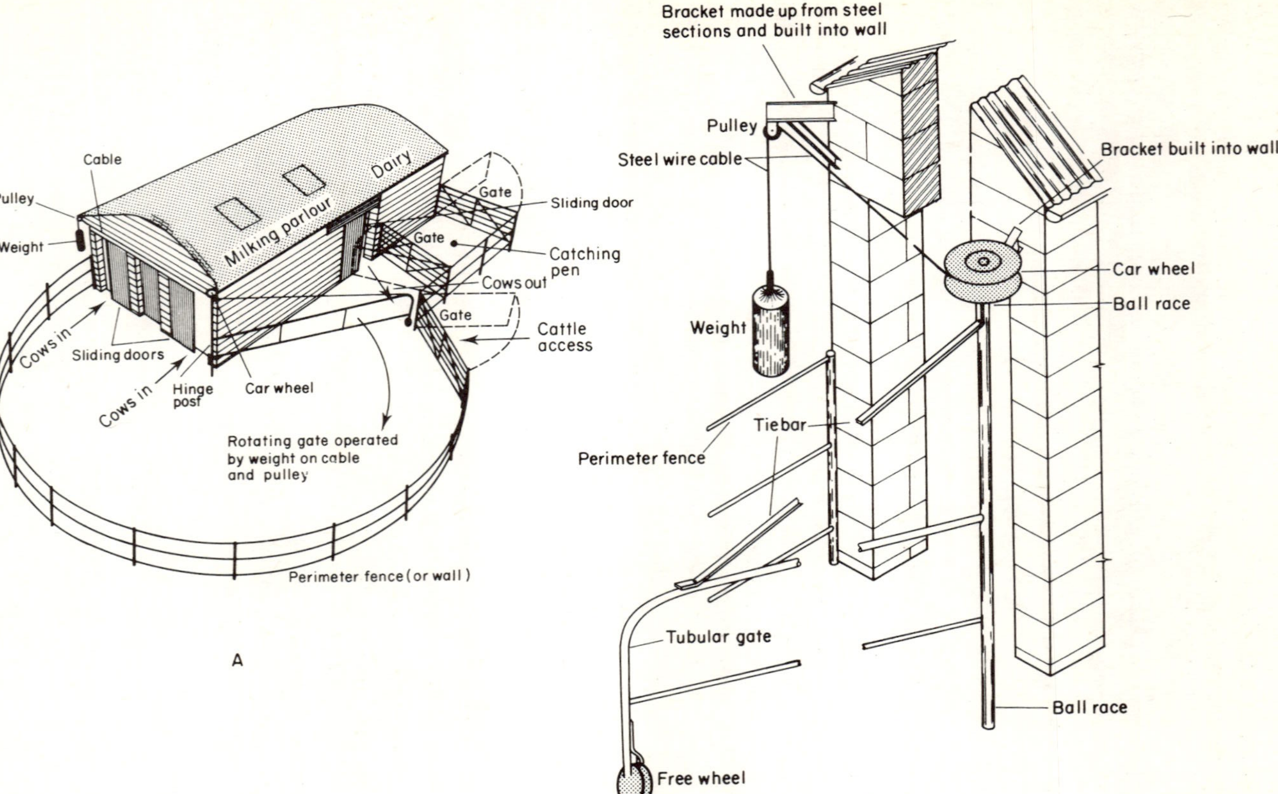

Fig. 10.9 Collecting yards, cattle control methods: (a) perspective view of circular collecting yard; (b) details of gate and operating mechanism.

With rectangular yards either a gate or wire can be used as a backing device which can be pulled up from the parlour pit. Electrifying wires to move cows up should not be necessary and are not desirable as they are liable to cause stress and nervousness among the cows. The speedy entry of cows into the parlour is likely to be controlled more by the person in the pit and the feeding policy than by the use of mechanical devices.[19]

Correct falls on the yard will make the scraping of slurry easier; in practice, where there are no site limitations, a fall of 1 : 30 is recommended and this should be away from the parlour. Sufficient drains must be provided, positioned clear of scraping routes. In a circular yard a drainage channel round the outside of the perimeter fence is most suitable.

Doorways

The following doorways must be planned for:

1 Entrance(s) for the cows from the collecting yard.
2 Exit to the dispersal area for the summer, to the bedded area in the winter or to a holding pen or box (for cows which require attention or observation), the doors being controlled from the parlour pit or work area. Exit passages which encourage cows to hang about should be avoided if possible.
3 Access from the parlour to the dairy.
4 Access to the dispersal and collecting areas from the parlour pit, where applicable.

After settling the correct positioning of doors, their width and operation must be considered. The following constructional details are recommended:

1 A suitable width for the entrance door would be 825–975 mm.
2 All corners at the entrance to be rounded to minimize damage to cows.
3 Strongly constructed doors, hung outside and sliding.
4 Self-closing sliders to be hung on an inclined track raised by at least 75 mm at one end. Weights can be used to close the door more quickly.
5 Rollers to be used instead of a bottom rail or groove of the sliding gear (less likelihood of freezing or other blockage). Rubber door-stops recommended.
6 A system of nylon ropes and pulleys to enable the doors to be opened and closed from the pit.
7 Well-lit entrances during the hours of darkness.

Water supply (see also Chapter 8)

For dairying a suitable and sufficient supply of water with adequate pressure for all purposes is required. It is essential to place sufficient taps in both milk room and parlour situated to reduce walking to the minimum; pipes should be lagged against frost damage.[20]

As gadgetry and electrics increase in parlours, keeping them clean and washing down needs more careful consideration. Most properly constructed building surfaces will withstand pressure washing but great care is needed with the electrics and components connected with feeding systems and the milking installation. Successful and effective cleaning with pressure hoses requires a careful balance between the volume and the pressure of the water used.[21]

Ancillary accommodation

Storage of concentrate foods

Usually all or some concentrate feeding is carried out in the parlour, as cows will come there more readily and rationing is made easier. Some supplementary concentrate may also be fed in the area outside the parlour or in purpose made cow activated out-of-parlour feeders in a convenient situation. Storage space and servicing facilities should therefore be provided as near as possible to where the cows are fed and in an accessible place for bulk delivery transport. The store can be provided by:

1 A room adjoining the parlour at the same level.
2 A loft over the parlour with chutes from self-emptying bins to fill feed hoppers.
3 Bulk storage bins above the stallwork in the parlour.
4 A single bulk storage bin outside the parlour to service smaller hoppers placed by each stall.

Concentrate feeds will usually be delivered in bulk and the delivery vehicle must be able to service the bins at any time; as it may be during milking time it should be possible to fill them without having to enter the collecting yard. Gravity filling of hoppers from bins does not usually present many problems although bridging of cubes can occur under some conditions. Mechanical filling by auger or chain and flight conveyor from a bulk store or bin is often the preferred method. The bulk bin may be more accessible for servicing and without a loft or storage bins over the parlour it provides a better environment for the operators.

The diversion box

Provision should be made for the separation of cows requiring A.I., veterinary attention or segregation for any other reason. This is most conveniently placed at the parlour exit, the door to the box or drafting gate being operated from the parlour pit or work area.

The milk room

The requirements for this will be discussed later in detail but there are some important points in parlour layout:

1 The milk room should directly adjoin the parlour with access from the pit or work area.
2 There should be good access and turning space if required for the bulk

tanker and where possible it is preferable that the tanker does not have to cross routes used by the cows for reasons of general hygiene and disease control.

Automation and mechanization

When the workforce is plentiful and moderately waged there is little incentive to mechanize or automate labour-intensive work. It is not until recently that attention has been given to the milking routine in larger herds to make capital investment on automation realistic. That is not to suggest that all investment on labour-saving can be justified and may not be so unless savings in time and effort and an increase in productivity are forthcoming. In the parlour it can enable the operator to utilize more units if they are available and to devote more time to other tasks in the routine which cannot be automated. Tasks in the routine which can be automated or mechanized:

1 Recognition of cows as they enter the parlour.
2 Operation of entry and exit gates or barriers.
3 Easy and accurate dispensing of concentrates.
4 Automatic cluster removal (ACRs) and recording milk yields.
5 Disinfection of teats.

The immediate and easy *recognition of cows entering the parlour* is essential to avoid any delays in dispensing rations and also as a means of identification for relief milkers. These marks may be needed for recognition from the front or rear or on one or both sides of the cows depending on the type of parlour being used. The Code of Recommendations for the Welfare of Livestock, Code No. 1 Cattle, recommends that the marking of cattle for identification should be done with care by competent operators so as to avoid unnecessary pain or distress to the animals.[22] The choice is between plastic or metal ear discs or studs and leg or tail bands embossed with numbers. Freeze branding is satisfactory and permanent and black dye is effective on white hair. Another permanent method is tattooing the udder.[23] There are also fully automated methods of recognition specifically for dispensing concentrate feedstuffs in or outside the parlour.

Cow entry and exit gates or barriers can be opened or closed by vacuum-operated rams.

Where it is decided to feed cows in the parlour, the *ease and accuracy of dispensing concentrates* is important. The choice of whether or not to feed concentrates in the parlour should be guided by the type of ration to be fed (nuts can be eaten more quickly than meal) and the speed of throughput expected from the parlour. Grouping of cows, provision of yard yokes, complete diet feeding or cow-activated out-of-parlour dispensers could be considered for avoiding feeding concentrates in the parlour altogether or for feeding reduced amounts.

Most dispensers in the parlour measure feed by volume and to aid accuracy of the ration delivered, the regular maintenance of any electrical or mechanical components is essential.

Operation of the dispenser can be:

1 Manually by rope or lever from the parlour pit.
2 A semi-automatic system. The operator identifies the cow on entering the parlour and then operates a dial control which automatically dispenses the correct ration to the appropriate manger.
3 There is a wide range of sophisticated programmed feeders available. Identification of the cows can be by the operator or by a fully automated system using microelectronics. In this system the cow is equipped with a unique identification disc round its neck which is activated by an interrogatory device when she puts her head into the manger. This identifies the cow and delivers the correct ration to the manger.

An automatic system of identification holds the key to other systems of automation.

Measurement of milk yields in pipeline systems is usually carried out volumetrically using flowmeters, calibrated jars or in automated systems with milk float sensors or strain gauges linked to electronic recording devices. This equipment is highly sensitive and requires regular checks for accuracy. Where records are manually recorded the scale or calibrated jar must be placed so that it can be read with speed and accuracy. Advantages with jars are the ability to inspect milk before it is added to the bulk.

The actual recording in small herds presents no problems but on a large scale the number of sheets of paper and time required would be prohibitive if attempted during milking so that often a tape recorder is used and the records transferred on to sheets after milking.

The advantages claimed for *automatic cluster removers* (ACRs)[24,25]:

a Increased labour productivity.
b Better working conditions.
c Elimination of risk of over-milking.
d Introduction is usually accompanied by a reduction in the cell count of the herd.

There are three main groups available: (i) manually activated; (ii) semi-automatic; and (iii) fully automatic. The manually activated type, as the name implies, relies on the operator deciding when the cluster should be removed and then operating a lever. The semi-automatic system has to be set to the automatic control position by the operator after milk flow has started. In this case the sensor does not incorporate an initial delay device. With the fully automatic remover the milk flow sensor incorporates an initial delay device so that the operator has only to apply the cluster and take no further action.

Milk flow sensors can be mechanical or electrical. In mechanical sensors milk passes through a float chamber; when the flow rate drops to below 0.2 kg/min cluster removal is initiated. Electrical sensors use a chamber but do not require a float. The presence of milk in the chamber completes a circuit between two electrical contacts. As milk flow drops the circuit is broken and after a delay time the cluster remover is activated.

Where recorder jars are used it is possible to incorporate automatic milk transfer and recording.

Disinfection of teats: electronically controlled teat spraying devices can be provided in the parlour exit. This forms an essential part of the mastitis control routine.

Other management problems

More attention has recently been given to the comfort of the milker, particularly in large herds where milking occupies several hours a day. One aspect of this is keeping sufficiently warm in the winter and cool in the summer. These conditions are difficult to control because of the continual opening and closing of doors creating a heat loss in winter, the general high level of humidity and the type of clothing worn by the milker; too much clothing is likely to restrict the operator's movements. It has been suggested that the best way to provide a comfortable air temperature is through ducts supplying either warm or cool air as the occasion requires.[26]

The control of flies in milking parlours is another aspect of management which can make milking a lot more pleasant for cows and operators. Control begins by the elimination of breeding places and killing maggots and adult flies where possible. Those that survive must be controlled in the milking house or efforts made to keep flies out. As there is a risk of contaminating milk only insecticides which are approved under the Medicines Act 1968 should be sprayed on to lactating cows or used in the milking parlour.

A safe and effective method of excluding most flies from the parlour is by the use of a fine spray of water at the parlour entrances. Cows have to pass through a fine spray as they enter the parlour, through which most of the flies are unable to penetrate.[27,28] (See also Chapter 6.)

LOOSE HOUSING

Loose housing dairy cows is compatible with modern systems of milking, the comfort and cleanliness of cows and can be labour-saving. It may be flexible in terms of cow numbers and some layouts can be adapted for use by other classes of stock if the need arises. When planning the layout the following points should be considered:

1 Type of structure.
2 Method of feeding and storage of fodder.
3 Stock comfort and cleanliness.
4 Litter storage and use.
5 Drainage and disposal of dung and slurry.

6 Stock handling and isolation facilities.
7 Relationship with the milking parlour, cow circulation and collecting and dispersal of cows from the parlour.

The distribution of types of housing is likely to be influenced by the probable rainfall of the area which has a direct bearing on the amount of straw available at an economic price, the disposal of slurry and the size of the herd. As herd size increases there is a greater need for a system of loose housing and whatever the choice, the cleanliness of cows must play an important part if cows are to be milked quickly with proper attention given to hygiene. Statistics available in 1981 suggested that over 50 per cent of herds in England and Wales are housed in cubicles and kennels. This figure, however, bears little relation to herd size or distribution. Certainly in the high rainfall areas housing cows in cubicles or kennels appears to be increasing. Advantages claimed are lower capital outlay, use of small amounts of straw or the possibility of using alternatives to straw and the greater comfort and cleanliness of the cow.

For many years it has been traditional to loose-house cattle in straw yards. In the main this was confined to fattening cattle and young stock, dairy cows being tied up in shippons or cowsheds. Yarding was well suited to beef cattle which would generally lie more quietly than a dairy herd and at a time when most dairy cows had horns, bullying and injuries could result. When dairy cows were dehorned housing cows in straw yards increased. Initially certain fundamental errors were made, e.g. cows being fed on the bedded area adding to the straw requirement, lack of knowledge of optimum space requirements and so on.

The housing area can be fully (Fig. 10.10) or partly covered, and may include a separate feeding area which may be in the open or under cover. A covered area may also be required for the storage of fodder and straw as a part of the layout.

The material used for the construction of the covered area of the housing will be determined by the long-term requirements. Among these will be durability, ease of maintenance and initial cost. Dimensions should be chosen to enable the unit to be used either for loose housing in a yard or for conversion to cubicles should the farming policy alter.

For the covered yard and in some cases for cubicle layouts materials available for the framework are wood, steel, reinforced concrete or a combination of these.

Many units have been built up around a central silo barn with lean-tos up to 9 m wide on one or both sides (a width of 9 m is unsuitable for conversion to cubicles). Siting for possible extension is important, as is the provision of adequate headroom for mechanical cleaning out. Allowance must also be made for a build-up of dung to a depth of 1 m or more, which may require alterations to the height of gates.

In-filling is usually in brick or blockwork between the stanchions to a height of 2–2.5 m and, where necessary, some form of cladding above this. An extension to the eaves on a cantilever or bracket giving an overhang of about 1 m protects the bedded area from driving rain. The importance of adequate ventilation to

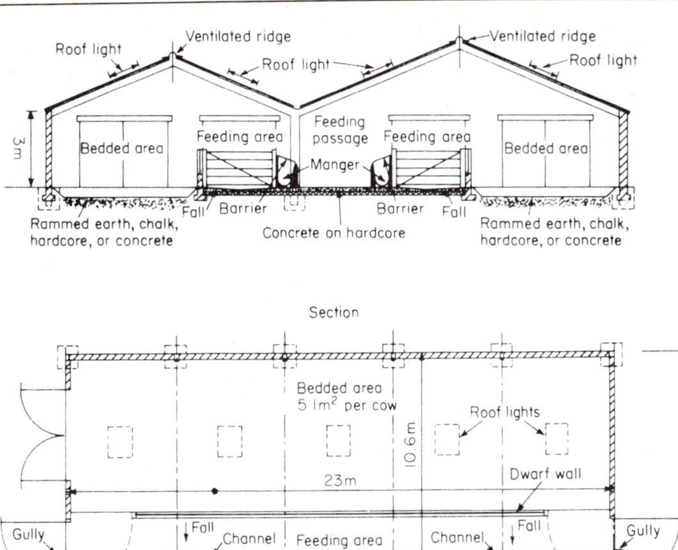

Fig. 10.10 Fully covered yard – 60 cows.

reduce the risk of respiratory conditions in dairy cows and young stock is now generally recognized. The use of space boarding above the blockwork is one method of obtaining a free flow of air. Suitable sizes are 125 mm slats with 25 mm gaps. The gaps may be less on very exposed sites. Other materials are also available to provide ventilation with protection against snow and driving rain.

Disappointing results have frequently been experienced with cows housed in straw yards and correct management is essential for success. The bedded area should be used solely as a place for cows to lie down and entry on to this along the length of one side and not through a narrow opening. This will prevent unnecessary trampling on straw and reduce litter usage. Feeding arrangements and water troughs should be sited on an unbedded concrete area which is also required for exercise.

The amount of space required for the bedded area is 3.7 m^2 per cow and at least 1.85 m^2 per cow of concrete exercise and feed area. Trough space required per cow is 600 mm. With a properly managed yard straw usage is likely to be about 500–600 kg per cow per winter of 150 days.

A completely different approach to housing dairy cows was pioneered in the early 1960s by Howell Evans. This combined features of both cowshed housing and yarding systems and which, with modifications, has become known as cubicle and cow kennel housing.[29] Cubicles are single stalls with a partition between each cow, constructed within a building and having a passageway of concrete or slatted floor construction. This allows access to the cubicles and also forms an area where slurry dung can be collected and cleaned away. Cows are not tied and are free to exercise, drink or feed at will. Feeding and watering facilities are provided in a separate area from the cubicle or lying area.

Kennels are an extension of the cubicle system each kennel being a cubicle complete with its own wall and roof. They are usually constructed in batches with end walls, so forming a building on their own. Construction can be in timber or metal.

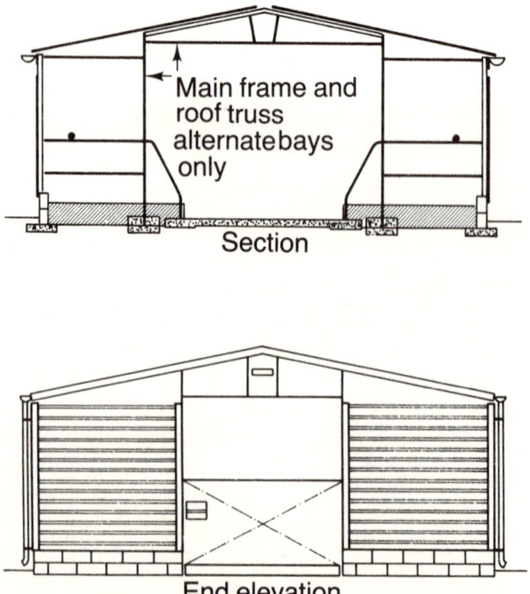

Fig. 10.11 Economical steel-framed cubicle shed.

The first cubicle sheds were designed for comparatively small numbers of dairy cows. As herd and shed sizes increased, various problems of management became apparent; these included refusals, injuries, lameness and mastitic infections of types hitherto rarely encountered.

A great deal of work has been necessary to define those aspects of design, construction, layout, dimensions, the type of floor and bedding, as well as other management factors which are jointly most likely to provide a cubicle shed which is successful in stock health, comfort and cleanliness (Figs. 10.11–10.13).

Despite some disappointing results this type of housing has several advantages which include:

1. Most cows keep cleaner than in other systems of loose housing.
2. There is economy of bedding material, generally at a lower cost than straw yards.
3. The bedded area can be constructed within a relatively cheap structure.

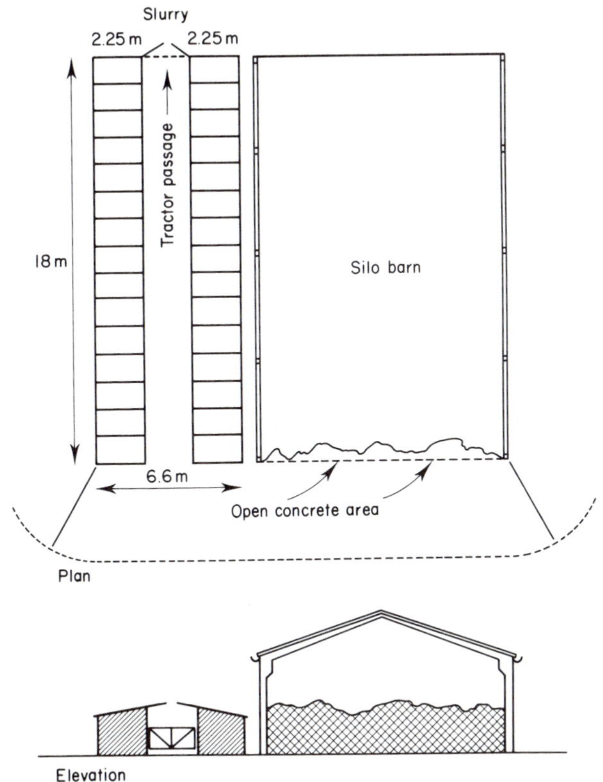

Fig. 10.12 Typical cow-kennel layout for 30 cows incorporating self-feed silage.

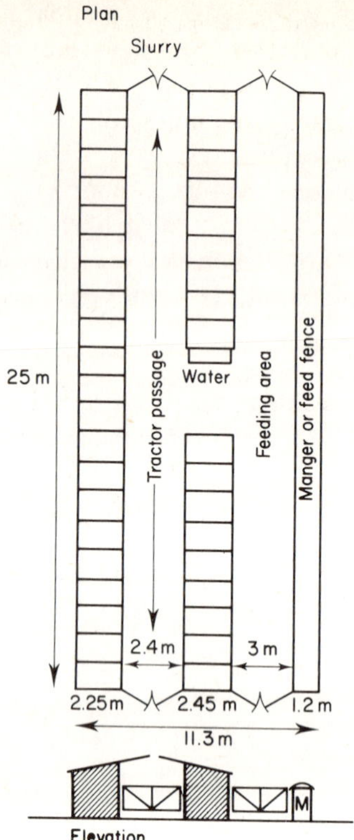

Fig. 10.13 'Cow kennel' layout for 39 cows–a design which can be extended as required.

4 With proper planning the system can be completely flexible including feeding arrangements and the possibility of extension.

In any system of cubicle housing the basic requirements in its design and construction are:

Construction of the floor-size and material for the bed.
Types of cubicle division and head rail.
Adequate ventilation to provide the correct environment.
Disposal of slurry.
Day-to-day management.
(See Fig. 10.14.)

Construction of the floor and bed. The size of the cubicle is important for dimensions which were adequate when they were first introduced may no longer be large enough for herds where, for example, Holstein blood has been introduced. To err on the generous side with dimensions is less likely to lead to difficulties with refusals. As the number of cows in a unit has increased, there

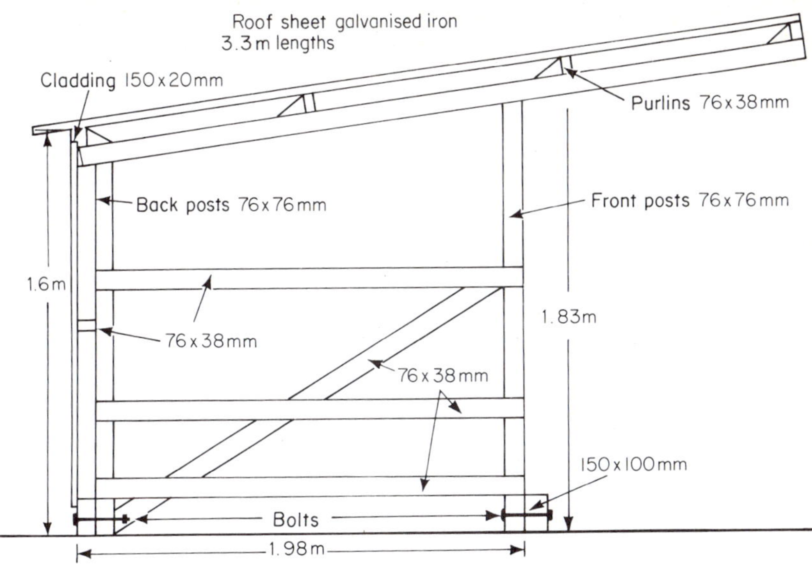

Fig. 10.14 Side view of a cow kennel with wooden frame and metal roof.

has been a tendency, on the grounds of cost, to allow too little space for cows to move around comfortably. Therefore the first rule is that the building shall be of adequate size to allow sufficient room for cows to behave as individuals and with cubicle beds large enough to enable the largest cow to lie down, rest and rise in complete comfort. Badly designed buildings are likely to create hazards and stress to cows and operators alike and thereby predispose stock to health problems. This may be seen where buildings have been adapted without sufficient thought given to the best environmental conditions. Suggested sizes for each cubicles are:

Average cow weight (kg)	Length (mm)	Width (mm)
Over 650	2240	1200
400–650	2120	1100
Under 400	2000	1000

It is usual for the passageway, which may service one or two rows of cubicles, to have a width of 2100 mm. When planning the layout no places should be left where dominant cows can prevent others from reaching vacant cubicle beds, the silage face, mangers or out-of-parlour feeders. All concrete areas should have a non-slip finish.

The original cubicle bed had a concrete or wooden heelstone some 150–225 mm high. The bed was then filled with a variety of materials, some of which were often available locally, e.g. sand, sawdust and chalk. These met with varying degrees of success. Disadvantages could be their high cost, lack of availability, and some required too much maintenance. With some there was evidence that they were connected with mastitic problems.

Whatever material is used the floor profile should be sloping slightly from front to back and be firm, safe, comfortable and dry. The type of base chosen will be permanent (e.g. concrete or bitumen macadam) or from materials such as chalk or earth which may require frequent or annual maintenance.

Concrete.[30] This provides a permanent and relatively maintenance-free bed which may or may not be insulated. It is usually formed from 100 mm of plain dense concrete over a hardcore base blinded with sand. Before laying the concrete it is advisable to lay a heavy duty P.V.C. damp-proof membrane on top of the sand. Fig. 10.15 shows the profiles of cubicle beds with and without a lip at the heelstone. The concrete floor can be effectively insulated with a 50 mm layer of polystyrene but the necessity for this is debatable. Some form of littering material is usually spread on top of the concrete; this may be long or chopped straw, sand or shredded newsprint. The method of slurry disposal is likely to influence a decision on this.

Opinions vary over the desirability of constructing a lip to the cubicle bed. Advantages of having a lip are that it helps to retain the litter and less will be pushed off the bed. But they are more difficult to clean and may allow dirty, wet bedding material to build up, which is undesirable. If an insulated cubicle bed is used without litter there should be no lip. Those without a lip should be given a wood float finish which will help to retain the bedding. Lipped cubicles should have a smooth finish.

Bitumen macadam. The cubicle is constructed as usual with a concrete heelstone 150–225 mm wide with a well-rammed hardcore base. A layer of 'dense' bitumen macadam is laid over the base to a depth of 75 mm with a fall of approximately 75 mm from head to heelstone. To allow for shrinkage the macadam should be slightly proud of the heelstone and the cubicle should not have a lip. For successful results it is essential to use the 'dense' type of material and to ensure that it is thoroughly compacted.

Other materials. These can be successfully used but this is less so than hitherto. They are dry stone-free soil, rammed chalk or sand. Regular maintenance is essential. The type of sand used is most important. It should be non-abrasive, be free from large particles, be non-staining and not of a muddy texture. Mushroom chalk free from flints and well compacted with a vibrating roller is also satisfactory.

With most cubicle beds it is usual to cover them with some form of litter to provide a warm comfortable bed. Requirements for litter are that it should be non-toxic and easily degradable, absorbent and cause no skin damage. Choice will be guided by price, availability and method of slurry disposal. Materials used are long or chopped straw, sawdust or shavings, shredded newsprint and

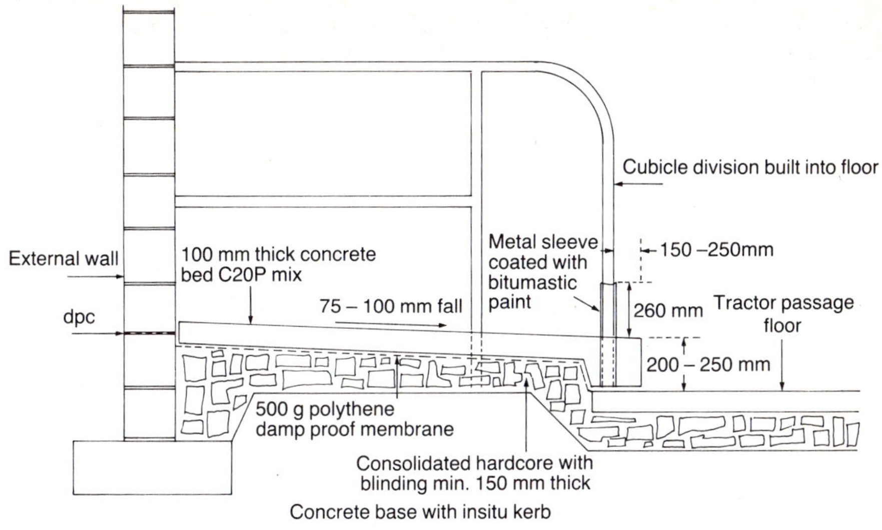

Concrete base with insitu kerb

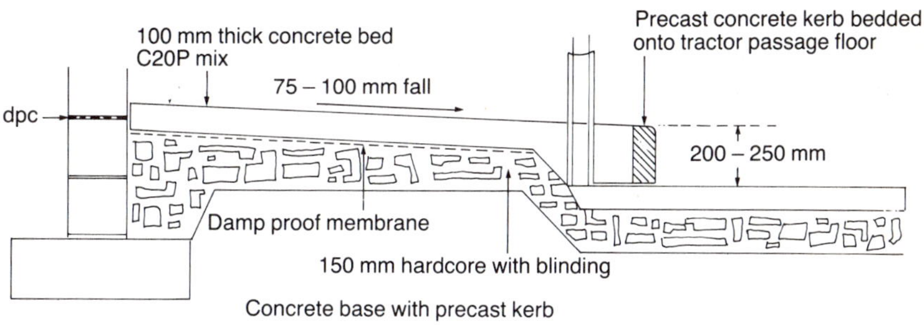

Concrete base with precast kerb

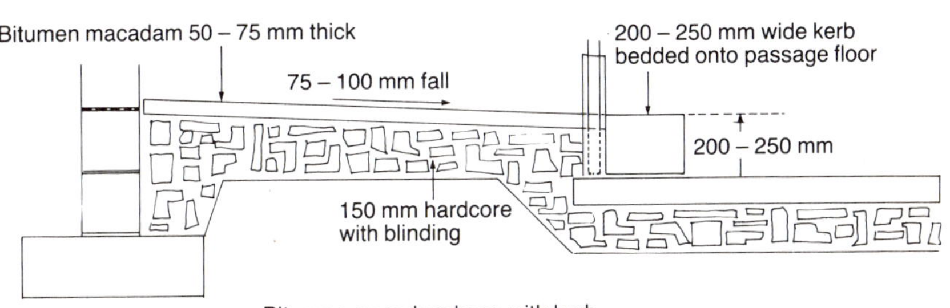

Bitumen macadam base with kerb

Fig. 10.15 Sections through alternative cubicle bases.

sand. Occasionally there may be local supplies of spent mushroom compost, bracken and quarry dust which can be satisfactory.

The use of chopped straw[31] offers several advantages. Less straw is used and there is a considerable saving in time and labour. It is also claimed that it keeps the bed drier and the cows cleaner. Several types of chopping machines are available. The amount of dust created can be unacceptable to the operator although dust control attachments are available.

Where sawdust or wood shavings are used it should preferably be from softwood, free from hard splinters and not have been treated with any toxic materials. It is absorbent and easy to handle but its use has been associated with coliform mastitis. Approximate requirements of litter per cubicle for a 180-day winter are:

Long straw	250 kg
Chopped straw	130–200 kg
Shredded newsprint	60–100 kg
Sawdust	100 kg
Sand	850 kg

Cubicle mats, carpeting and bitumen compound tiles[32,33]

Mats and carpeting are used on a concrete base and are claimed to improve cow comfort and reduce the litter requirement. Materials used for this purpose are rubber, polyester or P.V.C. Thickness varies and it can be laid as individual mats secured with studs or in carpet rolls. One type consists of three layers of different materials. Tiles made of thermoplastic bitumen can be laid on existing concrete beds and have given satisfactory results. Cubicle legs or other obstructions can cause problems in laying.

The kerb or step at the back of the cubicle is to prevent slurry being pushed onto the bed when the passageways are scraped and can also help to retain litter on the bed. These are usually rectangular blocks of treated timber or concrete about 75 mm in width and 200–250 mm high. The width of the passageway will usually be approximately 2100 mm but where a feed fence or manger is an integral part of the cubicle shed the concrete passage between the manger and heelstone should be 3000–3500 mm wide.

Cubicle divisions, headrails and brisket boards

Much of the success with cubicle housing will depend on the design of the cubicle divisions and their correct installation. Difficulties which can occur range from refusals to behavioural problems and physical damage to the legs and teats.

Since the introduction of this type of housing many different designs of division have been tried. They have been constructed of tubular or box profile steel or wood. Sufficient room and correct dimensions are likely to be most important;

there are many situations where different types of division have been used successfully.[34,35]

Suitable sizes for the bed have already been suggested. Fig. 10.16 shows some types of division and typical dimensions. These should be such that cows can rise and lie down without restriction, with safety and lie in comfort. To avoid the risk of cows getting trapped the height of the lower rail of the division to the finished level of the bed should be between 400–450 mm. If the rail is too low there is a risk of a cow trapping and possibly breaking a leg. A flexible lower 'rail' can be made from a polypropylene rope suitably tensioned. The recommended distance from the bed to the lower rail of the Dutch comfort cubicle division is 400 mm.

As with the cowshed, the aim with cubicles is for the cow to stand in the bed so that any dung falls into the passageway. To help to position the cow correctly it may be beneficial to fix a head rail or brisket board which will prevent her standing too far forward. The head rail may be fixed some 450–550 mm from the front of the cubicle although it is essential to choose the exact distance in relation to the height of the rail. The brisket board should be placed at the same distance from the front of the cubicle as the head rail and the kerb no higher than 100 mm to avoid injuries.

Ventilation

All stock buildings must be properly ventilated without draughts which is not always easy to resolve because cows are free to come and go at will in many cases to an open exercise or feed area. Siting of the building should be such that any openings are away from prevailing winds or sheltered where possible by other buildings. Many purpose made cubicle buildings allow only a small cubic air space per cow. These may be situated in areas of relatively high humidity where effective natural ventilation is not easy to achieve. Plenty of openings along the head walls and outlets at the ridge are essential. In contrast, cubicles placed in high general-purpose buildings can often be draughty; where the building is badly ventilated it is likely to remain damp. Damp bedding is conducive to the growth of bacteria some of which could be the causal organisms of mastitic infections.

Feed area

A part of most units will be a concreted feed area together with feed managers or barriers and this may be under cover or in the open. Many successful attempts have been made at feeding cows in cubicles. A simple structure to retain feed, prevent wastage and bullying and prevent animals entering the manger is shown in Fig. 10.17. This can be formed in either a single or double bank as required. The floor of the manger should be at or near ground level, which is the natural position for cows grazing, but by raising it slightly to 75–150 mm it will prevent liquid seeping into the manger. The width for single-sided mangers is at least 600 mm, and 1200 mm for double-sided.

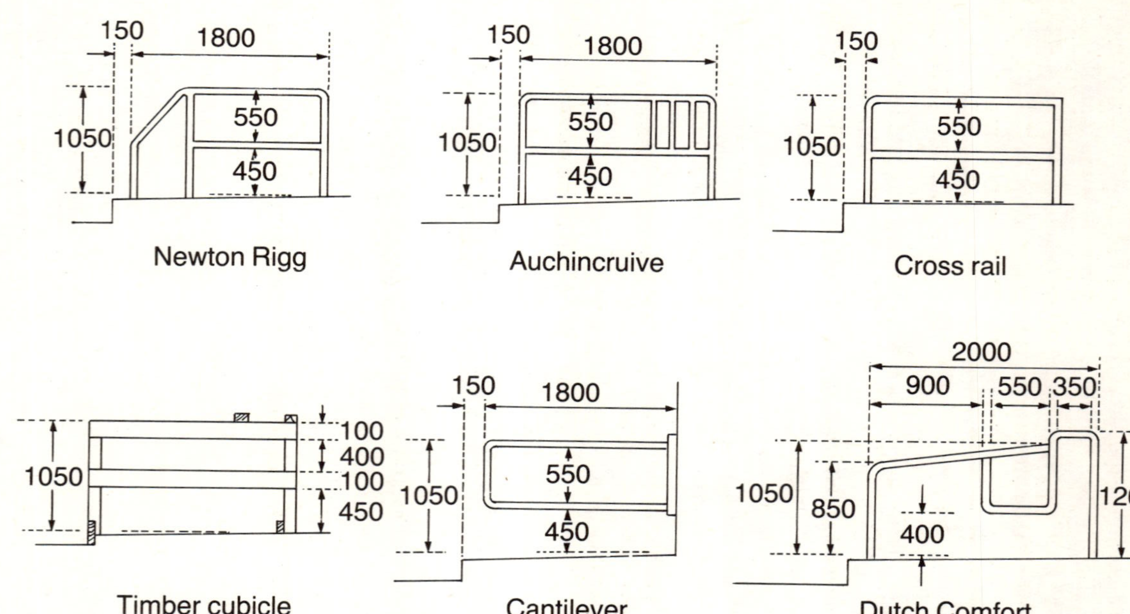

Fig. 10.16 Some cubicle divisions for dairy cows.

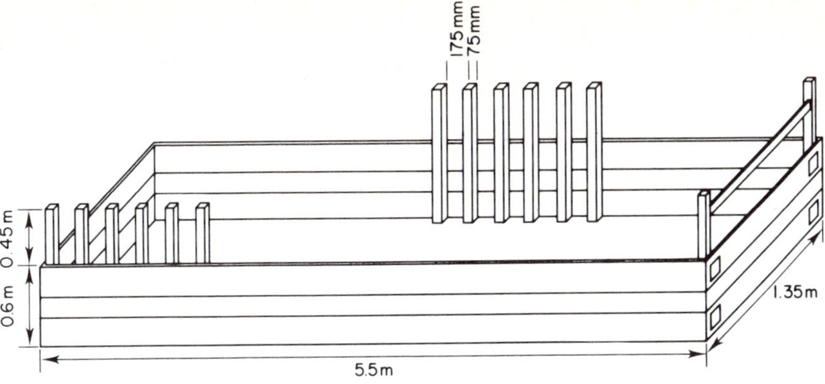

Fig. 10.17 The neck-slot type barrier.

The length of face for self-feed silage or manger space will be decided by the breed of cow and whether feeding is to be ad lib or rationed.

Feeding method	*Trough space or feed face per cow (mm)* Friesian	Ayrshire	Jersey
Rationed bulk feed fed once or twice daily	600–675	550–600	500–550
Ad lib	150	125	100

Other designs of feed barrier are shown in Figs. 10.18 and 10.19.

More recently round mangers have been used extensively and enable more cattle to be fed in a smaller concreted area. However, scraping with a tractor is difficult with this arrangement for feeding. Reference has been made to feeding in the cubicles. For the small herd where hand feeding is carried out this presents few problems. A small crib or feed area can be constructed in front of the cubicle for concentrates and a rack for feeding hay or straw. Movement of the cow can be controlled by a head rail. At the other end of the scale, particularly where there are two rows of head-to-head cubicles, mechanical feeding using a continuous belt making a central manger has been used successfully.

Disposal of slurry and drainage

In traditional systems of housing this presented few problems. With cubicle systems of housing and a greater awareness of the pollution of water courses, the disposal of slurry and liquid effluent requires careful consideration. Cubicle passageways and concrete feed and other areas should be scraped at least once a day and preferably twice. The collection, storage and disposal of dung and slurry can in many cases be solved by using capital equipment which may be expensive to install and operate and which may ultimately influence the system of farming policy. Whatever system of disposal is adopted, it has first to consider the requirements of legislation, both of public and animal health; there are

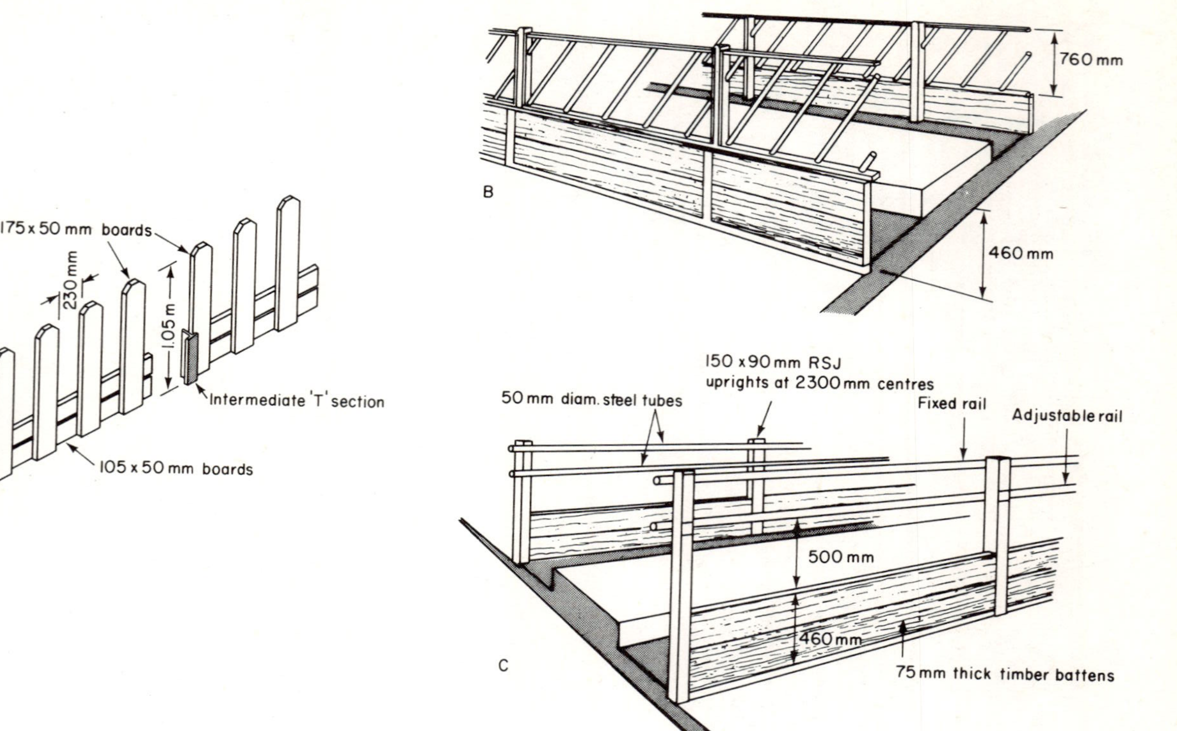

Fig. 10.18 Alternative forms of feed barrier. The tombstone barrier (a) and the diagonal feed barrier (b) are designed especially to reduce fodder wastage and bullying; the rail barrier (c) is especially designed for silage to be delivered from a self-unloading trailer.

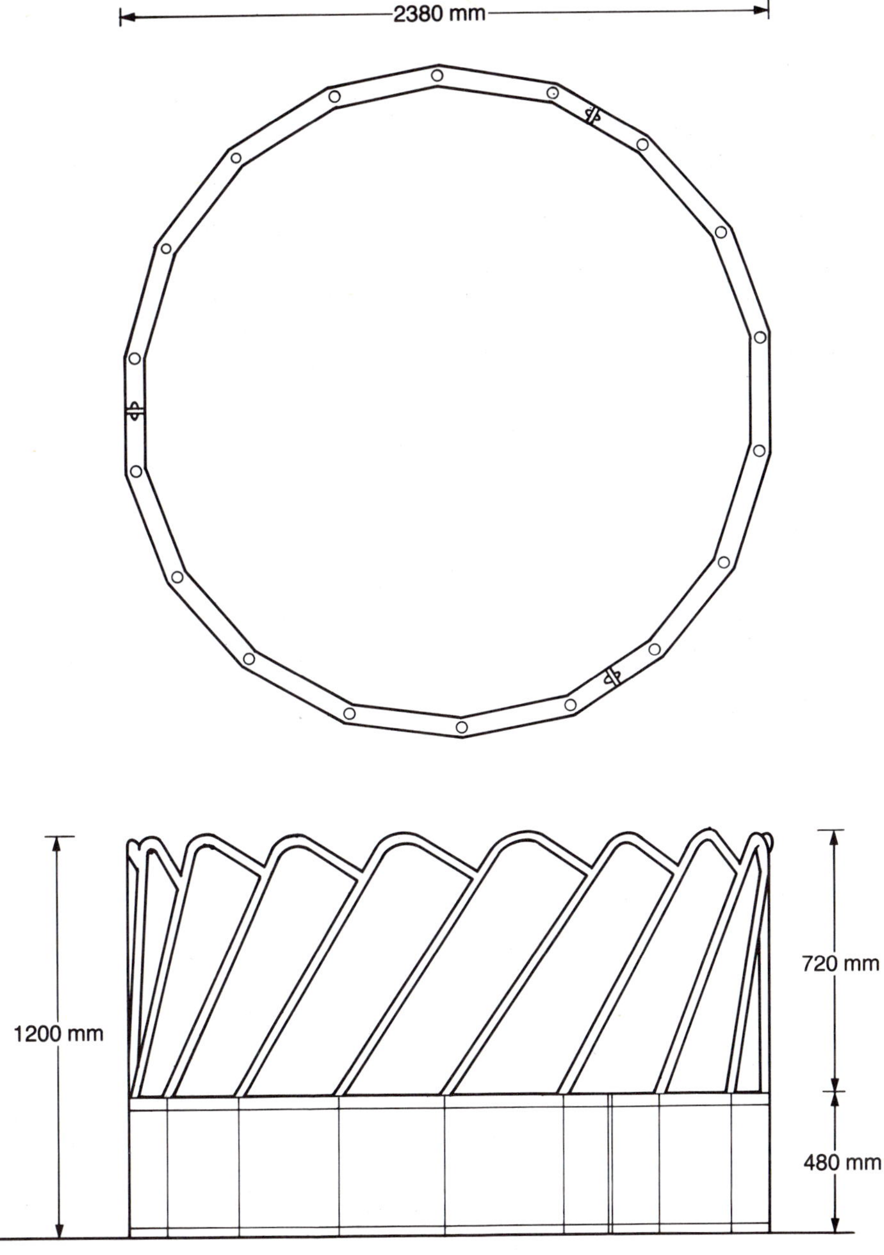

Fig. 10.19 Circular feeder.

also social considerations which may be the subject of legislation for both safety and the risk of causing a 'nuisance'. Proximity to villages, dwellings and water courses must decide the practicability of method of waste disposal and each case must be designed for a particular set of circumstances. There are several points in the day to day management of the cubicles to keep the bed clean, dry and safe. Daily maintenance should include:

1 Removal of dung pats from the bed.
2 Twice a day scraping of the passageways which should help to avoid slurry being carried on to the bed.
3 Littering the bed as required. Frequency will depend on the type of litter. Fresh litter should be delivered to the front of the cubicle bed. Where chopped straw or newsprint is used a dry compacted layer will help to retain the fresh litter when added.

After cows have been milked they usually like to return to the cubicle to lie down so that where possible these jobs should be carried out either before or whilst the cows are being milked. As the udder is vulnerable to infection just after milking a clean dry bed will reduce this risk.

The success or failure of any cubicle housing will depend to a large extent on the way in which the cows have been conditioned. Where cows are nervous and stressed the best design might possibly fail, resulting in injuries and behavioural problems. Where they are contented they are much more likely to adapt to any system even where improvements in layout or construction are possible.

Problems in the design of cubicle beds which can occur and their possible effect are as tabulated:

Cubicle designs	*Possible results*
Too long and/or too wide	Allows too much freedom of movement with soiling of beds and dirty cows
Too short and/or too narrow	Makes rising difficult which causes bruising to the hocks, pelvis and shoulders. These injuries can cause high refusal rates or cows lying back over the kerb. Where the cubicle is too short the cows tend to rise front first as there is insufficient room to move forward
Bottom rail too low	Possible injury to pelvis, shoulder and ribs and risk of leg injuries
Bottom rail too high	Injury to pelvis – rising front first
Head rail too far from the front	Injury to knees and teats. Lying back over the kerb and difficulty in rising
Low head rail	Injury to knees and neck and cut teats
Kerb too high	Bruised heels and high refusal rate
Badly maintained beds with broken concrete and protruding stones	Injuries to knees and hocks. Cut teats and general stress
Slippery base	Injuries to shoulder and pinbones and difficulty in rising
Rough and new concrete	Damage to hooves, knees and hocks

RELATIONSHIP OF THE MILKING PARLOUR WITH HOUSING AND COW CIRCULATION[36,37,38]

The smooth-running, maximum performance and good dairy herd management will, among other factors, depend on the relationship of housing, feeding, fodder storage and cow circulation with the parlour.

Some of the drawbacks that can be found in dairy units are:[39]

Badly designed and constructed cubicle divisions which can cause mechanical injuries to cows.
Cubicles too short and too narrow.
Uncomfortable muck-retaining cubicle beds.
Rough concrete cubicle passageways causing serious foot troubles.
Inadequate systems for scraping slurry from passageways.
Bad design causing cows to turn sharply on wet slippery concrete.
Insufficient feeding space.
Group size too large.
Inadequate facilities for segregating cows for A.I. and veterinary attention.
Badly ventilated buildings.
Insufficient slurry storage space.
Incorrect siting in relation to milking, housing and feeding.

In any layout the accessibility of the milk room for the collection of milk by the bulk tanker may have to be the point from which the pan is built. Other factors which will then require special consideration are:

1 The maximum anticipated length of trough space or feed face required.
2 Proximity of fodder and litter storage.
3 Compact concrete areas serving as many functions as possible, and designed for easy access for cleaning without hazards.
4 Good circulation of cows with well-designed collecting yards funnelling cows towards the parlour and suitable dispersal arrangements.
5 Early separation of cows for veterinary attention with handling facilities for treatment.
6 If the parlour is a part of an umbrella building, the relationship between the housing and milking area and the use of the building for stock other than cattle may be limited.

Cattle handling facilities will be discussed separately.

Fences

Fencing within the yard should be kept to a minimum. Around the yard dwarf walls with rails above contain dung and slurry when the concrete area is scraped. Inside the yard holes can be left in the concrete to form sleeves for posts as required. Hurdles may often form a suitable temporary fence. Squeeze gaps can be left at suitable points to allow operators to enter or leave yards without opening gates. Gaps of 300 mm are satisfactory.

The farm dairy

A dairy or milk room will be required for handling and processing milk and for the cleansing and storage of utensils. The situation of the milk room will be subject to the following considerations:

1 Accessibility for collection by the bulk tanker.
2 Relationship with the dairy complex.
3 Isolation from any form of contamination.
4 Availability of services.

The basic requirements have already been discussed and all dairies will have installed bulk tanks. Access by the tanker is especially important. Adequate turning space for the tanker and farm roads sufficiently strong to bear the weight if necessary of a fully laden tanker are essential.

FACILITIES FOR HANDLING CATTLE[40,41]

With the general increase in herd size, there is more need to provide facilities for the segregation and treatment of dairy cows. A well-planned system should mean a saving of time for the stockman and veterinary surgeon as well as being safer for both operators and stock and causing less stress.

The basic units which have to be considered are a diversion box to separate individual cows on leaving the parlour; a race and crush for the treatment of animals on a herd basis and to provide isolation; and calving boxes.

The diversion box for separating off one cow at a time is best arranged at the parlour exit after the cow has been milked. This can be achieved by using a shedding gate or door which can be operated from the parlour pit or work area by remote control. It is an advantage to have individual stalls in the diversion area for veterinary treatment or artificial insemination.

The cattle handling unit

The requirements for this are gathering pens, a forcing funnel, race and crush. It is an advantage to have a shedding gate after the crush.

The layout should be situated as close as possible to the parlour. Often concrete collecting yards can be used as the gathering pen, which will reduce costs and areas of concrete to be cleaned and will also fit in with the cows' normal behaviour pattern. General requirements are:

1 Access to the head and rear of the animal.

2 Animals securely restrained for the safety of stock and operators.
3 Crush preferably under cover.
4 All services available, i.e. electric light and power and hot and cold water.

For the gathering pen about 1.4–1.85 m^2 per cow should be allowed, which for a herd of 40 cows will require an area of about 60 m^2. The forcing funnel can have one side in line with the race and the other side at an angle of 20–30° to guide the cows into the race. A splay on one side only will guide one cow at a time into the race, whereas a double splay may allow two together to try to enter.

The handling race should be designed to hold up to four adult cattle, which will require a length of just over 9 m and have a width of 675–700 mm. In practice it may be difficult to obtain such a length and therefore necessary to reduce the number of cattle held to two. Construction can be in tubular or sawn timber uprights and rails or a combination of both. For tubular uprights a diameter of 75 mm is suitable with rails of 50 mm diameter. Uprights in timber should be 125 × 125 mm with rails of 125 × 50 mm. The height of the race should be approximately 1500 mm, with the bottom rail 250 mm from the ground and three more rails to make up the required height. Access to animals along both sides is desirable.

The requirements for a suitable 'crush' have been suggested and are listed below:

1 All parts of the animal must be accessible and the animal must be securely restrained.
2 The head, neck, feet, udder, flanks and rear of the animal should be accessible for inspection and treatment.
3 The crush should be adjustable to take all types of cattle.
4 The design and construction should not be such as to cause injury to cattle or handlers.
5 It should be relatively quiet and firmly secured.
6 It should have a free-standing roof if it is outside a building.

Most farms will purchase a proprietary crush. Many tubular steel designs with removable panels are available and it may be possible to incorporate them into the handling system so that the crush can be portable and used for outlying young stock when required. At the end of the crush a shedding gate is desirable to sort out cattle for further treatment or dispersal.

A cattle-handling layout has been designed by the West of Scotland Agricultural College (see Fig. 10.20) which incorporates most of the features referred to above to ensure the steady movement of cattle in safety for both cattle and operator and to enable the whole area to be kept clean, having services available for washing down and a supply of electricity for a hand inspection lamp, clippers, hot water and dehorning.

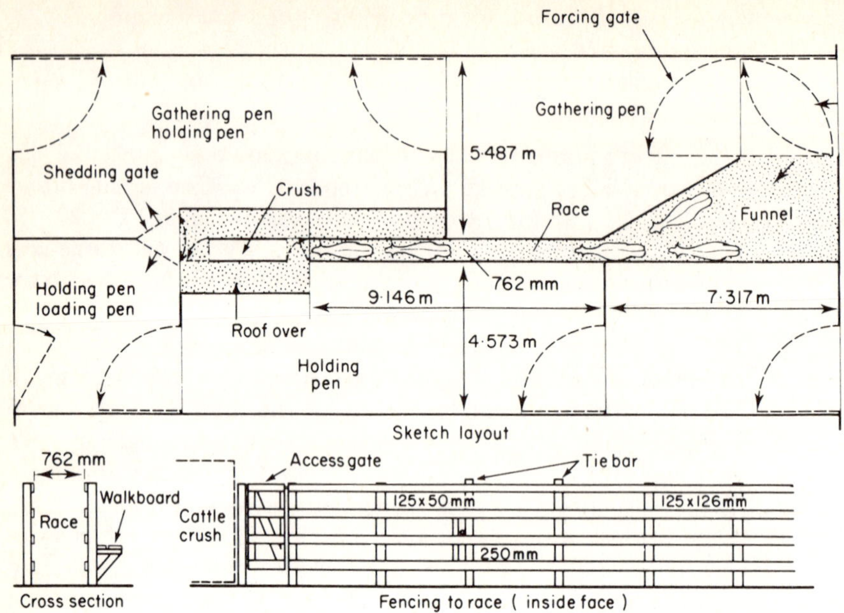

Fig. 10.20 Cattle-handling facilities.

Calving boxes and isolation facilities[42]

Cattle may need to be isolated for various reasons. It may be for reasons of injury, for example, or calving cows and those cattle which have to be kept in isolation to prevent the spread of disease. It is essential that cattle really can be kept isolated and that healthy animals are kept away, that drainage, straw and dung can be disposed of separately and without causing any danger of infection to other stock, and that the boxes can be effectively cleaned and disinfected as required. A suggested size for an isolation box is 4200 × 3600 mm and 2600 mm high, and a guide to the number required is one box for every 25 cows in the herd.

Plenty of light and ventilation will be required, and as the box may be housing sick animals, insulation of the roof and floor will help to keep the box more comfortable. Division walls where a series of boxes are being constructed should preferably be taken to full height. All internal walls should be cement-rendered smooth to a height of at least 1500 mm and preferably to full height.

It is important to include some method of securing cattle either by ties, a head yoke or a holding gate. A nose-ring may also be an advantage for restraining animals which are difficult to handle. A suitable construction is shown in Fig. 10.21. Facilities for milking cows need to be available, and where the boxes are some distance from the milking parlour, a separate vacuum pump could be necessary and provision made for disposal of milk.

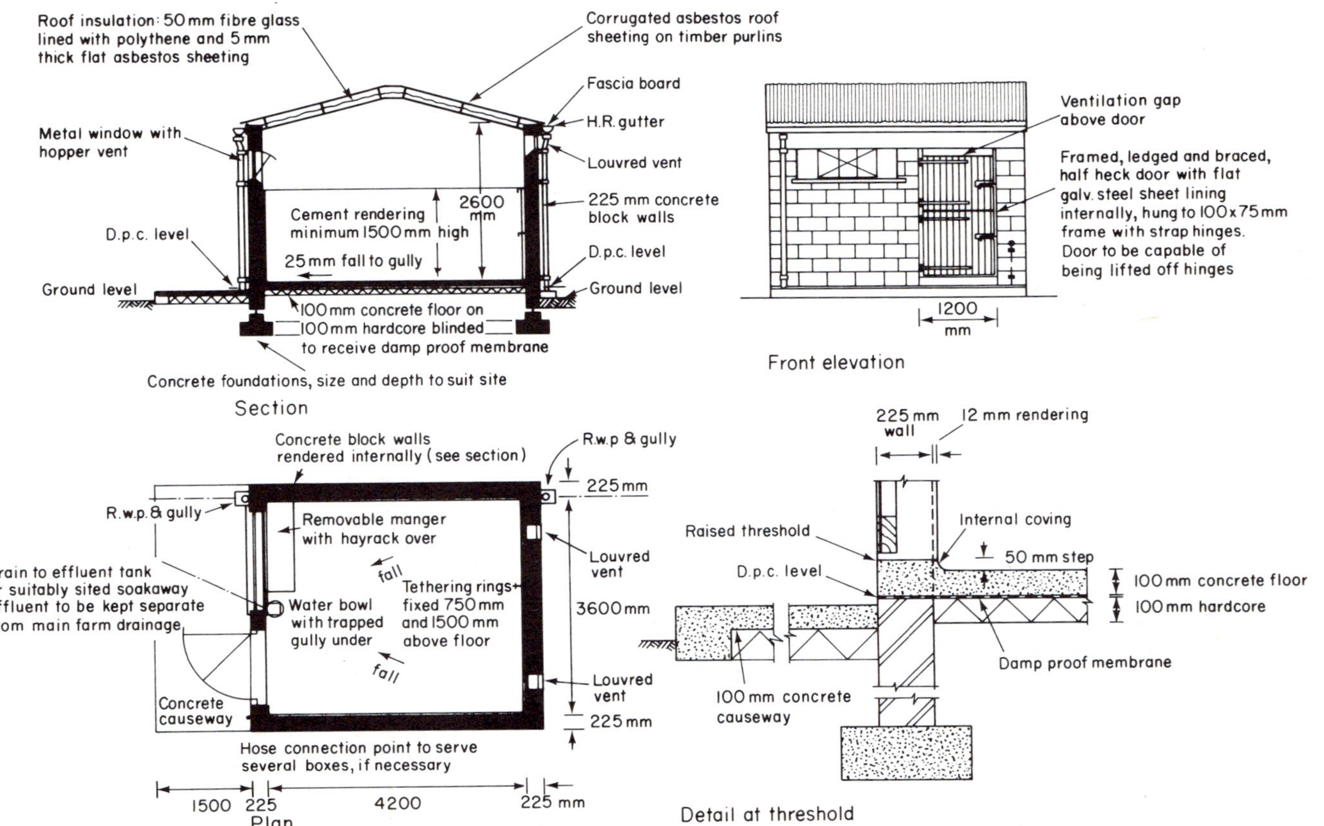

Fig. 10.21 Isolation box for cattle.

As it may be necessary to move a carcase from the box, or an animal may lie across a door and be unable to rise, special attention should be given to this aspect. Doors should be at least 1200 mm wide and be hung to open outwards and such that the door can be lifted off its hinges. A half-heck stable-type door is recommended so that animals can be observed without having to enter the box.

The requirements for calving boxes are similar, although there is not likely to be the same need for segregation, and the number required in a herd will depend upon the calving pattern and the management of cows after calving. One box for every 20 cows in the herd is suggested where the calvings are evenly spaced throughout the year. Some units have provided an open yard which can be divided with sheeted gates into pens for the calving cow and eventually form a suitable yard for followers when not required for the cows.

Care of feet in dairy cows is essential to avoid falling milk yields and severe culling. Most lameness starts in the feet, and the causes may be interlinked. While husbandry factors are important, the shape and soundness of feet are inherited characters, so that it is important to breed from bulls whose progeny have feet without defects and are sound and long-lasting. The quality of the horn of the foot can be influenced by the quantity and composition of the feed. High-protein feed increases growth rate and tends to produce softer horn, and deficiencies of vitamin A will also cause deterioration in horn quality. Another most important environmental and husbandry factor is the conditions for the cow underfoot. Standing in pools of slurry for long periods, travelling a lot in muddy lanes or standing in badly poached kale fields are all predisposing causes for softness of the feet and susceptibility to injuries. Feet which are soft allow small stones, grit or other sharp objects to break the skin and produce a suitable condition for invasion by bacteria which may cause foul-in-the-foot.[43,44] The texture of concrete floors can also cause soreness in the feet, and this appears to be particularly so when the floor is laid with a rough surface and when the concrete is 'green'. In most cases the soreness disappears as the concrete 'cures' and there is some surface wear.

In order to reduce some of those conditions which lead to softness of the feet and thereby lessen risk of infection, the construction of tracks for the movement of cows from the parlour to the grazing area has been tried on many farms.[45] There are also other advantages apart from the one of cows' feet, these being the quicker movement of cows, cleaner cows and less poaching of grassland. The tracks can also be used during silage making and for transporting slurry in winter. The tracks can be constructed from various materials, some of which could be available locally. The base will usually be hardcore, and this can be topped off or blinded with chalk, quarry, dust or other materials which do not contain large or sharp particles. A more permanent but more costly surface could be a 75–150 mm concrete roadway. The width of the tracks does not appear to be critical, a suitable width being 3–4.5 m, and it is possible for wider tracks to have a range of uses. One of the essentials to obtain as long a life as possible with as little maintenance is to ensure that water is kept off the track by allowing sufficient camber with drainage channels along one or both sides of the track where necessary.

The regular use of a foot-bath[46,47] will help to harden the horn of the hoof as well as acting as a preventative against infection. The foot-bath can be constructed in either single or double sections. Where there are two sections the first will contain clean water to act as a foot-wash prior to treatment. Foot-baths are usually sited at the parlour exit but can in practice be situated in any position where cows must pass through them. Suitable dimensions are: width 900–1050 mm, length 2100–2400 mm and depth of a minimum of 75 mm. The bottom of the bath should be shaped in corrugated ridges running the length of the bath to splay the claws of the hoof. The width from the top of one corrugation to the next should be 50–60 mm. Non-slip entry to and exit from the bath are important. It should be possible to drain the solution from the bath quickly so that it can be scrubbed out and flushed. Drainage should only be allowed to discharge at a point where it cannot pollute any water course. A 3 per cent copper sulphate or 10 per cent formalin solution is usually used, and it is important that the bath be kept clean.

THE BULL PEN

An essential adjunct for the dairy farm is safe, strong and comfortable accommodation for the bull. Fig. 10.22 shows a double pen designed by the West of Scotland Agricultural College which incorporates the following essential features:

1 Adequate covered space and a good exercising area, giving a completely healthy environment.
2 Sliding doors between the box and yard which can be remotely controlled from pulley ropes outside. There are also sliding doors into the feeding passage, which enables complete security to be maintained.
3 A feeding passage conveniently placed so both pens can be serviced in safety and under cover.
4 The exercising yards incorporate service pens and there are two steel stanchions screening off a small corner of the yard as a refuge in the event of emergency while the yard is being cleaned out. The service pens are safety devices consisting of a short passage approximately 1 m wide internally and separated from the yard, except during service, by a 'control' gate approximately 2.1 m long and 2 m high. This gate is hinged in such a way that the cow may be admitted to the service pen from outside the buildings while the bull is confined to the yard.
5 The design shown here should be strongly built; solid double brickwork is recommended. It should be rendered on the inside. A tethering system by overhead cable is often utilized. This consists of a strong steel cable stretched diagonally from a point about 1.7 m above floor level at the feed

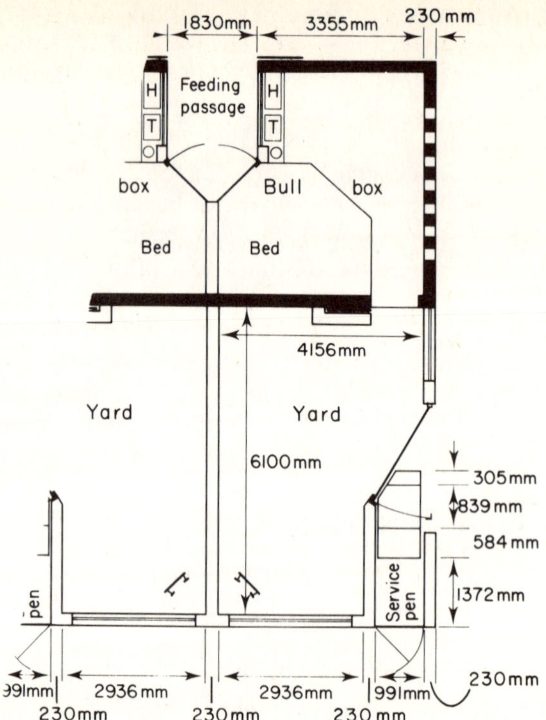

Fig. 10.22 A well-designed pair of bull boxes.

trough across the pen and exercising yard to a point about 1.9 m above ground level at the far corner of the service pen. The bull is tethered to this cable by a chain fastened at one end with a slip-hook to his nose-ring and to the cable at the other end by a free-sliding runner-ring. In order that the weight of the tether chain is not taken on the nose-ring, the slip-hook is also attached to a short chain harness led round the horns and down through the ring. The tether-chain is long enough to allow the bull to lie down and use the service pen but is short enough to prevent him reaching at least two corners of his box and yard, respectively.

REFERENCES

1 Harrison, R. (1979) *Planning Dairy Units*. Farm Buildings Information Centre, Warwick.
2 MAFF (1984) *Farming and the Countryside*. Farm Buildings Booklet 2331.
3 MAFF (1984) *Milking Pipelines in Cowsheds*. Leaflet No. 795. London: HMSO.
4 Addison, J. N. (1970) Mechanical cleaning of cowsheds. *Agriculture*, London, **77**, 11.
5 Fyfe, J., Murray, R. D. and Ross, S. A. (1979) *Milking Parlour Selection*. West of Scotland College of Agriculture, Technical Note No. 23, Jan. 1979.

6 MAFF (1983) *Choice of Milking Parlour*. Booklet 2426. London: HMSO.
7 MAFF (1983) *Static Abreast Parlour Milking*. Booklet 2425. London: HMSO.
8 MAFF (1982) *Herringbone, Trigon and Polygon Parlour Milking*. Booklet 2411. London: HMSO.
9 MAFF (1984) *Buildings for Static Herringbone Milking Parlours*. Leaflet No. 789. London: HMSO.
10 MAFF (1970) *The User's Guide to Modern Milking*, No. 1: *Herringbone Parlours*. London: HMSO.
11 Mate, J. (1982) Covering notes. *Dairy Farmer*, November.
12 Adams, S. C. M. (1983) *Wall Finishes at NAC Dairy Unit*. ADAS Unit, NAC, Newsletter 1983.
13 Gustafson, R. J. (1983) Here is one way to solve stray voltage problems. *Hoard's Dairyman*, **128** (6). USA.
14 Gustafson, R. J. (1983) How to prevent stray voltage in new milking parlours. *Hoard's Dairyman*, **128**, (9). USA.
15 Gustafson, R. J. (1983) Poor grounding can cause electrical headaches. *Hoard's Dairyman*, **128**, (12). USA.
16 Meneer, R. R. (1977) Lighting in Farm Buildings 1 and 2. *Farm Buildings Digest*, 12(1) Spring; 12(2) Summer.
17 MAFF (1982) *Repairing farm floors*. Leaflet No. 825. London: HMSO.
18 Rose, M. (1973) Good yards speed parlour throughput. *Dairy Farmer*, March.
19 Seabrook, M. F. (1984) The psychological interaction between the stockman and his animals and its influence on performance of pigs and dairy cows. *Veterinary Record*, **115**, 84–87.
20 MAFF (1982) *Precautions Against Freezing*. Leaflet No. 797.
21 MAFF (1981) *Washing Down Milking Parlours*. Leaflet No. 628.
22 MAFF (1983) *Codes of Recommendations for the Welfare of Livestock: Code No. 1, Cattle*. Leaflet No. 701. London: HMSO.
23 MAFF (1983) *Cow Identification*. Leaflet No. 600. London: HMSO.
24 Lowe, F. R. (1981) *Milking Machines*. Oxford: Pergamon Press.
25 MAFF (1982) *Automatic Cluster Removal and Milk Transfer*. Leaflet No. 826. London: HMSO.
26 O'Neill, D. (1977) Man-comfort at milking. *Dairy Farmer*, June.
27 Walsh, F. (1975) Chemical fly control. *Dairy Farmer*, July.
28 MAFF (1983) *Fly Control for the Dairy Herd*. Leaflet No. 656. London: HMSO.
29 MAFF (1983) *Design and Management of Cubicles for Dairy Cows*. Booklet No. 2432.
30 Barnes, M. M. (1983) *Concrete in Cow Cubicles*. Farm Note 12 (2nd edition). Cement & Concrete Association.
31 Millman, J. (1984) Straw chopper machines. *Livestock Farming*, June.
32 Kelly, M., Bishop, J. and McKerrow, A. J. (1983) Bitmac and Mooker tiles for cubicle beds. *Farm Building Progress* No. 72, April 1983, p. 23.
33 Tasker, R. J. (1980) Cow cubicle bed treatments. *Farm Building Progress* No. 62. Oct. 1980, p. 3.
34 Cermak, J. (1983) Comfortable cubicles for profit. *Big Farm Management*, Feb. 1983.
35 Hollinshead, Peter (1984) Cubicle design – variations on the theme. *Livestock Farming*, June.
36 Harrison, Ronald (1979) *Planning Dairy Units*. Farm Buildings Information Centre.
37 Weller, J. (1970) *Planning Farm Buildings*. F.B.I.C.
38 MAFF (1984) *The Cattle Industry and Welfare in Great Britain*. Booklet No. 2482.
39 Gaisford, M. (1983) Cow comfort counts. *Farmers Weekly*, 22 April 1983.
40 Shepherd, C. S. (1972) *Layout and equipment for Handling Dairy and Suckler Cows*. West of Scotland Agricultural College Advisory and Development Service.
41 MAFF (1980) *Cattle Crushes and Handling Facilities*. Booklet No. 215.2
42 MAFF (1982) *Isolation Facilities for Cattle on the Farm*. Leaflet No. 807.

43 Chancellor, G. (1983) Ideas on the hoof. *Dairy Farmer*, October.
44 Prentice, D. E. and Neal, P. A. (1972) Some observations on the evidence of lameness in dairy cattle in West Cheshire. *Veterinary Record*, **91**, 1–6.
45 MAFF (1981) *Cow Tracks for the Dairy Herd*. Leaflet No. 744.
46 Shepherd, C. S. and Walker-Love, J. (1980) *Footbaths for dairy cows*. West of Scotland Agric. College. Technical Note 125.
47 MAFF (1983) *Footbaths for Dairy Cows*. Leaflet No. 841.

FURTHER READING

Kilgour, R. and Dalton, (1984). *Livestock Behaviour*. London: Granada.
Fraser, A. F. (1974) *Farm Animal Behaviour*. London: Baillière Tindall.
MAFF (1980) *The Storage of Farm Manures and Slurries*. Booklet No. 2273.
MAFF (1980) *Slurry Handling*. Booklet No. 2356.
MAFF (1983) *Equipment for Handling Farmyard Manure and Slurry*. Booklet No. 2126.

11

Calf Housing

The provision of correct housing conditions for calves has always been important but, as methods are becoming more intensive and rearing units bigger, the risks from bad housing become infinitely greater. Calves thrive well when kept singly or in pairs in loose boxes, but when specialized buildings are used great care is needed in detailed design. Ventilation, space, drainage, pen size, fittings and materials must all be carefully considered to avoid environmental extremes, poor hygiene, damp and draughts, and other housing defects.

THE ENVIRONMENT

As explained in Chapter 3, recent investigations have shown that the calf is able to withstand a very wide range of temperatures and in practical terms the calf house temperature is not critical since even freezing conditions will not be detrimental to health or productivity. Good calf housing is much more an amalgam of isolation between groups, keeping small numbers in one air space, maintaining dry conditions both on the flooring and in the air, with relative humidity below 90 per cent if possible, and the elimination of stressful fluctuations. The valuable practical application of modern knowledge on the environmental and health requirements of calves by Dr Dan Mitchell of the Farm Electric Centre, National Agricultural Centre, Stoneleigh, suggests a simpler and more economical approach to calf housing is the correct one and even the veal calf, traditionally kept at temperatures between 20 and 25°C, may be maintained at a much lower temperature than this range, without suffering any disadvantage yet promoting its better growth.

The totally enclosed house

Great importance is attached to correct ventilation which must not inflict chiling cold or draughts. Ventilation can advantageously be on simple lines. Inlet ventilation is normally provided by inward-opening bottom-hinged hopper windows along both sides of the building. They should open about 300 mm below the eaves and be placed evenly around the house – about one-third of the length of the wall as opening windows is sufficient, each window being about 1200 mm long and 600 mm deep (see Chapter 5). Double glass is strongly recommended, not so much for the reduction in heat loss but because it will prevent condensation. In the most exposed areas of the country, farmers may prefer to have some small, baffled ventilators between the windows so that the latter can be completely closed in cold and windy weather. Outlet ventilation is easily effected by box-type outlet chimneys with flat tops (Fig. 11.1).

Natural lighting is provided if hopper windows are used. No great areas of glass are needed in the calf house but, wherever roof lights are preferred or are used of necessity, double thickness is desirable. With artificial lighting, a light point (incandescent bulb) every 3 m along the house is sufficient. The veal calf house normally has artificial lighting only (Figs. 11.2 and 11.3).

To help eliminate temperature extremes and also keep the surfaces free from condensation, insulated construction may be preferred, but it is not essential (see Chapter 3).

To assist in correct environmental control, the building needs to be kept within modest proportions: the very large building is to be avoided and the roof should be kept low. Where a larger building is to be adapted as a calf house – and it can generally be done on the lines suggested for new buildings – it is strongly recommended that it is divided into smaller sections by complete cross-partitions. In planning calf accommodation, it is most important that the building can be closed completely at times, disinfected and rested. Separation into at least two units – one for the very young, another for the older calf – is desirable, as not only are different environments needed but the disease risk is reduced in this way. If a building is to take all ages of calves, it is often very difficult for it to be completely vacated and rested but this is very nearly an essential if disease build-up is to be avoided.

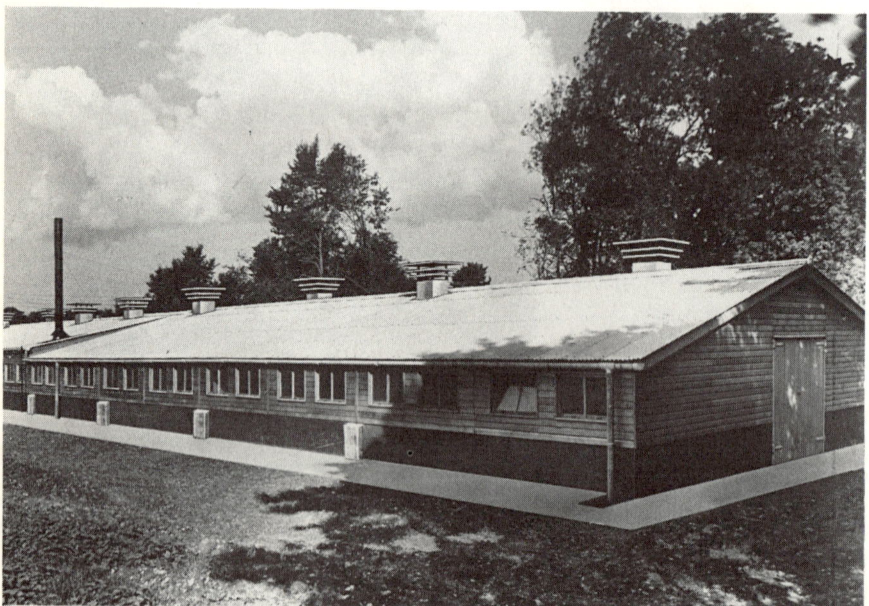

Fig. 11.1 Exterior of totally enclosed house for calves.

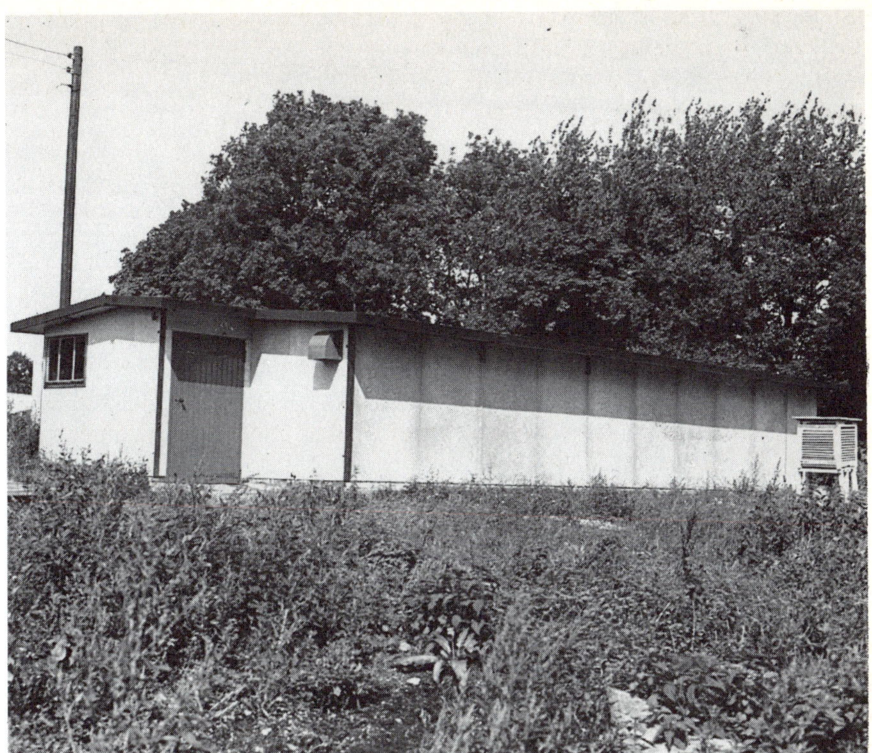

Fig. 11.2 Exterior of windowless controlled environment calf houses for veal production.

PENS AND LAYOUT

Generally, the best layout for a totally enclosed house is to have the pens of a calf house on each side of a centre passage not less than 1.2 m wide (Fig. 11.4). Drainage can then be to shallow channels on each side of this passage discharging to a gully at one end.

For the first few weeks, individual pens are preferred for calves, but they are not essential and pens containing three or four can certainly be used (Fig. 11.5). A satisfactory space allowance for single pens is 2.2 m^2 per calf up to three months, but rather less is possible and pens as small as 1.4 × 0.9 m or 0.75 m are sometimes used, giving areas as small as 1.2 m^2 and 1 m^2 per calf. The smaller sizes are not usually liked so much, and good dimensions are 1.5 × 1.2 m for the young calf up to six weeks. Space allowances should be increased up to 3.7 m^2 by six months and 4.6 m^2 by twelve months, when 'traditional' straw-bedded pens are used though rather less is often given satisfactorily. For example, there are excellent pens taking calves to four months of age, allowing only 2.3 m^2 per calf. A reduction of up to 50 per cent in the dimensions given would appear to be permissible. This flexibility is important as many calf houses

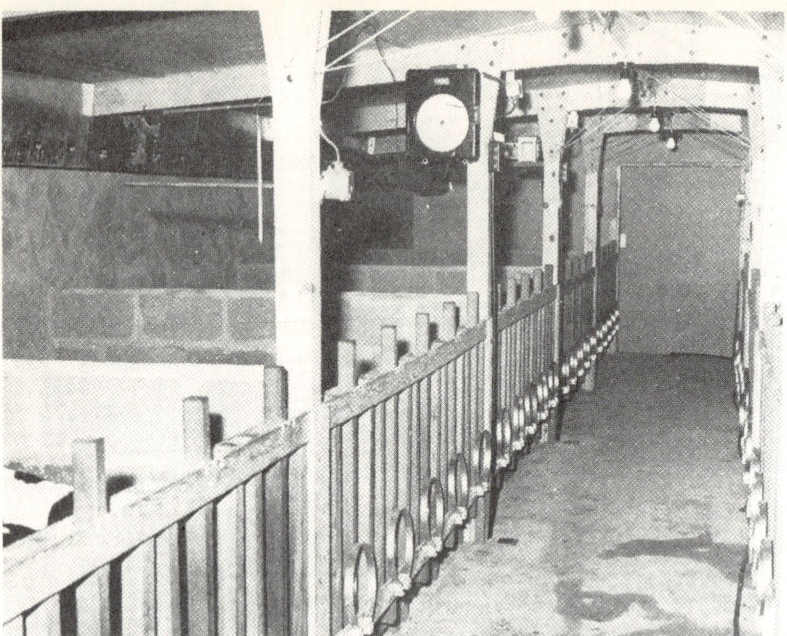

Fig. 11.3 Veal calf house with community pens. Drainage under slats falls to a gully at the rear so that the passage remains dry.

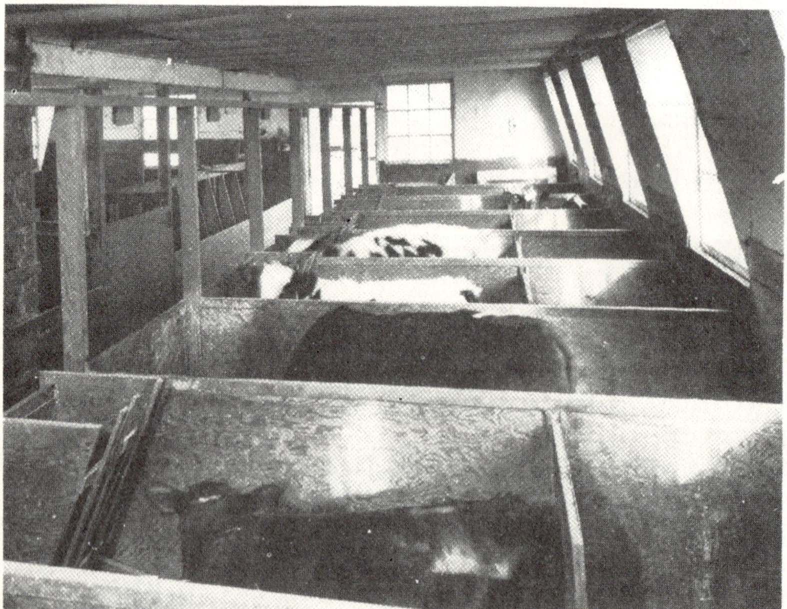

Fig. 11.4 Enclosed calf house with individual pens and solid partitions, often preferred for the 'bought-in' calf with a high disease risk.

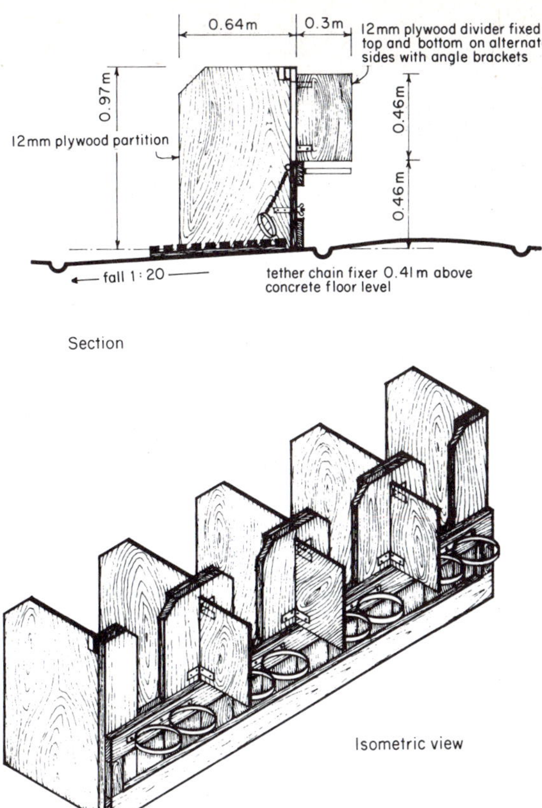

Fig. 11.5 Section and isometric view of a tethered feed fence for calves kept in small groups. (Designed by Dr D. Mitchell.)

are adapted buildings so that it is helpful to know that a certain amount of latitude is possible without taking undue risks. An alternative pen arrangement which may be favoured is to place two rows of pens back to back in the centre of the house with side passages alongside the walls. This puts the calves well away from the walls and windows and makes for easier and more uniform environmental control and in general appears to provide a healthier environment.

In some cases the use of slatted floors for young calves is favoured. Portable pens that can be easily assembled, to take young calves up to 2–3 months of age, have also been used which can be dismantled for cleaning and disinfection, and placed in any suitable box or building, and thus allow the utmost adaptability and avoid specialization (Fig. 11.6). Slatted floors are often made of 50 × 50 × 32 mm slats spaced 38 mm apart. On top of the slats 13 mm wire mesh may be placed to stop the bedding (long straw), if used, falling through.

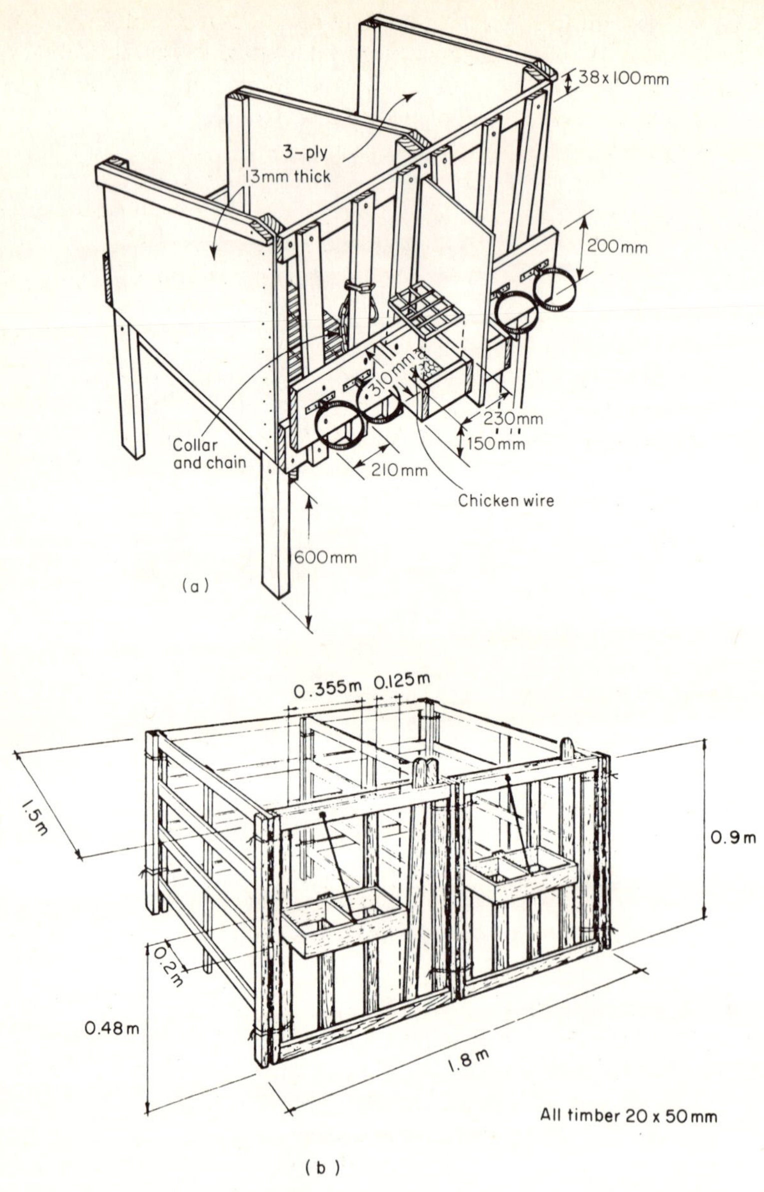

Fig. 11.6 Individual calf pens. (a) A portable pen with either a raised slatted or a wire floor. (b) A timber-railed pen developed by BOCM.

Such slats can be used in portable pens or as a top floor over an existing concrete one to assist drainage.

As an alternative to the slatted or solid-sided pen, the very simple construction of the BOCM pen is an example of an arrangement that is favoured in small units or for home-bred stock where the disease risk is less (Fig. 11.6). However, perhaps the best arrangement of all is the new tethered feed fence, developed and designed by Dr Dan Mitchell, as an alternative to the individual pen for the first few weeks of life. It prevents inter-sucking and gives separate feeding for each calf and excellent access. It may also be used after the tethered stage as a feed fence and pen front for calves up to twelve weeks of age. Layouts for the tethered feed fence are similar to those with individual pens (Fig. 11.5).

Useful pen division sections are, in fact, made up economically in exterior grade plywood. The front of the pens can be made in timber or galvanized metal with access by the calf through openings to food and water containers outside. The whole front should be made so it may be easily taken apart. Where several calves are kept together the front should have yokes so that the animals can be secured for feeding, and usually some time afterwards. Hay racks should be provided, with 50 mm spaces between the slats. They may be fixed on the inter-pen partititions near the front. Automatic water bowls should also be fitted as near the front of the pen as possible so that spillage passes straight outside and is drained away.

ALTERNATIVE CALF HOUSING

The monopitch calf house

The arrangements described previously are those used in totally enclosed housing but the monopitch house is an alternative and rather cheaper and very often healthier scheme. At its simplest it consists of a series of pens, open-fronted and facing south, with a sheeted gate across the front. Temporary pens can be placed in each unit for the individual housing of the calves for the first few weeks. These are removed later and the calves are then reared as a group (Fig. 11.7). When the period is over, at the age of 3–6 months, or later if desired, the entire pen is cleaned out with a tractor. An excellent arrangement is shown in Fig. 11.8. It has been the authors' experience that this arrangement in general is capable of producing calves that are much healthier than those kept in totally enclosed buildings due, no doubt, to the isolation of groups inherent in the design. Running costs are less as there is no mechanical environmental control.

The straw bale house

Another arrangement for cheap housing is the house made of straw bales or pens of straw bales inside a covered yard. Straw bales give excellent warmth, isolation, dryness and freedom from draughts. They can be destroyed after every few batches so ensuring hygiene is maintained. A suitable design of a straw bale shack is shown in Fig. 11.9 which demonstrates a cheap, effective, disposable housing system for calves from five or six days to weaning at 5–7 weeks. The calves are individually penned in wooden pens, the rest of the building being

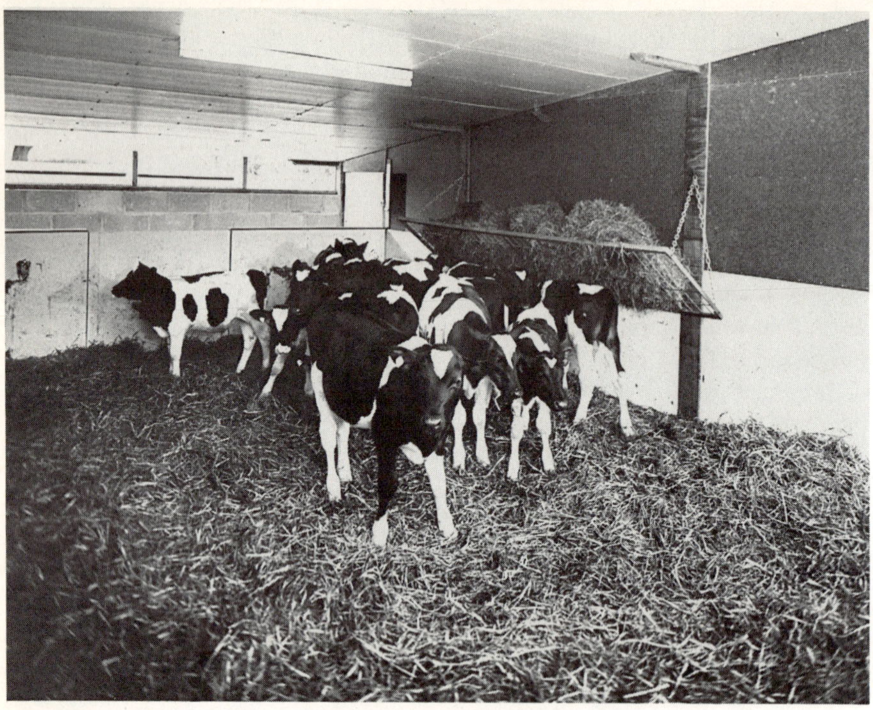

Fig. 11.7 A group of calves in a Mono-Pitch House. With approximately 12 calves only in this house and with plenty of bedding this forms an ideal environment.

of straw bales, timber trusses and metal roof sheets. The entire building is quite easily dismantled and re-erected with new bales.

The importance of good hygiene must always be remembered; many points in design have been suggested to assist towards this end. The more the building is rested and cleaned the better. Also, from the health and productivity aspects, the smaller the calf house is, the easier it can be to control the environmental conditions and keep disease at bay.

FURTHER READING

Calderwood, R. T. (1972) Calf housing. *Scottish Agriculture*, **51**, (5).
Calf Rearing (1959) Supplement to *Farmers' Weekly*.
Calf Rearing (1962) Supplement to *Farmers' Weekly*.
Calf Rearing (1962) London. Survey, British Oil and Cake Mills.
Calf Rearing (1963) *Farmers' Weekly*.
Good Calf Management (1961) *Farmer & Stock-Breeder*, London.
MAFF (1965) *Beef Production*. London: HMSO.
MAFF (1965) *Housing of Calves*. London: HMSO.

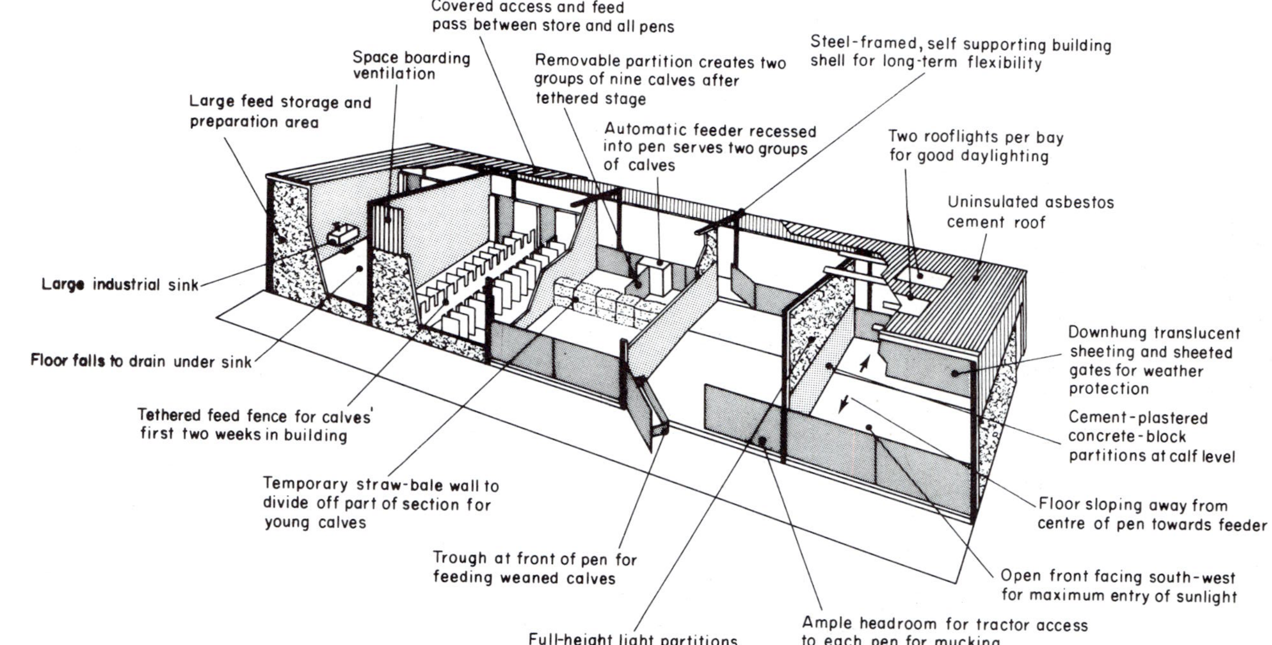

Fig. 11.8 Monopitch calf house.

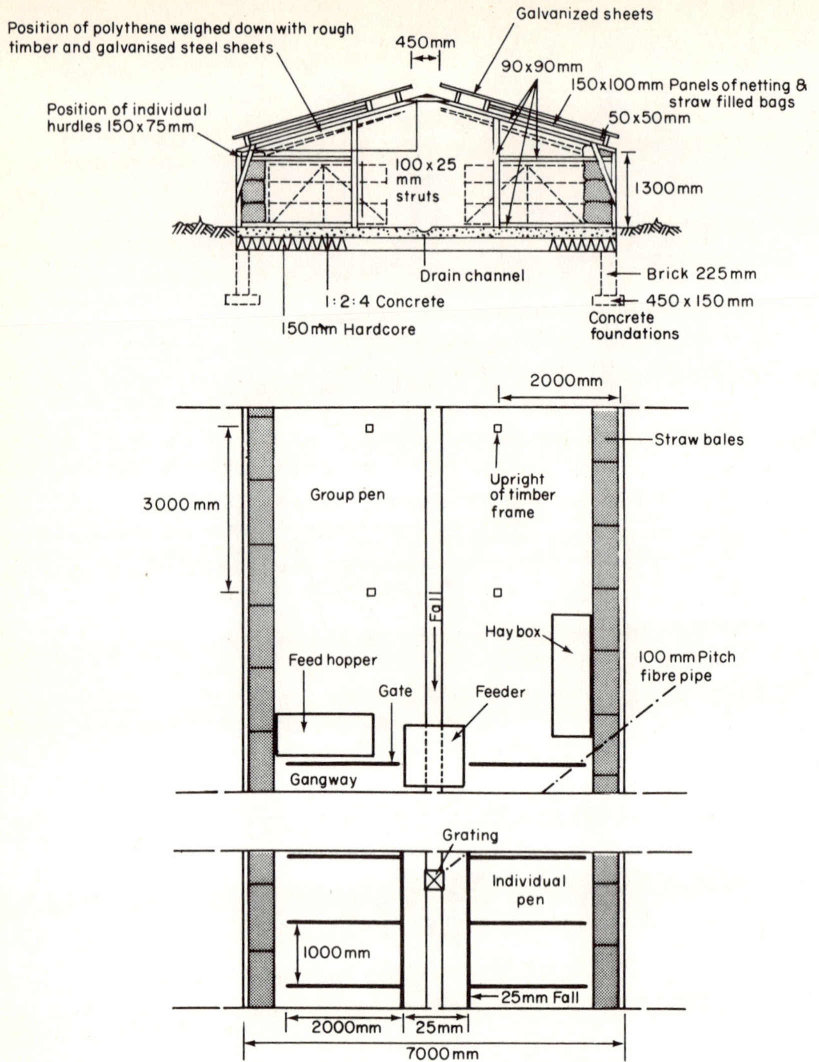

Fig. 11.9 Straw bale calf shack.

Mitchell, D. (1976) *Calf Housing Handbook*. Aberdeen: Scottish Farm Buildings Investigation Unit.

Preston, T. R. (1960) *Calf Rearing*. MAAF. London: HMSO.

Rearing Healthy Calves (1964) Supplement to *Farmers' Weekly*.

Roy, J. H. B. (1955) The calf, its management, feeding and health. *Farmer & Stock-Breeder*.

Webster, John (1984) *Calf Husbandry, Health and Welfare*. London: Collins Professional & Tech. Books.

12

Housing Beef Cattle

The production of beef[1] can involve two or three different enterprises and the system and aims of these are so diverse that at first sight housing may appear to be relatively complex. After the rearing stage, however, the requirements are less exacting and cattle will thrive well under a variety of conditions.

Apart from individual experiments, housing has until recently ben confined to traditional lines which were evolved from the availability of local building materials, type of feed, amount of bedding available and climatic conditions. Many 'rearing' farms are situated in marginal and hill areas where, through lack of capital, farmers have not been in a position to provide suitable fixed equipment. Stock buildings may be inadequate for wintering cattle which, together with a poor layout, may make labour-saving impossible. However, grants have done much to assist in the provision of improved stock accommodation and other amenities on these farms.

The traditional methods of beef production can be roughly classified into three enterprises which, on some of the larger farms suitably situated to produce high-quality grass and bulk feeds for winter feeding, may be integrated to take the cattle right through to slaughter. The enterprises are:

1 Rearing.
2 The store period.
3 Fattening.

Within the last few years greater interest has been taken in systems of beef production based on the quick fattening of calves from dairy or dairy cross-breeds, and these will be discussed separately, as there are certain fundamental differences in the aims of these procedures.

REARING

Calf housing has already been dealt with in detail but, whilst the same basic principles apply to beef calves as to dairy breeds, the systems of rearing are, normally, different. For example, with beef calves a traditional method is to single- or multiple-suckle them on nurse cows for anything from 3 to 6 months. The building must therefore be planned so as to allow the calves to be near the nurse cows, without neglecting the warmth, light, drainage facilities and cleanliness of the building required for any system of calf rearing.

A suitable system can be arranged from a shed having dimensions similar to those for a double-range cowshed. The nurse cows are then tied up on standings on one side of the shed, and calf pens are constructed to replace the standings on the other side, leaving a central passageway through the length of the shed. This passageway should be of sufficient width to allow a tractor and trailer to be taken through the shed so that both calf pens and cows standings can be cleaned out with the minimum amount of labour. The calf pens can be constructed of removable tubular rails so that the size of the pens can be adjusted according to the number and size of calves being reared. The usual allowance of floor space for small calves is 1.8 m^2 per calf. Pens should be fitted with hay racks and mangers.

At present it will be more usual to loose-house the single suckler herd either in cubicles or kennels or fully or part-bedded yards. This will enable the stockman to take advantage of labour-saving methods of feeding and cleaning out. The buildings will be similar to those for any yarded stock, divided into suitably sized pens with the same space allowances. A calf creep area should be provided which can be separated off with removable barriers and provided with small hay racks and portable feed containers for concentrates if required.

As with all systems of yarding, adequate ventilation is essential and ample straw will be required to maintain a high standard of cleanliness.[2]

THE STORE PERIOD AND FATTENING

In some areas it is traditional to tie up fattening cattle, but yarding is equally suitable and labour economies are probably easier to apply to this method of housing (Fig. 12.1). Details of construction of yards are in general similar to those for dairy cows, and in many districts yards or cattle courts have for many years been the accepted method of housing stores and fattening cattle. The layout usually consists of an open yard around which open-fronted sheds, and very often the threshing barn, are grouped to provide shelter. The present trend is towards fully or part-covered yards with an open area for feeding. The amount of straw required for litter is usually high, although in the arable areas farmers may regard the use of straw an advantage, since it is available in abundance, and the production of dung an adjunct to the arable enterprise. In addition racks and mangers are often inconveniently situated for feeding. Yards may be fully or part-covered with an open area for feeding. In the latter case it is usual to concrete the open area and arrange cribs and racks along the outside to provide shelter and facilitate feeding. This arrangement has two principal advantages: a smaller covered area is required, which cuts down initial outlay; and the straw required for litter will be less where cattle are fed outside the covered area, provided the feeding area is kept clean. In a good layout it should be possible to mechanize cleaning, thus avoiding a laborious job. Suggested space allowances per animal are given in Table 12.1.

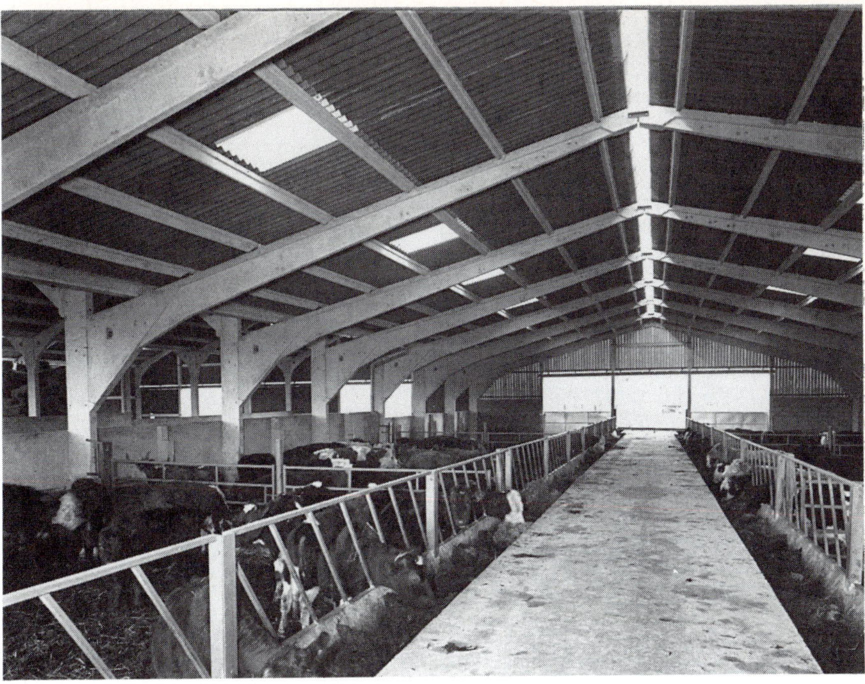

Fig. 12.1 Interior of a straw yard for beef cattle. Note the good ridge and gable ventilation, and troughs.

These allowances refer to totally covered yards and the figures can be reduced where an outside area for feeding is allowed. Details of planning which have to be borne in mind (see Chapter 10) are the construction and positioning of cribs for ease of feeding, together with access to roadway or feed passage. Also important is the provision of adjustable gates to allow a build-up of dung and sufficient drinking troughs. The usual requirements for health of stock must be provided, including adequate light and ventilation. Better stockmanship is possible where groups of cattle are kept in small numbers, although the cost of labour for feeding will probably be higher, as will the initial capital outlay on buildings.

Table 12.1 *Space allowance per animal*

Type of animal	Area per animal including manger (m^2)	Manger length per animal (mm)	Depth back from manger (incl. manger width) (m)
6 months old	4	600	6
1 year old	6	680	8
2 years old	7	680	10
Bullocks (dehorned)	9	760	12
Bullocks (horned)	12	850	14

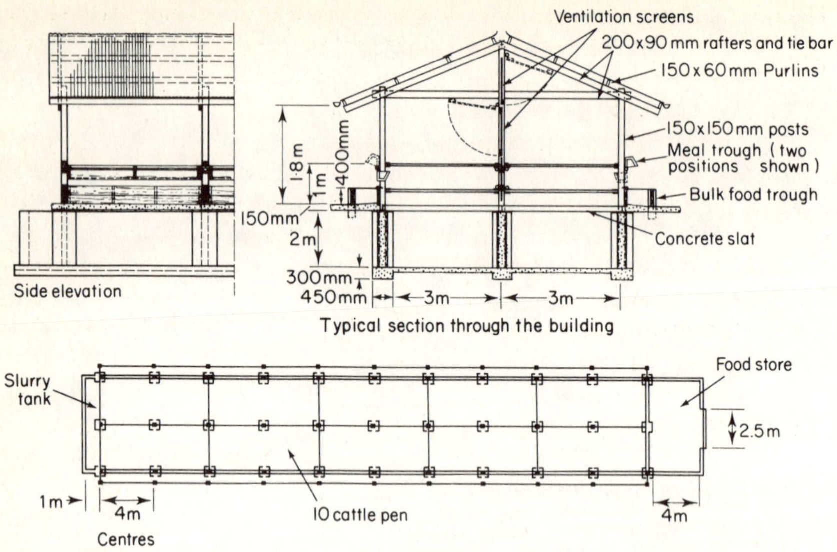

Fig. 12.2 Slatted floor–beef house.

Stores can be quite successfully out-wintered if there is no risk of poaching the ground and sufficient natural shelter is available. However, in most districts it is essential to house stock for at least some part of the winter.

Beef cattle can be satisfactorily housed on slatted floors, and there are now many slatted floor units in use. They have been found suitable both for young stock and fattening cattle (Fig. 12.2), given correct density of stocking and spacing of slats, and provided that the building is well ventilated and free from draughts. Advantages claimed are economies in bedding and space, and the quietness and cleanliness of stock. Slats can be installed in existing buildings and, as density of stocking on slats can be much heavier, more animals can be housed within the same area. The structural requirements for new buildings will be similar to those for cow yards, although warmer temperatures may be necessary, in which case some form of roof insulation and controlled ventilation will have to be installed.

Soutar[3] has suggested dimensions of slats and areas for various classes of stock, these figures being applicable to both hardwood and concrete slats:

Table 12.2 *Dimensions for slatted floor units*

Class of stock	Area per beast (m^2)	Slat size (mm)	Gap between slats (mm)	Trough space per beast (mm)
Calves (up to 4 months)	1.1	50–38	32	380
Yearlings	1.4–1.8	100–75	38	380–510
Beef steers and heifers (over 508 kg)	1.8–2.3	130–100	38	600
Cows	3.2–3.7	130–100	38	600–750

The most suitable dimensions for suckler cows and calves have not yet been found, but in the light of existing knowledge recommendations would be for an area of 3.7 m^2 of slats together with a solid floor calf creep of 0.7–0.9 m^2 per calf. Slat size would be 100 mm slats with a gap of 33 mm.

Because of the high rate of stocking more control of the environment is essential. Full stocking ensures the cleanliness of the slats; if stock numbers fall below the optimum it will be necessary to shut off some part of the yard. The use of slats can assist in increasing stocking. Another new method of keeping beef animals is to use a cubicle system, as shown in Fig. 12.3, which has the advantages of economy of space and bedding and is a system of great popularity with its most enthusiastic followers.

BULL BEEF

The confirmation by experimentation that entire bulls put on weight more efficiently and quickly than steers suggests that increasing numbers of animals of this type will be reared. However, there are greater dangers to the stockman with this system and it is advocated that the bulls are kept in small groups of about 8–10 only. Once the group has been established they must not be changed.

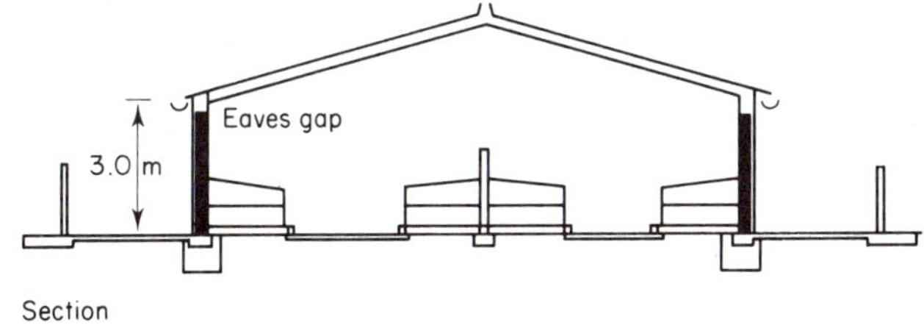

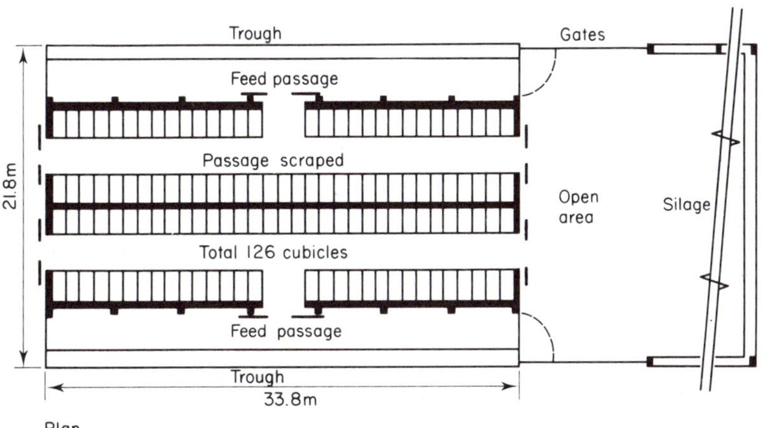

Fig. 12.3 Beef feeding house with cubicles and self-feed silage.

Pen divisions must be especially strong and at least 1.5 m high and adjustable if there is a build-up of muck. Walls must be stronger too; for example, reinforced 225 mm concrete blocks or 255 mm brickwork are satisfactory arrangements with piers at 2.4 m intervals. Gates and doors must be childproof, and consideration should be given to the provision of refuge areas in pens and a 'squeeze-way' into or out of the pen sufficient in size for the stockman only. Feeding and bedding servicing should be carried out from outside the pens.

BABY BEEF

This system, which can provide an additional enterprise on dairy farms, meets a demand by butcher and consumer – a finished beast of 432–457 kg at about 12 months old. Success is dependent on obtaining the right type of calf and adopting an early weaning system. Intensive and specialist buildings are not essential for this type of enterprise, although the usual conditions for the health of the animals are required. With this system, which utilizes barley as the main ingredient of the ration, it is usual to house the stock from birth to slaughter, and many animals are successfully kept in the slatted floor layouts previously mentioned. In big units there can be a serious risk of disease build-up unless the rearing unit is periodically rested. This system can be successfully used with Friesians or Friesian-cross with a beef breed.

For the veal trade, in addition to Friesians and Shorthorns, Ayrshire calves and suitable crosses of these breeds are satisfactory.[4] Calves are ready for slaughter from about 113–136 kg liveweight, and should reach this weight in up to 14–15 weeks. As the calf is growing rapidly, more specialized housing is required than for baby or barley beef. Warmth and controlled ventilation are important. It is an advantage to keep calves singly or in small groups to avoid vices such as sucking navels and licking each other. Crates, with slatted floors and sides of three-ply or other suitable material, have been used quite successfully. The timber work should be creosoted at least once a year to act as a disinfectant (see Chapter 6).

TOPLESS CUBICLES

The arrangement of providing cubicles for cattle without a roof has had a limited following in all parts of the United Kingdom but more especially in the southwest. Topless cubicles are chiefly used for wintering fattening and store cattle and beef cows (though dairy heifers are also held this way). Their main advantages are that the structure is cheap, there is a saving on bedding, and the beasts keep free from respiratory disease. Management can be simplified with easy feeding arrangements and adequate slurry disposal. The stockman has poor working conditions with this system and there are risks for the stock during the worst blizzards of the winter, but in the several years of their use they have given generally good results.

An essential feature is the construction of a suitable bed which must remain well drained under the wettest conditions. There are two methods used to cope with this. Either the bed is solid with a good fall to drain off all liquids, or it is made porous so the liquids drain through. The most favoured system is the latter which consists of a base of large stones, topped with 37 mm graded stone about 75 mm thick. This is then covered with sand, shavings, straw or sawdust. The whole site should have a good layer of hardcore underneath, not less than 300 mm deep. Land drains should be laid under the cubicles parallel to the dung passage to take away liquid seeping through.

All those who have used topless cubicles have stressed the importance of placing them on a sheltered site; if a natural shelter of trees or buildings is available so much the better, otherwise an artificial windbreak should be constructed round the cubicles. This should be about 2 m high and made of a solid wall or fence or of spaced boarding.

REFERENCES

1 MAFF (1970) *Beef Production*. Bulletin No. 178. London: HMSO.
2 Loynes, I. J. (1985) Suckler cows – housing the single suckler herd. *Farm Buildings & Engineering*. Vol. 2, No. 3.
3 Soutar, D. (1962) Design for beef. *Farmers Weekly*, 30 November.
4 Shillam, K. W. G. (1961) *Veal Production*. National Inst. for Research in Dairying. Paper 2419.

FURTHER READING

Allen, D. M. and Kilkenny, J. B. (1984) *Planned Beef Production*. London: Collins.
Beef Cattle Housing (1973) *Proceedings of Farm Buildings Staff Seminar*. Craibstone, Aberdeen.
Beef Housing Manual (1978) Stoneleigh, Warwickshire. Farm Buildings Information Centre.
Bowden, W. E. (1962) *Beef Breeding, Production and Marketing*. Land Books.
Cooper, M. McG. and Willis, M. B. (1972) *Profitable Beef Production*. Ipswich: Farming Press.
Fraser, A. (1959) *Beef Cattle Husbandry*. London: Crosby Lockwood.
McFarlane, D. (1966) *The Intensive Housing of Cattle for Beef Production*. Stoneleigh, Warwickshire. Farm Buildings Information Centre.

13

The Housing of Pigs

FARROWING ACCOMMODATION

Full details of the climatic requirements of the sow and piglet have been given in Chapter 3 where it was emphasized that the modern sow as we have bred her is a clumsy mother, so that a protective crate or other device is considered essential to prevent her cumbersome movements crushing the piglets. At the same time, the piglets must be encouraged to spend their resting periods away from the immediate proximity of the sow, and this is best done by providing nests close to the crate or as part of the crate itself. Ideally, artificial heat and light sources should be placed above or around the nest to attract and warm the piglets. Also, the pigman must keep a watchful eye on the sow and piglets over the farrowing period and it is therefore essential to provide easy inspection facilities.

For all these reasons the totally enclosed specialized farrowing house is preferred. Nevertheless, every farmer should be aware of the error of making the house too big. Sows and piglets need hygienic surroundings, which mean that an essential requirement is periodic depopulation, and disinfection of the building. Also sows need quiet surroundings and this is achieved far more satisfactorily in the smaller building. The aim is to have a unit of a maximum of 16–20 pens within a building, and preferably less. But the limiting factor is that it must be small enough to be emptied of all stock regularly.

The farrowing crate unit

The simplest farrowing crate consists of a pair of three parallel rails. The top rails are set 530 mm apart, as also are the centre rails. The bottom rails are 750–800 mm apart, depending on the type of sow and to allow adequate room where she lies down. The bottom rails are a minimum of 250 mm from the floor and the second row is 300 mm above the bottom row and 300 mm below the top. Thus the crate has a total height of 850 mm from the floor. There are escape nests on each side, a minimum of 530 mm wide. Thus the total width of the crate is 1.6–1.65 m, or with dividing walls approximately 1.8 m. The walls at the outside of the nests and at the front of the crate can be solid, and there is a gate at the back for access by the sow and the attendant. On the inside of this gate there should be a semi-circular metal bar 250 mm from the base extending 230 mm inside the gate. This will prevent the sow backing right up against the gate and crushing the piglets. In many crates the position of the bottom rail is adjustable to allow for variations in height and width, depending on the size of the sow. There are many proprietary crates on the market with their own unique features and the final choice made by the farmer is very much a case of individual preference (Figs. 13.1 and 13.2).

It is desirable to have a cover of plywood, hardboard or asbestos sheet over each nest to conserve heat and reduce floor draughts, and also a heat source – either an electric infra-red lamp or gas heater. Great care must be taken with the fall in the floor to make sure that any water or urine runs towards the back and away from the crate and the creep.

There are also so-called 'blow-away' units, which are designed on the principle that piglets dislike cold draughts. When the sow is standing the unit, which is fitted to the side of the farrowing crate, blows cold air under the sow. This creates a draught which the piglets find uncomfortable to lie in. The cool air blower is triggered by breaking an infra-red beam across the farrowing crate when she stands. On lying down, the sow gets out of the path of the beam and the draught stops. This allows the piglets to suckle in comfort. Being portable

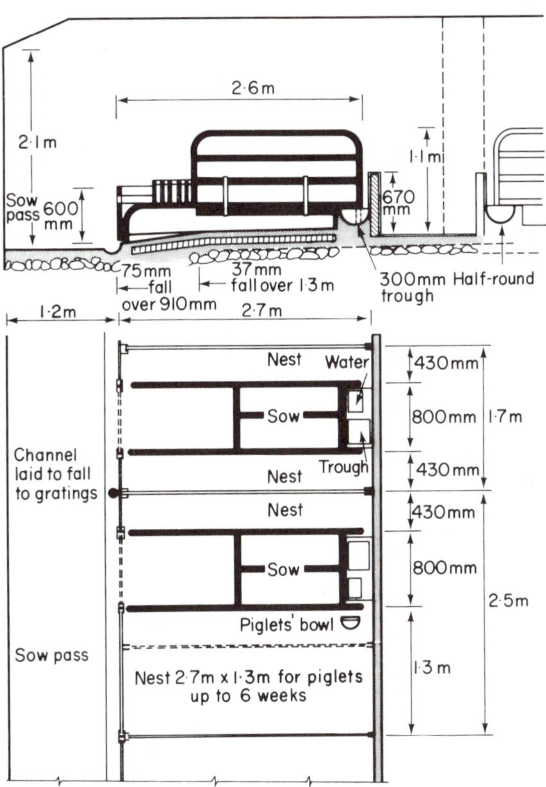

Fig. 13.1 Pitmillan-type farrowing pen.

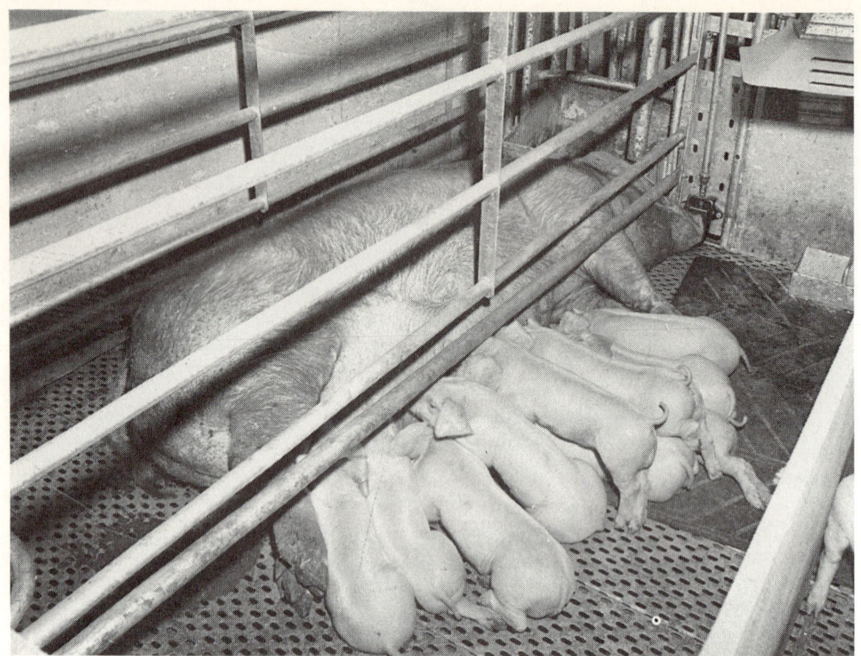

Fig. 13.2 Fully slatted farrowing crate using punched steel.

the unit is moved from crate to crate soon after farrowing, usually 72 hours after is sufficient.

As sows vary in size, the gate at the back of the crate is sometimes made to fit in a number of runners situated at distances measuring from the front 2.3 m, 2.2 m and 2.1 m. Another refinement is to have several metal bars across the top of the crate to prevent the sow rearing up. This fitting is best left portable so that the bars can be used as and when required.

As the sow may not be in a crate more than 14 days, it is not considered important for her to have exercise. Indeed, many of the most successful units consist of a row of crates, single- or double-sided, with a feeding passage in the front and a small passage for cleaning and movement of the pigs at the back. To ensure easy access to the creep to attend to the piglets, the walls adjoining this portion need be only 530–600 mm high to retain the piglets.

The most popular type of farrowing units are based on the Ritchie farrowing crates in Pitmillan type pens (Fig. 13.1). These are fixed crates with creep areas on each side with low walls allowing easy access to the piglets. The nests are 430 mm wide on each side. If the piglets are removed early before there is feeding in the creep, or if the latter is to take place, the creep on one side is increased to 1.3 m. Sows and litters may be kept in this accommodation up to six weeks after farrowing. It should also be mentioned that some farmers prefer the piglet creep to be in front of the sow; this has the merit of encouraging the piglets to an even safer position and also making inspection and handling easier.

Slatted-floor farrowing pens

There has more recently been a considerable following for farrowing pens with either part-slatted (perforated) or entirely slatted (perforated) flooring. In the case of the latter a suitable slat has been either a 75 mm or 100 mm concrete one with a normal gap of 12–20 mm but with an enlarged gap of 20–28 mm in a 0.18 m^2 area behind the sow. For the first week after farrowing, the area behind the sow is covered with expanded metal to prevent the baby pigs catching their feet in the gap (Fig. 13.3).

Two forms of part-slatted pens have been tried with success. In one case 75 mm slats have been used with 12 mm gaps and the rear half of the pens only is slatted. In the other case a similar area is used but with expanded metal, 44 mm long and 12 mm across, with the grid supported every 25 mm by metal cross-pieces. It is best to use galvanized metal. Those who have used this system have established the importance of keeping the piglets, and indeed the sow, warm since there is no bedding, or at the most a modest amount for the piglets in the early stages. It is also especially important if concrete is used, that the slats should be impeccably finished, otherwise both the sows and the piglets will suffer. The most recent innovation for slatted floors is to use panels of polypropylene plastic which give a very 'kind' surface finish for the pigs.

One very useful method of satisfying the requirement for a slatted floor farrowing arrangement consists of a raised and portable platform farrowing

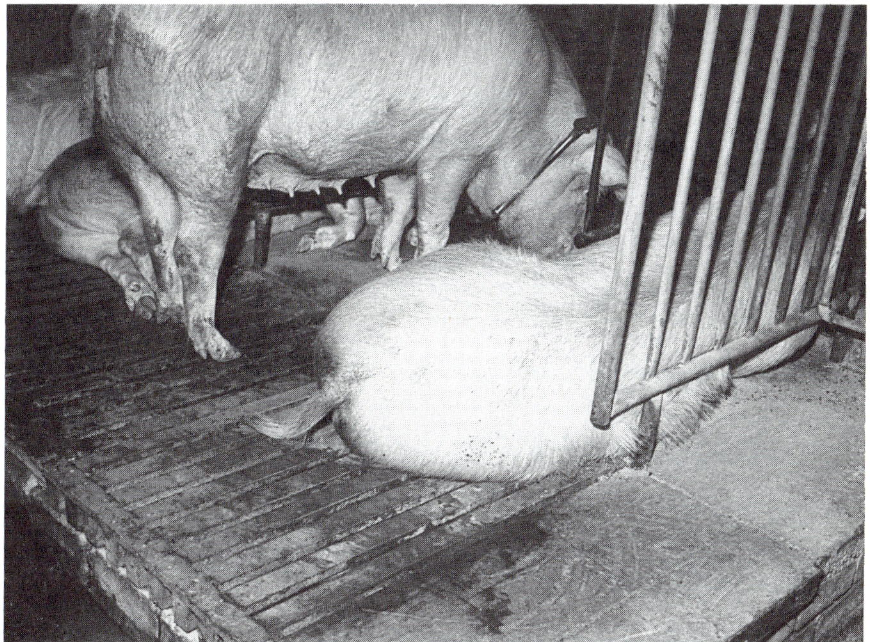

Fig. 13.3 Tethered sows on slatted floors; a popular system but with risks of injury from badly finished flooring.

unit on tubular steel legs. The floor is perforated except for a recessed mat 20 mm thick and 1 m square under the sow's udder and with boarding in the creep box which is placed in front of the sow.

The Solari farrowing pen

A simpler approach to the farrowing and rearing of pigs is epitomized in the design that aims to keep litters warm and comfortable by providing a limited air space and freedom from draughts and keep the sow's movements under control by the judicious use of farrowing rails and a limited area for the pens.

The pens in the Solari house consist of a range of units each 1.5 m wide and 4.95 m long. The height at the back of the pen is 910 mm, rising to 2.4 m at the front. In the front there is only a wall and a door, both 1.2 m high, leaving a 1.2 m high open area above to allow free air circulation. There is a creep of 750 mm depth the whole way across the back, formed by a simple steel grille. Farrowing rails are fitted extending 1.75 m in front of the creeps and there is a space of 830 mm between them, and the sow lies voluntarily in this area. This leaves the rest of the pen for exercising, feeding and dunging (Fig. 13.4).

The rear part of the pen floor only is insulated to encourage the sow to lie in this area and there is a good fall from back to front of 130 mm. The farrowing rails are 150 mm from the floor while the side ones are 250 mm. All the equipment is easily demountable: when the pen is used for farrowing, all the equipment will be in place; after ten days the rails will be removed, leaving only the creep grille. Should it be desired to continue using the pen thereafter, the creep may also be removed.

Adaptation for porkers

An adaptation of this pen for use from birth to finishing is to place a slatted or weld-mesh area in the front which is covered during the farrowing and rearing stage but uncovered afterwards when the sow is removed. A pen can take up to 20 porkers, so the cost of this accommodation is extremely economical. Its disadvantages are that environmental controls are incomplete and labour requirements are quite heavy. Inspection and access are more difficult than in the totally enclosed house, the pigman has no protection while tending the pigs and access to the nest and creep are behind the sow and therefore more difficult.

FARROWING OUTDOORS

The easiest farrowing accommodation to manage is certainly the indoor totally enclosed unit but the merits of outdoor farrowing are not inconsiderable. In general, outdoor units are healthier, due to the isolation and they are also much cheaper in capital costs though maintenance can be high.

A hard-wearing unit for outdoor farrowing is the 'ark' shape. The Craibstone ark, designed by the Farm Buildings Department of the North of Scotland

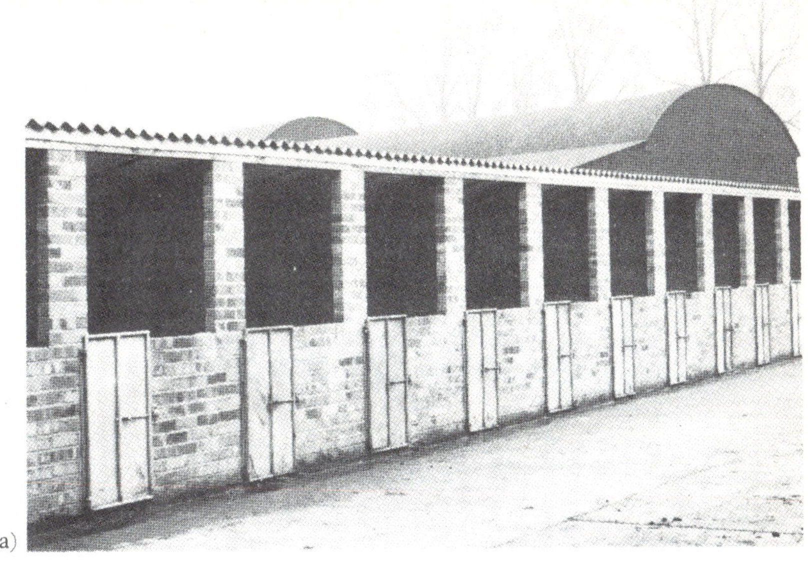

(a)

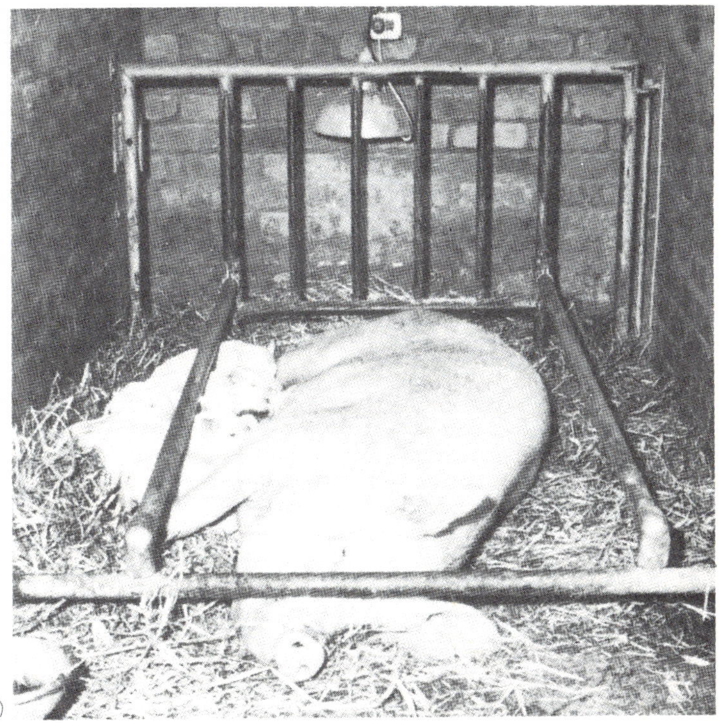

(b)

Fig. 13.4 The Solari farrowing and rearing pen: (a) exterior, (b) interior.

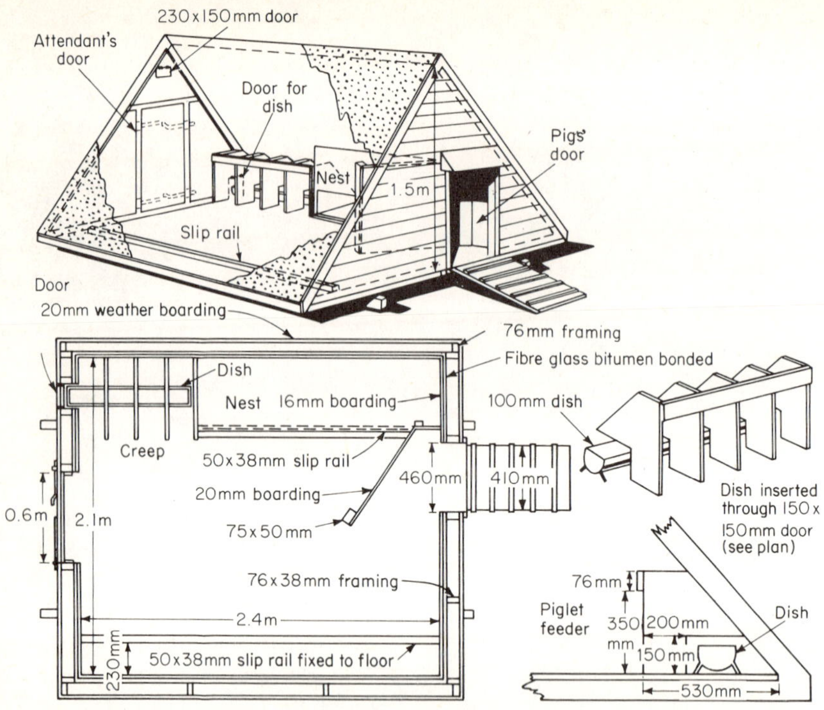

Fig. 13.5 The Craibstone ark. An excellent design for outdoor rearing.

College of Agriculture, is an excellent example. Dimensions are 2.4 m long, 2.1 m wide and 1.5 m high (see Fig. 13.5). The shape of the hut itself forms an escape for the piglets where the roof meets the floor and it is also a shape that makes for economy and rigidity. Some of the essential features of outdoor farrowing huts, of which several types exist, are well shown in this hut and should be incorporated in any farrowing unit.

The first essential is sound, two-skin construction which ensures warmth and freedom from draughts. Next, really good baffling is placed inside the door to deflect wind from the nest. All huts must incorporate a nest and creep feeding and watering arrangements when the building is to be used for rearing. To keep the piglets warm in their nest, straw is packed on top of it or artificial heating is commonly provided by the use of portable gas heaters.

Access to the sow and litter is by a door at the back, 600 mm wide at least, and 1.05 mm high. The fittings on the door must be extremely tight fitting to give a complete seal when closed. In the Craibstone ark there is also a small observation door up to 300 mm square in the back that is used for quiet inspection without disturbing the sow. It is usual to fit wooden battens to the floor 50 mm wide and 37 mm deep along the sides, 230 mm from the edge to prevent the sow's feet jamming the piglets against the wall and causing them injury.

Rectangular hut with creep

Another common type of farrowing hut is of rectangular shape and measures 2.4 m long and 1.65 m wide with a further 600 mm extension at the back to form the special creep. The height at the front is 1.2 m graduating to 910 mm at the back. As well as baffle doorways, creeps and nests, there must also be a farrowing rail 250 mm from the floor and 250 mm from the wall. With both farrowing huts and arks there may be a fold unit in front, usually about 3.6 m long. Alternatively the sows may run in paddocks or very occasionally be tethered. To inspect the pigs the roof may be constructed to be raised or may slide open.

There are also some circular farrowing huts with central creeps and nests which have been popular, especially in New Zealand, for many years.

MULTI-SUCKLING PENS

One of the major problems of pig husbandry is the serious check that takes place when piglets are weaned and mixed at the same time. One approach is the farrow-to-finish pen where pigs are taken from birth to finishing in the same pen. Another, known as the multi-suckling pen, is to mix 3–5 sows and litters together, usually at about three weeks of age, and thereby form a 'weaner pool' which includes the dams. After about two weeks the sows are removed and the group of 30–50 weaners are left for a further period, nearly always ad lib feeding, until ready for the finishing stages of fattening.

There is no doubt that weaners mix much better if they are still receiving their mother's milk. Considerable flexibility is possible with the housing, which may be totally enclosed or yarded. Successful examples are shown in Figs 13.6 and 13.7, the first being an open-front yard and the second a totally enclosed, deep-strawed building.

Minimum specifications are as follows. Adequate space, at least 6 m^2 for each sow and litter. Plenty of bedding is preferable under most systems and a large creep for the piglets of not less than 0.2 m^2 per piglet gives plenty of food and water space. The creep should also be warmed and covered in the usual way. Individual feeders for the sows are recommended wherever possible, but they are such a costly item that they may have to be dispensed with. Both the designs shown can be tractor-cleaned, the yards by access from the front after the feeders are removed and the totally enclosed pen by access from the side after removing the pen divisions when each batch has gone through. At present the multi-suckling system is less popular in the pig industry in general but continues to be practised by a large number of enthusiasts in many areas of the world who appreciate the intrinsic merits of the system.

EARLY WEANING ACCOMMODATION

Weaning at 21 days or sometimes a day or two younger is now successfully carried out. Under the correct environment and housing conditions the

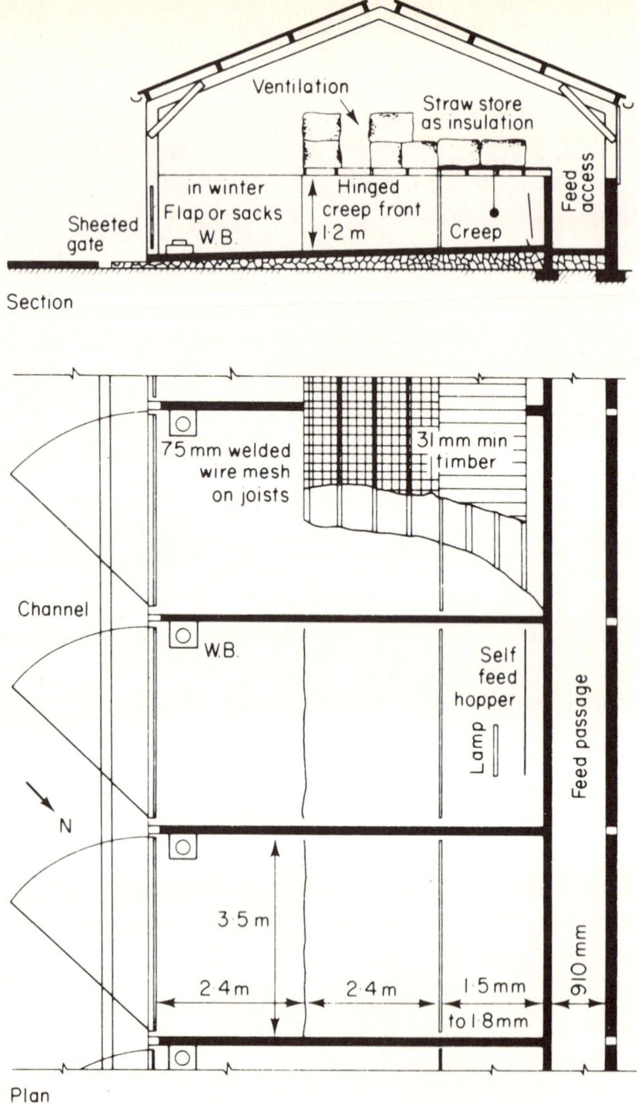

Fig. 13.6 Weaner pools and yards for four sows and litters (floor-fed sow cobs).

predictably uniform growth of the piglets represents a very notable advance in pig husbandry techniques and the sow will be able to produce more than two litters per annum.

It must be strongly emphasized that at three weeks of age the piglet's resistance to infection is lower than at any other time in its life, since it has lost most of the 'passive' immunity it had from its mother either *in utero* or via the colostrum,

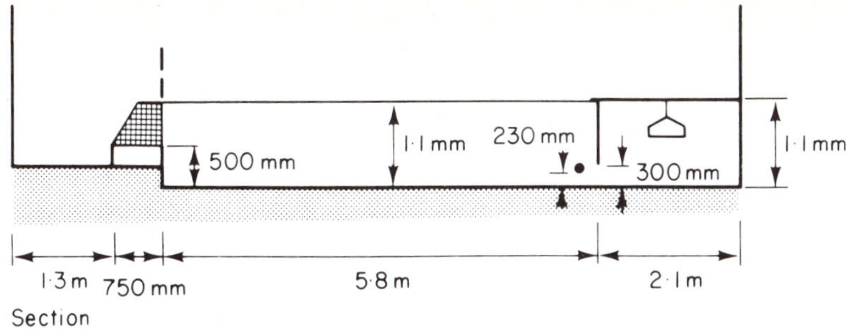

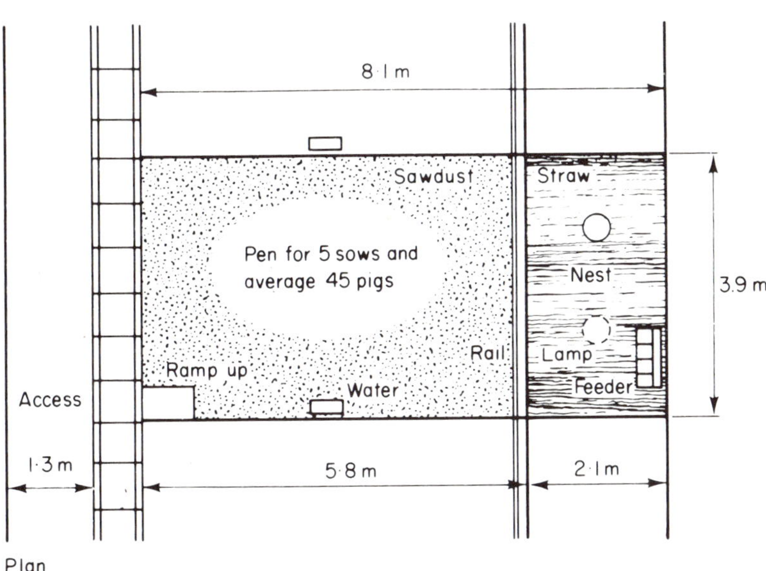

Fig. 13.7 Scottish design of rearing pen for five sows and litters.

and yet has not developed the 'active' immunity which will be produced later. The need to 'batch' groups of piglets through an early weaning unit on an all-in, all-out arrangement is essential and helps to ensure that the groups are not too large.

The second essential for piglets weaned at three weeks is that they are reared on as clean a floor surface as possible with a system that ensures they have as near absolute freedom from pollution by their own dung and urine. This implies that the lying areas must be absolutely clean and the dunging area, if separate, should be either perforated or, if solid, should be so frequently cleaned that the chances of pollution are minimal or, as some farmers have practised for many years, the piglets are reared on a deep bed of straw which is constantly 'topped-up' to keep the floor warm, dry, dung-free and comfortable.

Provided that the above essentials are satisfied, systems using a completely perforated floor (the 'flat deck' system) or partly solid and perforated or all-solid flooring with or without bedding, can be utilized. Thirdly, the temperature should initially be about 24°C but whilst it is acceptable for it to be a little lower (between 21° and 27°C) at this stage, the more important issue is to keep it uniform. In practice, the question of air movement is almost as critical as that of the temperature. The air movement rate suggested in Table 3.1 is low, and since some ventilation should be maintained at all times, this can only be achieved with the utmost care in the design and control of the ventilation system itself.

In 'flat deck' systems for early weaning as opposed to the kennel arrangement, heating will be used. For cheapness of running costs gas is usually chosen and the regulation system should be linked with that of the fans to make sure they act in unison.

The correct procedure is to let the fans operate thermostatically down to a minimum setting which will correspond to the minimum given in Table 13.1. Then, if the temperature tends to fall below the optimum temperature artificial heat should be switched on with the thermostat to keep the temperature at the right level and the ventilation will be safely operating at the minimum level.

THE KENNEL SYSTEM

There is a choice between two major systems – either the kennel and outdoor verandah, or the all-indoor (Figs. 13.8 & 13.9). The former has a solid bed and usually a perforated floor for the verandah. The kennel and verandah was the first system developed and represented a major breakthrough, since it is a technique which gives reasonably consistent results. Its advantages are considerable: low-cost housing; isolation between small groups; warmth without artificial

Table 13.1 *Lower critical temperatures for housed livestock*

Type of livestock	*°C**
Adult cattle	0
Young calves	15
Farrowing sows	15
Newly born piglets	27
Fatteners	18
Adult poultry	7
Broilers, 3–7 weeks	16
Day-old chicks to 3 weeks	21

*Air temperatures below which intensively housed livestock should not be allowed to go.

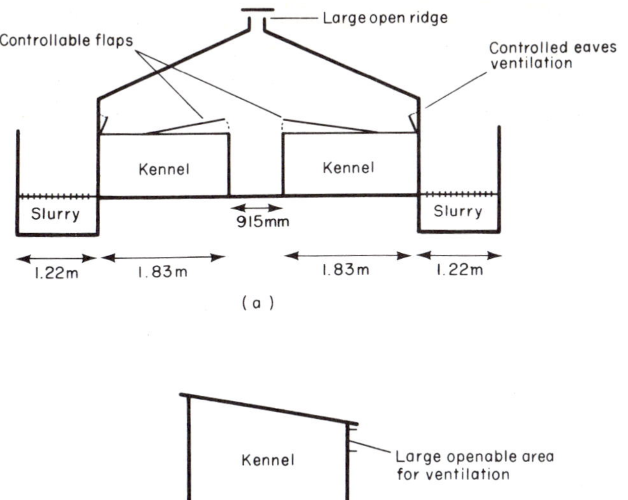

Fig. 13.8 Kennels for early weaning: (a) covered kennel housing, natural ventilation; (b) outside kennels, natural ventilation.

heating and ventilation; good muck disposal from the pigs, ensuring the essential criteria of separation of pigs and muck. Nevertheless, the system has disadvantages. In order to ensure warmth the piglets do need to be penned closely; if this is in any way done at all excessively it can lead to uneven growth and difficult inspection. The variation in the environment, which is inevitable in housing like this between the different seasons, means that careful and individual care of the kennels is required.

Perhaps the most important feature to emphasize is the need to be able to control ventilation adequately in all kennel arrangements. With the outdoor kennel there must be ventilators at the rear to give controlled air flow, especially in the hot weather, while for the kennel placed inside a covered yard not only should there be ventilation from top flaps on the kennel, but also the house itself should be well ventilated.

A critical factor in the successful rearing of pigs from three weeks onwards is achieving the correct balance between the numbers in the group and the space they are allowed. Many trials have been conducted on pigs of all ages and in summary they have shown (1) over-stocking retards growth; (2) small groups do better than large ones; and (3) the litter group is the ideal. Therefore if the benefits that are undoubtedly obtainable by three-week weaning are to be realized, it is essential that the very large groups which are often seen should be avoided. Indeed they form probably the most frequent basis of criticism of

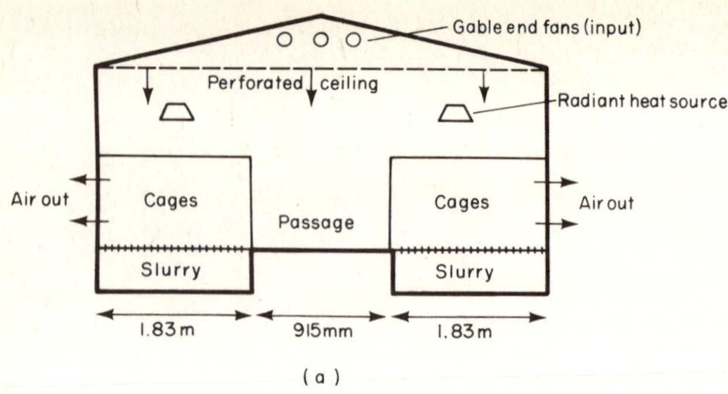

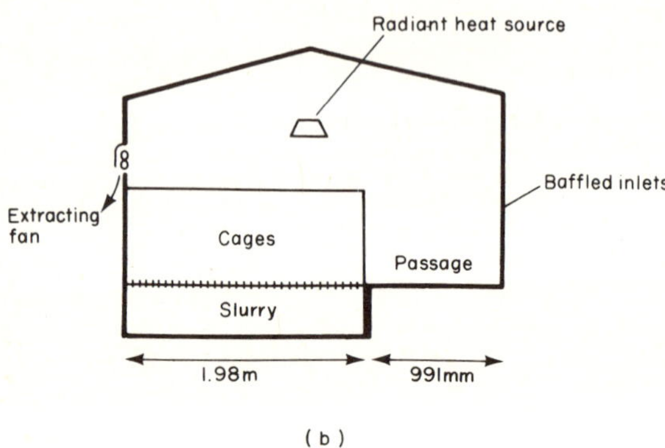

Fig. 13.9 Two-deck cage systems for early weaning: (a) double row pressurized; (b) single row extraction.

such housing. This is especially common in the kennel arrangement since it is here there is an in-built temptation to crowd the pigs in large groups in low-roofed kennels to ensure a high temperature. For example, it is not uncommon to have 50 piglets in one pen, but the troubles they can produce range from uneven growth, poor food conversion and vices such as tail biting to scour, pneumonia and rhinitis. In general, while a small group is ideal and often obtainable with flat decks, up to 25 seem perfectly acceptable, with the absolute necessity where larger numbers are used, of providing rather more space to compensate. The optimum total floor area should be approximately 10 kg liveweight of pig to each 0.1 m^2 of floor space. If the flooring is partly solid and partly perforated, then the living area may be reduced by about 25 per cent, but an extra area for dunging must be added on top of this.

The 'flat deck' house (*Figs. 13.10 & 13.11*)

The relative simplicity of the 'flat deck' totally perforated floor has much to commend it since it can ensure a completely clean floor. There are four main

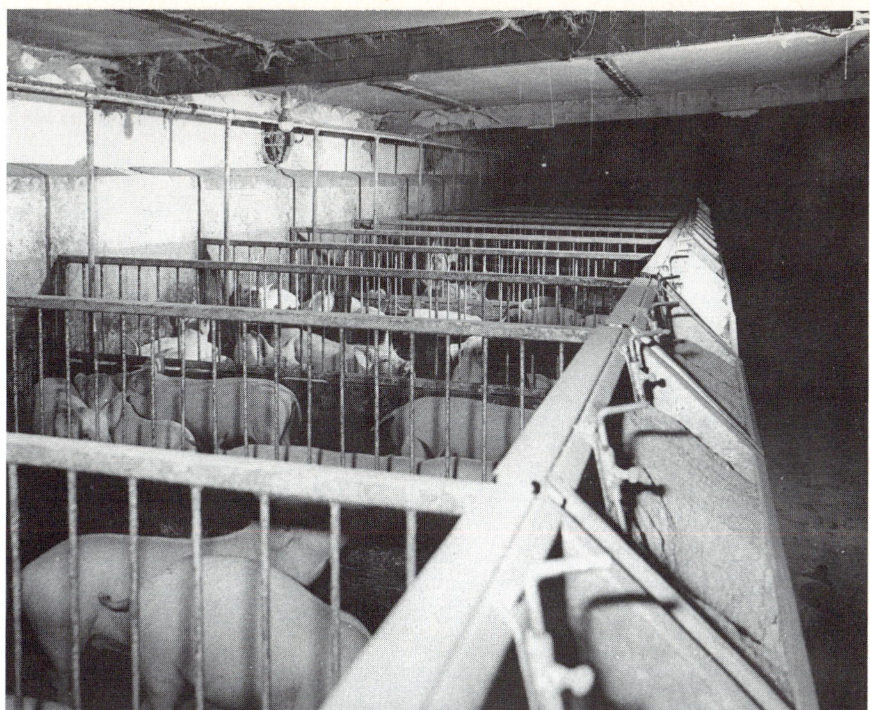

Fig. 13.10 Flat-deck cage for early weaning.

types of flooring so used. Punch-perforated steel floors with a very smooth finish are costly but kind on the pigs' feet and can be long-lasting. A cheaper flooring is expanded metal.

The welded mesh floor has the biggest area of void and is probably the cleanest but can be the least comfortable and most damaging, whereas the perforated steel floor has the largest solid area, may be a little dirtier, but is usually the most comfortable. In all cases galvanizing of the steel has the advantage that it greatly increases the life of the metal floor, which will otherwise not last many years. The most recent floor is one of polypropylene plastic and this is proving most successful so far. A trough space of 100 mm per pig is sufficient with one drinker per ten pigs. Whilst nipple drinkers are perfectly satisfactory, it is an added advantage if, for the first few days, there is a water trough with more accessible water.

Cage rearing

A few pig farmers rear piglets away from the sow from about seven days. Piglets are grouped by weight, nine at a time, in cages of three, four or five tiers high. Each cage measures 1200 mm long × 600 mm wide and 390 mm high and has a floor of 12 mm × 12 mm × 12 gauge wire mesh or plastic. Such cages are placed

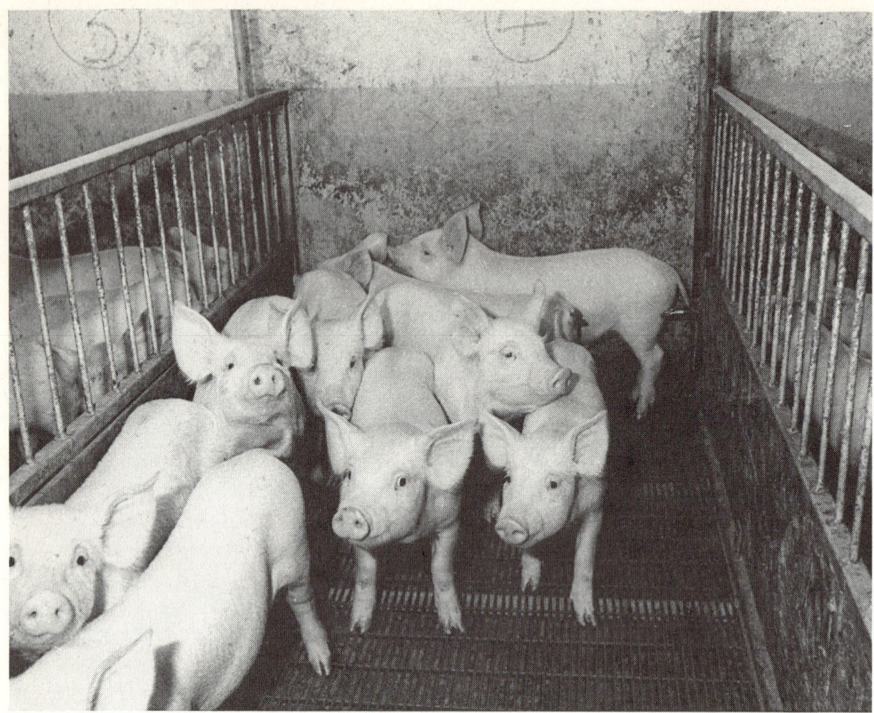

Fig. 13.11 Close-up of 'flat-deck' cage pen with wire floor.

in housing kept at 27°C and in subdued light. The piglets remain here until about 7 kg weight, after which they are usually moved to flat deck cages.

FATTENING ACCOMMODATION

The totally enclosed house

While there are several fundamentally different forms of piggery for the fattening stages in the pig's life, probably overall the most popular is the totally enclosed piggery, where the environment is under complete control and all attendance to the pigs is under cover. A basis of design and the most familiar world-wide is the Danish-style layout (see Fig. 13.12). It consists of a central feeding passage 1.2 m wide, side dunging passages 1.05 m and a pen of 3 × 1.8 m, to hold 10–12 pigs to bacon weight. This conventional arrangement is probably the most expensive in layout and cubic area per pig of all designs but it remains an adaptable design and is particularly suitable for the small pig keeper. It has the advantage that the pigs are kept in small groups and management can be of a high standard. Feeding is simple and can be carried out easily with a trolley or overhead conveyor; dung cleaning may be by hand or squeegee, or by mechanical

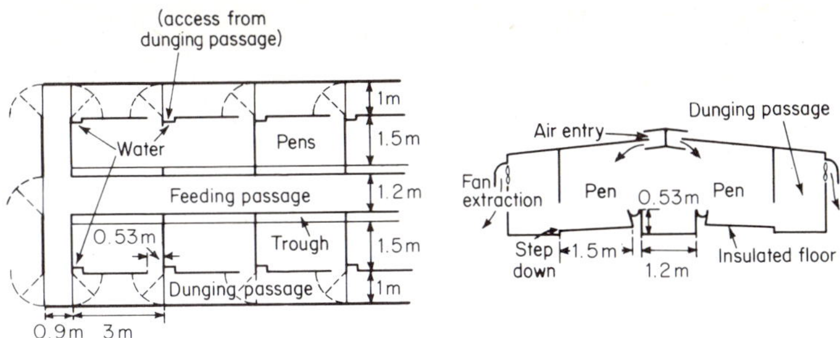

Fig. 13.12 Danish-type fattening house with screened-off dunging passage.

means. Straw may or may not be used, as desired. It is advisable to screen off the dunging passage from the pens, leaving only a pop-hole between the pen and the passage. This greatly improves environmental control as the pigs in effect lie in a building within a building. In such a design, making use of good insulation and mechanical ventilation taking in fresh air from the ridge, temperatures within the range 20–25°C may readily be maintained. Only the central part of the house needs complete insulation. It is always best to place a number of complete partitions across a Danish-type piggery and aim to have not more than 200 pigs within a common air space and 800–1000 pigs in one building.

Wide-span totally enclosed house

In an important attempt to produce a more economical piggery, though of the same basic layout, and where trough feeding is required, a wider span building may be employed by running the troughs between the pens. In the Danish layout the cross-section is approximately 7.9 m, 2.1 m being taken up by the dunging passage, 3.9 m by the pens and trough and 1.2 m by the feeding passage, making, with the walls, a total of 7.9 m. If, however, a wider span of 13.3 m is used, the dunging passages may each be 1.5 m, making 3 m in all, the central service passage may be 1.2 m and the pen depth may be 4–5 m on each side to take 15 pigs to bacon weight. The depth of the pen behind the trough may be 1.7 m, the trough 300 mm and the catwalk serving the trough 300 mm (see Fig. 13.13). The economy of this design is apparent when it is noted that whereas in each metre length of a Danish house six pigs can be kept, in each metre of this type the number of pigs is double. When automatic floor feeding systems are used, no trough is needed and with any automatic feeding systems the catwalks between the pens may be omitted. The extra space will allow for 1–2 extra pigs per pen. A popular modification is to make the dunging passage 2.1 m wide to allow tractor cleaning.

Central dunging passage

In order to reduce labour or activities associated with dung cleaning, the installation of one centre passage, rather than a centre feeding passage, allowing

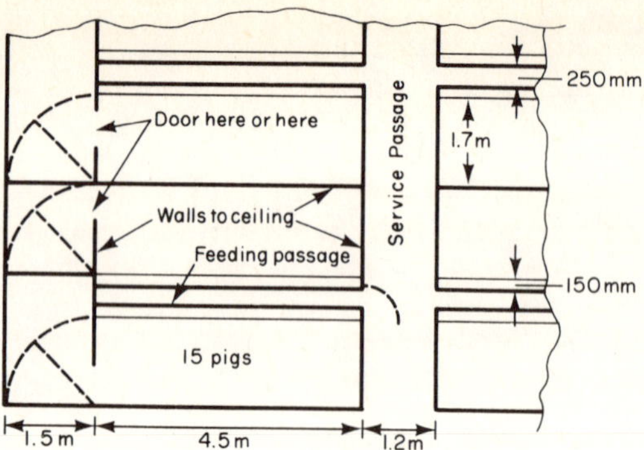

Fig. 13.13 Fattening house suitable for large unit, built as single- or double-sided unit.

access by the pigs from each pen to half the length of the passage opposite their pen, is an improvement on the traditional design (Fig. 13.14).

Ventilation can be quite simply by extraction of stale air over the dunging passage. It is noteworthy that the pigs have no contact at all with the outside walls of the house; this is quite an important point as the floors may well be warmer, much heat being lost laterally from the pig when it lies against the outside wall of a building. Nowadays, too, it has some real advantages, as many houses will be made out of prefabricated design, and lighter and less robust walling can be used although it will, of course, be well-insulated and vapour-sealed as in any other design. Also, with a centre passage there is considerable saving in cost; instead of two runs of dung passage there is only one, and the cost of this is little more than half, as the width need be increased only slightly.

Floor feeding with over-pen catwalk

This design has lent itself to further economies in building costs by the elimination of the side feeding passage. This is a very attractive proposition as it reduces the width of the buildings by over 2 m.

Feeding can be carried out by installing catwalks over the pens at the height of the pen division. A design of this type can be fitted into buildings of many shapes and sizes. For example, a single-sided unit could fit into a building as narrow as 3.6 m with 1.05 m dunging passage and 2.4 × 2.7 m pens, taking 15 pigs to bacon weight. At the other extreme pens could be 3.5 × 1.8 m taking up to 20 pigs in a building of approximately 10 m span. Units of this type are clearly suited in particular to adaptation in irregular-shaped buildings, and have especially useful application to those farmers using automated feeding systems of any type, but such is the concentration of pigs that they require a very high standard of husbandry.

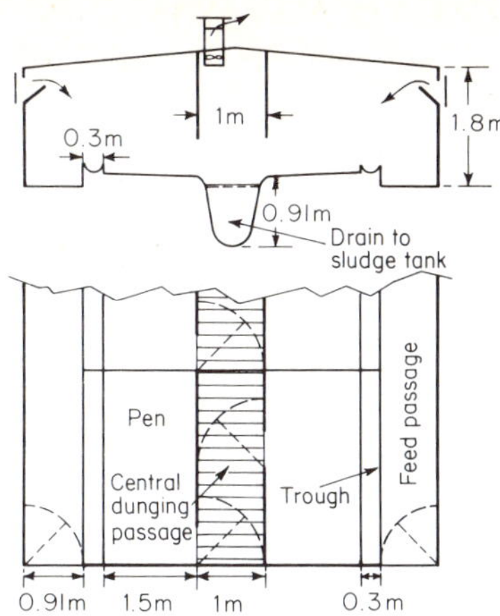

Fig. 13.14 House with centre dunging passage, using slatted floor.

Totally slatted floor

Pioneered in Scandinavia, the fattening piggery with totally slatted floors has a strong following. Although relatively expensive it is simple to manage and eliminates a major problem in slatted dung passage arrangements of persuading the pigs to dung in the right place. An excellent Scottish design is shown in Fig. 13.15. This not only incorporates four slurry channels and pens of modest size (400 pigs in 20 pens) but also has a pressurized ventilation system that moves the air from an overhead duct, then over the pigs to under the slats and thence out.

The Jordan system

A method of housing pigs that is economical and cuts across many of our preconceived ideas of what constitutes a good environment for pigs was evolved by Mr J. Jordan of Northern Ireland. The design was originally produced primarily as an aid of relieving respiratory distress in pigs and the secondary result has been that pigs have been found to thrive generally under such conditions.

The design consists of a row of buildings, like a row of loose boxes, closed all round except for a half-heck doorway in front and also a window area alongside the door and under the eaves of approximately 0.74 m^2. This is fitted with sliding glass panes. The construction is uninsulated, the roof and walls being of 100 mm thick reinforced concrete. Under such conditions the condensation can be enormous but this constitutes what is considered an essential part of the system. The ideal floor area for the building is 2.4 m frontage and 4.8 m depth, making a total floor area of 11.9 m^2 and being sufficient for 20–25 pigs. The floor is given a considerable fall from front to back of 150 mm and in the front of the pen, running right across the front, is a 600 mm-wide slatted floor area with 750 mm-wide manure channels underneath.

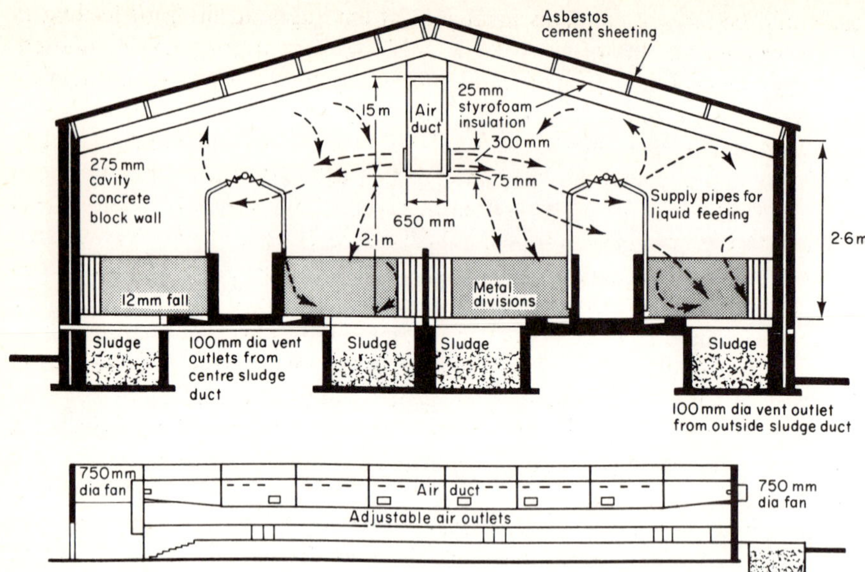

Fig. 13.15 Feeding piggery with pressurized ventilation and under-slat outlets.

The cost of housing pigs on this system is favourable but it requires the greatest possible skill in management. Many of those who have tried it have failed; reports exist of pigs being killed by heatstroke and by poor control of the ventilation. Those who have copied the system and have failed usually neglected important features in management and design and those who are considering this arrangement should study the Welfare Codes (see p. 62), which deprecate any conditions which deliberately cause stress.

Stocking densities

An important question in the design of fattening accommodation is how many pigs should be penned together. The evidence is that groups of fatteners are best in lots of not more than 15–20, with 10 perhaps as the ideal.

It is essential that when pigs are lying in the pen they comfortably cover the floor, otherwise there is a considerable risk that dirty habits will develop and muck will be deposited in the pens. The problem arises as to how one can ensure this when a weaner will occupy only about $0.18\,m^2$ of floor space when recumbent, whereas a baconer occupies some $0.46\,m^2$ and a heavy pig $0.50–0.55\,m^2$. Several solutions can be offered.

One is to design a pen with a sliding front so that the area can be enlarged as the pigs grow. Another solution for baconers and 'heavies' is to have pens of two sizes, one for the growing stage from weaning to say 16 weeks and the finishing pens from 16 weeks (45 kg) to finishing. If it is desired to have 15 pigs to a pen, the area of the grower pen would be 2.4×1.8 m and the finishing pens could be 3.6 × 1.8 m. This arrangement envisages ad lib floor feeding in the grower stage and floor feeding in the finishing stage. If troughs were inserted, 12–13 pigs only could be penned under this arrangement. For bacon production two finishing pens would be needed for every grower pen.

Another arrangement is to have a weaner pool at 6–8 weeks approximately in which young pigs are placed in fairly large pens, 20–30 to a unit. They can be allowed 0.18–0.27 m^2 of lying area and kept there until 45–54 kg. At this stage the best ten are taken off to the finishing pens, when they can be divided off into well-balanced groups in the finishing pens. One such weaner pool pen may therefore serve three finishing pens. It is likely that the mixing of several litters at weaning creates a 'stress' from which the pigs may take some time to recover under intensive conditions, and it is for this reason that the deeply bedded yard with warm kennel lying area is more popular allowing up to 0.74 m^2 per pig. The same system can be used if multiple suckling is practised but without the severe weaning stress of several changes at once.

When the pigs do muck in the pens, it is always a help to clean and disinfect the floor and then place a barrier across part of the pen so that when they are lying down they really do fill the available space. The great limitation on the shape of the pen is that with pigs being trough-fed 230–380 mm of linear space has to be allowed to each pig so that pens are usually long and narrow. With floor feeding, such limitations are removed and much more economical buildings and conversions can be made but, as mentioned previously, floor feeding is often unsuccessful up to about the age when pigs reach 45 kg liveweight.

Dung disposal: enclosed piggery

In the totally enclosed piggery there are various ways of dung disposal. With solid-floor passages, the construction is cheap and the dung may be disposed of in solid or semi-solid form. Bedding may be used or not, but frequent cleaning is advisable; it cannot be considered acceptable to allow a build-up of dung inside a totally enclosed piggery as the evaporation of moisture and ammonia will make the internal atmosphere very unpleasant and the effect on the building structure undesirable.

The traditional method for a Danish piggery with solid floor and side dunging passages is to clean out with a shovel and barrow and provide trapped drains to take off the excess fluid. With such a design the dung is in solid form and bedding is optional. This method of cleaning can be mechanized by using a small horticultural cultivator with blade attachment and by pushing the muck through from end to end. While this can be used with side dunging passages, it is easier still with the arrangement of a central dunging passage and pens on each side so that there is one movement only of the machine through the piggery. An alternative is to have a solid floor dunging passage with a step down from pen to passage of 75–100 mm, omit the drains, but have a virtually flat floor so that the passage can be cleaned out with either a mechanical scraper or a squeegee that is made to fit exactly the width of the passage (Fig. 13.16). This

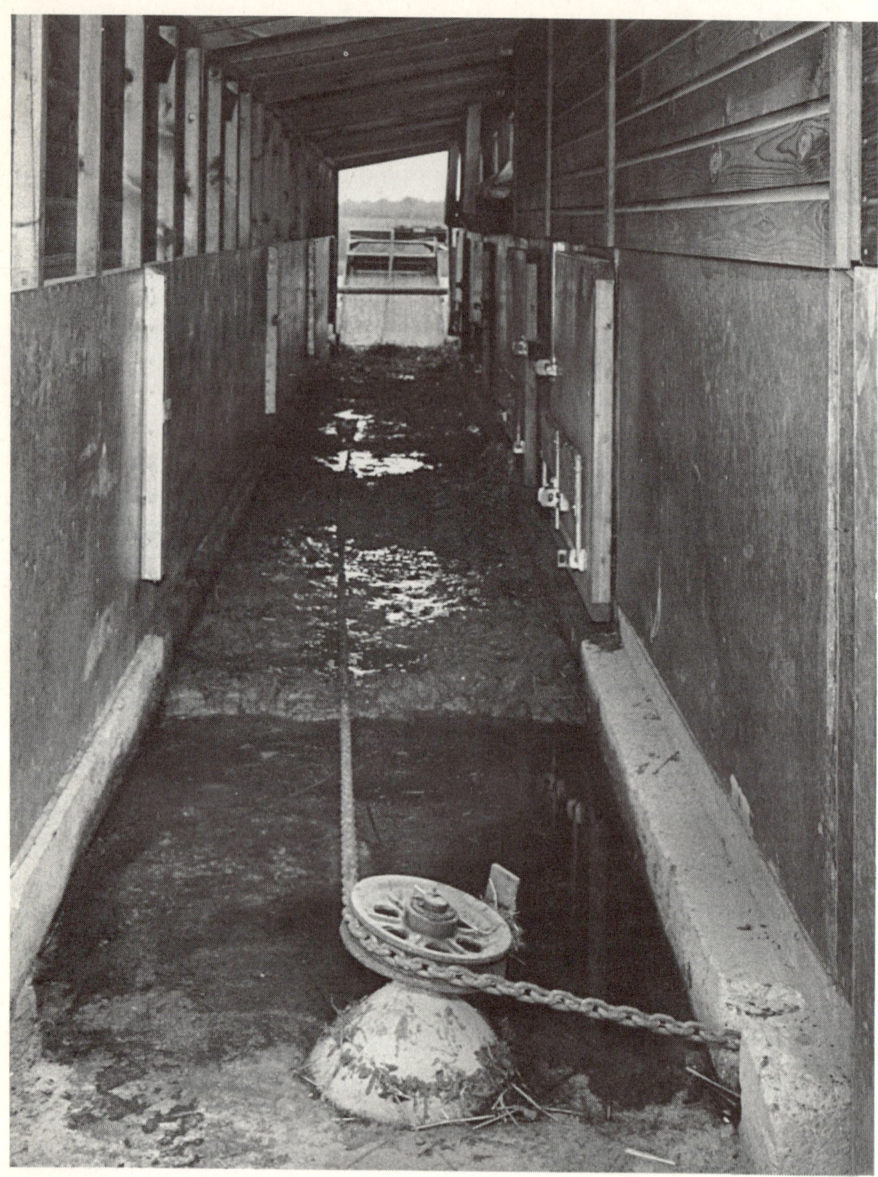

Fig. 13.16 View along a dung passage equipped with mechanical dung scraper. The scraper blade can be seen at the far end and the chain and pulley are clearly visible in the foreground. Note the dung passage is separated from the pens.

is used in piggeries without bedding or with very little and produces an end product in slurry form that can be dealt with as a liquid.

The easiest arrangement for dung disposal is the slatted floor with a channel or slurry pit underneath. Apart from its virtually automatic nature it is also probably the most hygienic, as the dung and urine pass to the channel below and have no inter-pen contact. Clean pens, however, must be maintained and research has shown that pens approximately twice as deep as they are wide favourably influence this requirement. In addition there should be a slatted area at least 910 mm or more in depth and approximately 0.55 m^2 of uninterrupted floor area for each bacon pig. Finally, the house temperature should not exceed 21°C if possible.

The slurry may be allowed to accumulate under the slats and be pumped out periodically through drainpipes fitted at intervals and opening to the outside. The pipe must be fitted with a cap to prevent draught blowing into the pen from under the slats.

In calculating the volume required for slurry, an allowance should be made of approximately 0.08 m^3 of slurry per pig per week with whey feeding (which produces the maximum) down to 0.04–0.05 m^3 per pig per week with meal feeding.

Alternatively, a drain may be placed under the slats to take the slurry to a tank at the end or ends of the building. This channel is usually 600 mm deep, 910 mm wide or less at the top, sloping to 300 mm across at the base, which may have a half-round glazed pipe. A fall between 1 : 120 and 1 : 180 is required and should not go outside the range. At the end of the channel, where it enters the tank, a sluice-gate of metal in wood runners is provided so that the sludge may be periodically run off into the tank.

Some piggeries, however, do not provide a sluice-gate and it seems to work just as effectively with slurry trickling slowly into the pit. The sludge in the tank can be dealt with in a number of ways.

Fattening piggeries with yards

Whilst the totally enclosed fattening house represents the most popular choice at present and provides designs of general application throughout the country, under some circumstances piggeries with outside or covered yards may be strongly advocated. The advantages of such designs are several. A 'yarded' piggery is cheaper; the section of the building which needs to be well insulated is of more modest proportions and so the cost of materials and erection can be reduced. Also, some will consider the environment obtained by such designs basically healthier, for the dung and urine are outside the warmer part of the building. Ventilation measures can therefore be on simpler lines. The yard itself can be left uncovered but this arrangement is only suitable for areas where the climate is mild and frosts infrequent or less severe. Covered yards are best in all other locations.

The greatest problem with piggeries with outside yards is how to keep them warm and free from draughts in the cold weather. For this reason the size of individual unit within the building must be kept small and each unit must be completely separate from the other units to prevent through-draught. Also the siting and aspect of the building are critical factors. Open yards should always be of southerly aspect. Good baffle arrangements between the yard and the pen are necessary, and if fans are used, though this is rare, a reverse-acting ventilation system which blows the air into the piggery and out through the pop-holes is desirable to reduce the risk of floor draughts.

Single-side yarded piggeries

We may take as our pattern of the yarded piggery a good design of a single-sided deep straw piggery with covered yard and individual cleaning. The design consists of a service passage running along one side of the unit, the wall containing double-glazed dead lights. From this passageway are catwalks at right angles serving pens on each side, each one being 4.8 m in length and 1.8 m deep, assuming that a trough is used.

There must be doors along the service passage between each pair of pens to prevent draughts blowing in the pop-holes at one end and out at the other. This part of the building is well insulated and can be ventilated by installing a push-in ventilation system by a duct running in the angle between the roof and the north wall with the fans at each end. An alternative is to place fans in the north wall and force air into the pens, with a baffle placed in front to protect the pigs from direct draught. The walls between each pair of pens are taken to the roof and may be load bearing and support it.

The yard is separated from the pen by a cavity wall. A pop-hole not more than 750 mm wide and 1.05 m high allows access for the pigs. Above the pop-hole may be a half-heck door to make for easier access between the pen and the yard, facilitating such operations as the weighing of the pigs and a curtain and baffle arrangement is needed to prevent excessive wind blowing in to the pens.

The depth and extent of the yard will depend on the amount of straw it is required to build up. The length of the yard must be limited to keep the covered area to economical proportions and the building as compact as possible, while the width will be some 2.1 m with feeding passages arranged in this way. A 600 mm drop to the yard, with ramp for access by the pigs, will give a build-up of 3–4 months, depending on the amount of straw used, while a 300 mm drop will last about 6–8 weeks.

Open yards

A single range of pens leading to uncovered yards is often used for whey-fed pigs in southern areas or swill-fed pigs in the northwest (Fig. 13.17). While the

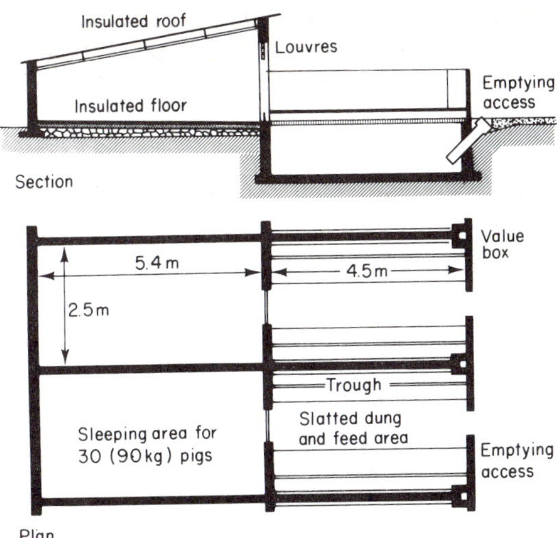

Fig. 13.17 Cottage-type piggery with open feeding/dunging area.

control of the conditions is not complete, with cheap and highly nutritious feeding pigs will thrive. The whey and swill feeding are fed in the yards and the copious and very liquid dung is squeegeed or hosed into a drain to run to a sludge tank, or the outside yard may be slatted and the pigs lie in warm insulated kennels behind the yard. With solid-floored yards the cleaning can be carried out more easily and frequently by running a tractor straight through the yards with scraper blade attachments. This is done by providing gates between the yards that swing back, enclosing the pigs in the pens and giving a clear run for the tractor.

Double-sided arrangements

An alternative approach with yarded piggeries is to have a covered yard allowing some build-up of muck, a central passage with troughs on each side and kennels at the back for the pigs to lie in. The cleaning out is carried out by swinging the gates back to the kennels and pushing through with tractor and blade attachment.

An original design of this form was produced by the late Mr Stephen Horvat of Suffolk (Fig. 13.18) and various refinements which are now popular are referred to as Suffolk houses: the centre area is uninsulated and naturally ventilated. The kennels at the back are well insulated and have flaps to control the air supply. Plenty of straw must be used in the yard and cleaning out should be frequent to maintain a healthy and dry atmosphere.

Several adaptations of the design have been produced, as the general arrangement of the 'Suffolk' house has a large following. The cost is less than

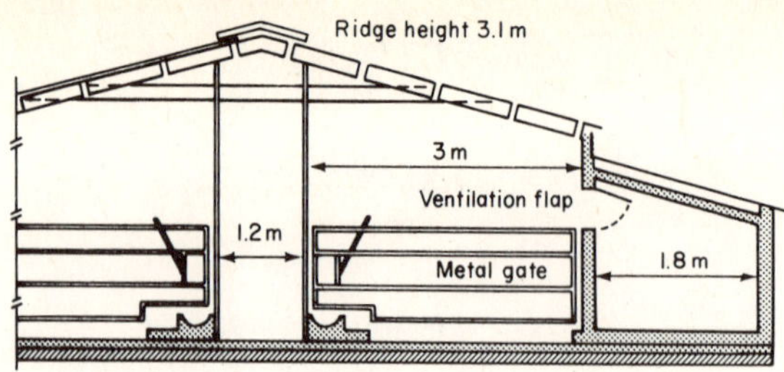

Fig. 13.18 Suffolk-type fattening house, with insulated kennels, covered yard and push-through mucking out.

that of a totally enclosed piggery with troughs, probably varying from three-quarters to two-thirds of the cost.

Nowadays the 'Suffolk' type of house is frequently built in the form of kennels under a covered yard (see Fig. 13.19). Another very popular but rather similar alternative is the zig-zag house with kennels in the centre of the general-purpose building giving access on alternate sides to feeding and dunging areas twice the width of each kennel (Fig. 13.20). Both these designs use straw, and also store it above the kennels; cleaning may done daily or 2–3 times a week by tractor and scraper.

Mono-pitch fattening houses

Open-fronted units similar in concept to the 'Solari' farrowing house described on p. 250 are frequently used for fattening pigs. There are many minor variations but the essentials are a simple design, space for up to 20 pigs in each pen, a warm lying area at the back and exercise, feeding and dunging at the front. All feeding systems can be used and dung cleaning operations vary from strawed floors and hand cleaning out to slatted dunging areas and slurry disposal. If the general rules referred to are followed, the result can be very successful. An absorbing study of the effect of different forms of fattening piggeries was carried out in Nebraska. This showed quite clearly that the open-fronted mono-pitch fattening piggery gave the best all-round economic return compared with all other designs. The evidence is clear. Experiments over at least a quarter of a century in countries as climatically diverse as Sweden, Great Britain, Ireland, Canada, USA and South Africa show that simple designs that 'insulate and isolate' can give consistently good results.

THE HOUSING OF SOWS AND BOARS

The strawed yard

A traditional, comfortable and healthy way of housing in-pig sows is to keep them in a completely covered yard. It keeps them well protected from bad

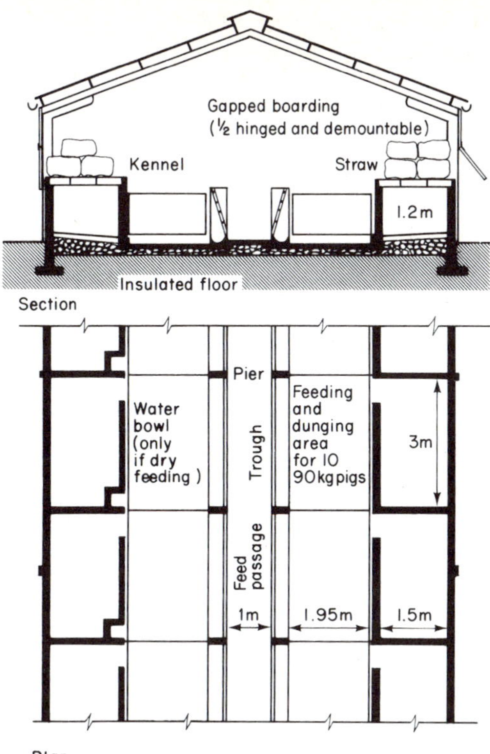

Fig. 13.19 Suffolk-type piggery in a covered yard.

weather, allows plenty of exercise and makes the provision of good stockmanship easy. Individual feeders can be provided and a suggested layout is shown in Fig. 13.21. The system is based on a line of feeders down one side of the yard which is raised above the general level of the yard itself – the further the raised area the greater can be the build-up of muck before cleaning out is necessary. A drop of 750 mm will allow a build-up of approximately 3–4 months.

A suitable yard on these lines can be provided by having a span of 9 m and dividing it into bays of 4.5 m along its length. This gives a total area of 42 m^2 per bay, which is suitable for eight sows. This is a convenient number to keep together as the likelihood of fighting and bullying rises as the numbers kept together increase. Along one side the individual feeders have a length of 2.1 m including the trough, so that the actual lying and exercising area is just over 3.7 m^2 per sow.

Gates and fences between the sections of the yard should be easily removable to allow for cleaning. The construction of the yard will be simple and uninsulated, but extra comfort can be provided by storing much of the straw on a platform above the strawed area, thus also making good use of the free space of the yard. Alternatively, the straw can be stored to one side of the yard under a lean-to

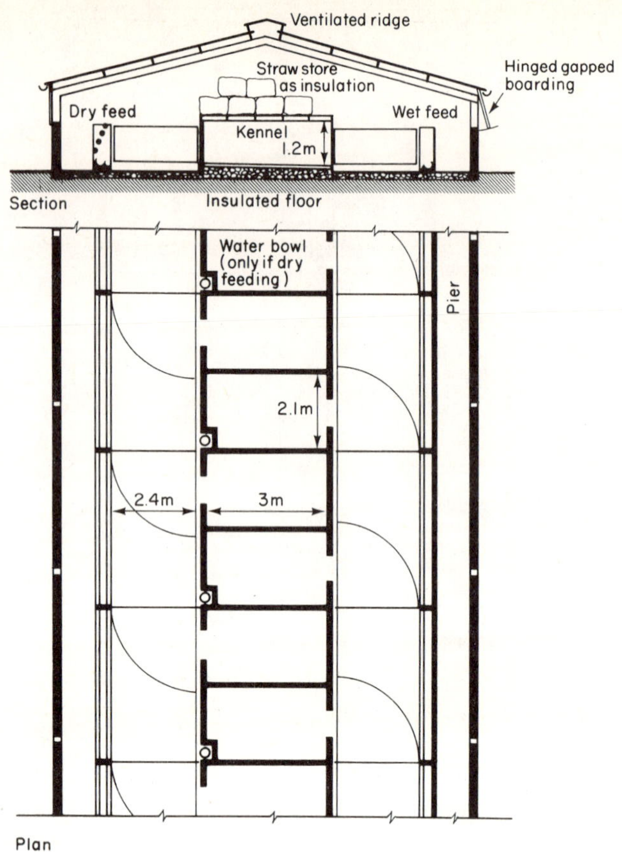

Fig. 13.20 'Zig-zag' fattening house.

extension. In both cases the straw can be thrown down on the floor quite easily.

The ventilation of the yard is an important aspect that requires some careful attention. A yard of this type can be closed in on three sides, i.e. the back and the two ends; the ridge must be left ventilated, either by using a capped open ridge or by installing chimney-type ventilating trunks. The front of the yard should face south and have an overhang of 1.5 m on the roof, which will give the pigman protection in feeding and also protect the yard from undue entry of snow or rain.

The base of the yard should be on concrete: this will not only assist in its cleaning, but also prevent the dangers of disease build-up which can always be a serious problem where ground is used continuously to house livestock. The base of the walls of the yard can be of solid brick or concrete construction, and the remainder of the wall above this to the eaves of the yard can be in spaced boarding to give good ventilation.

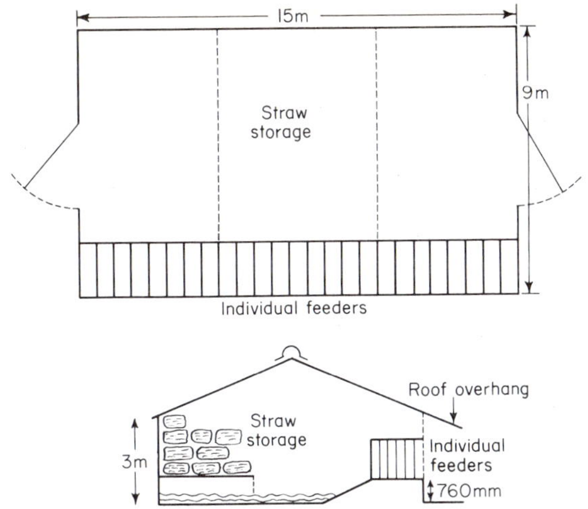

Fig. 13.21 Totally covered yard for 25–30 sows. Each sow needs about 3.7 m^2 of floor area, but it is best to keep the sows in small, evenly matched groups of about ten sows.

Partly covered yard

A cheaper system and one probably little inferior in practice, is to have only part of the yard strawed and covered and the remainder composed of a concreted yard for exercising and feeding, and containing individual feeders (Fig. 13.22). The simplest layout is similar to that in the totally covered yard, with the lying area at the back in the form of small kennels allowing 0.93 m^2 of lying area per sow, and a concreted area in front of 2.8 m^2 per sow. At the far side of the unit will be the individual feeders served by a concrete apron.

The sleeping area can be modestly constructed with an overall height of 1.5–1.8 m and will need insulation to prevent condensation and undue temperature fluctuations. To keep the sows dry and warm there should be a narrow step up into the pen and a small sill; the entrance need be only 750 mm wide and half-heck doors can be used for further ventilation except for a sliding shutter at the back of the pen measuring 750 × 300 mm for a unit of eight sows.

Some breeders concerned with the number of foot and leg troubles that occur when sows are kept on built-up litter, may prefer this latter design, as the exercising on hard concrete may produce a healthier reaction on legs and feet.

SOW STALLS

When sow stalls were first introduced as a method of housing sows about 25 years ago, they were a totally revolutionary method but now over half of the dry sows in the U.K. are housed in this way. Stalls are rather similar in size to a farrowing crate and allow the sow only to stand up and lie down; she can

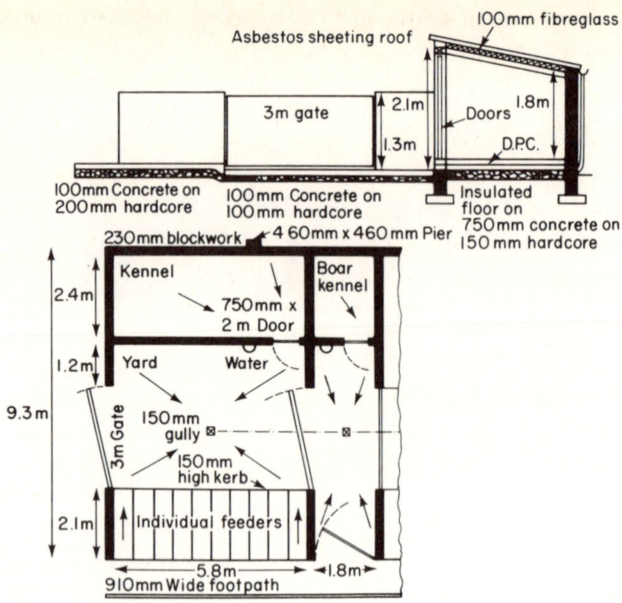

Fig. 13.22 Sow yard with individual feeders.

neither turn nor exercise. The idea originated in Scandinavia where the practice was to tether the sow in a stall, like a cow stall, with collar and chain round the neck, a trough in front and timber or metal partitioning. Such stalls are 750 mm wide, 900 mm high and 1.97 m long. Sows can be kept in this accommodation from the time they are weaned from their piglets until they return to the farrowing pen, the only time they leave being for service. Alternatively, they may go into this accommodation after being safely in-pig, the previous 'dry' weeks being spent in a yard or paddock adjoining the boar accommodation. This is the preferred system at present.

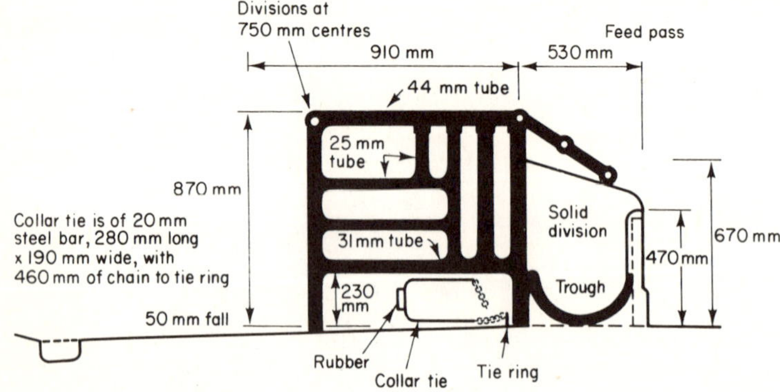

Fig. 13.23 Stall for tethered sow.

Stalls may be placed in simple narrow buildings some 4.2 m wide, although it is more usual to have them in two or more rows. The system has the advantage that it ensures each sow has a fair share of food, freedom from fighting and bullying throughout pregnancy, and uniformly equable conditions.

The Scandinavian system of tying the sows by the neck has found increasing favour in the U.K., as in other countries. A suitable design is shown in Fig. 13.23. The short tubular stall divisions are cheap and the open area at the back allows the sows considerable movement and makes cleaning out as easy as possible with a solid floor. Bedding may be used if desired. There is also a system of girth tethering which is preferred by some, since it allows a greater degree of movement.

There is also an alternative arrangement with sows kept in confinement stalls without tethers. Tubular steel divisions are usual and may consist of horizontal rails only or a combination of horizontal and vertical rails (see Fig. 13.24). Stall fronts are also normally railed and occasionally fitted with gates to allow easier movement of the sow. Rear gates may be solid, which is best when a partially slatted floor is used to retain any surplus dung, or when bedding is used with a solid floor. The doors at the back may slide vertically or be hinged. With solid floor stalls vertically sliding tubular gates or chains are used at the rear, the former being designed to clear the floor, so that cleaning out is facilitated.

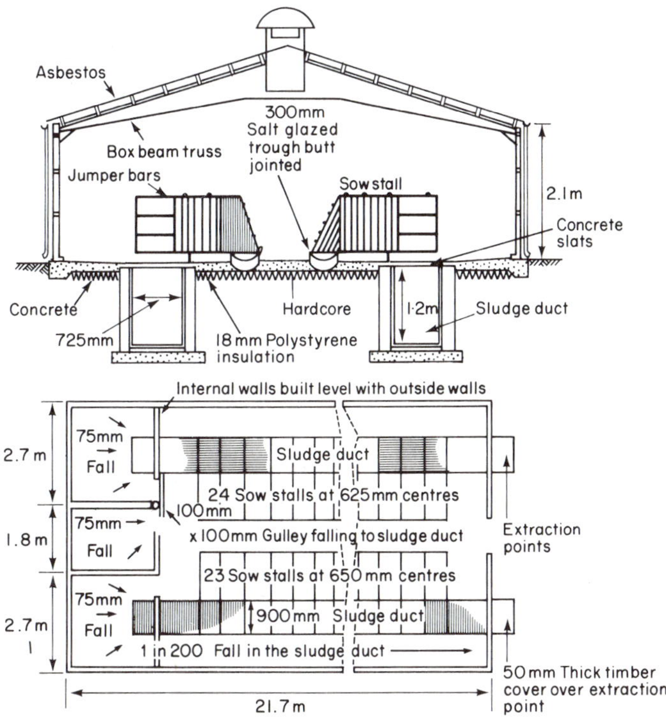

Fig. 13.24 Sow stall house, with boar pens.

If a raised trough is used, the length of stalls is 1.95 m from the rear gate to the front edge of the trough itself forming an extra 375 mm, but if a sunken floor trough is used, a total length of 2.02 m is sufficient.

Raised troughs, required for wet feeding, should be half-round, glazed fireclay not less than 300 mm wide, but floor troughs 300 mm wide and 50 mm deep are otherwise preferable and can be lined with tiles. Ad lib drinkers are usually mostly installed, with one drinker being shared by two sows. It is best to have the water level controlled by a tank and float valve at the end of the row to minimize the working parts. Nozzle drinkers are also frequently used.

Floors may be solid or the rear part may be slatted. The solid floor should be well insulated and non-slip, the front half being level and the rear half sloped well back with a fall of 25–50 mm. With a slatted rear end the front half falls the same amount to the rear, 910 mm which is slatted. A commonly used slat is concrete, 60–70 mm top width and 21–25 mm gap. The slats are best laid at right angles to the stall divisions.

If two rows are used, they should be housed face to face rather than back to back, as in the latter case the sows strain to see what is going on behind them. The sow stall house itself must be very well insulated and ventilated, bearing in mind that often the sow will have no bedding, she will be fed frugally under modern techniques, and there will be no heat generated from exercising. Extreme temperatures and dampness will therefore be potentially very dangerous.

At present there is still considerable development taking place in the search for the ideal housing for the sow. Sow stalls have certainly enabled individual attention to be given to the sows, but some people do not agree with the restriction on the movement of the sow and also object to the unclean state of the sow's hindquarters in litter-less pens.

Two interesting approaches have been evolved which keep sows in small groups. Sow cubicles consist of a group of three or four 2.1 m long × 600 mm wide free-choice cubicles for feeding and lying with a communal dunging area behind them of 1.8 × 1.8 m. The unit would normally be placed under a covered yard with gates between dunging areas, which could be mechanically cleaned (Fig. 13.25). Cubicles may also be placed in an outside hut with separate or communal dunging areas; one design has a door that can be opened and closed by the sow. These are most useful techniques to give a stress-free environment at minimum cost and with easy management.

Electronic sow feeding system

Within the past three years a new arrangement has emerged for managing dry sows based on the straw yard principle. This is a computer-controlled system providing automatic individual rationing of group-housed dry sows. A central computer with keyboard and printer controls one or more feed stations. Every sow wears a collar carrying an individually coded responder. When a sow enters a feed station an interrogator located underneath the front of the trough identifies her as the responder comes within range. If she has food due to her it is disposed

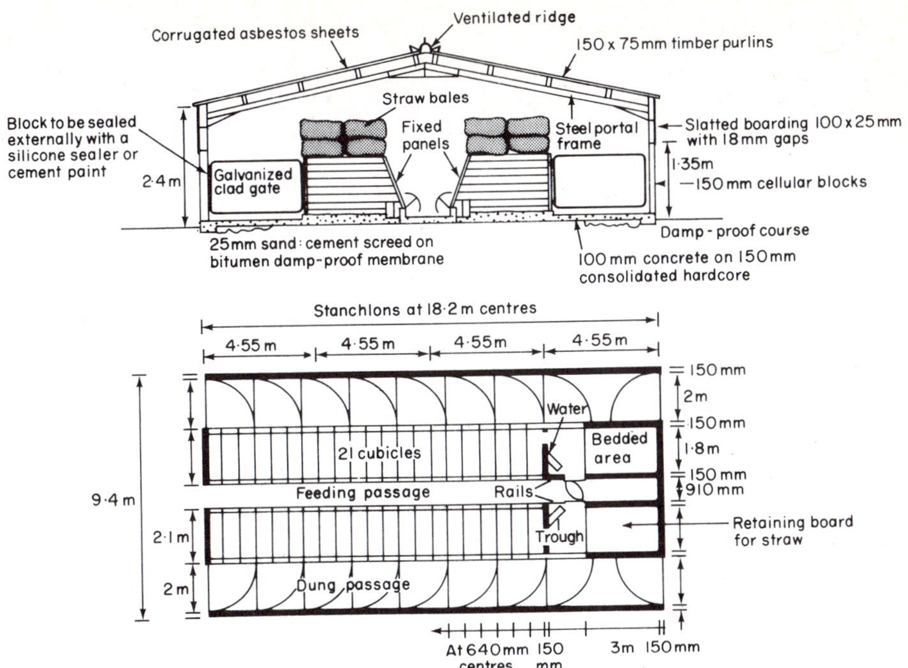

Fig. 13.25 Sow cubicle systems developed by BOCM Silcock Ltd. Boars are housed in bedded areas.

by an auger and rotating cup. While feed is being dispensed, gates at the entrance to the station automatically lock shut behind the sow to prevent bullying and unless she chooses to leave the station they stay shut until she has eaten all her allocated ration. If a sow which has already had her full ration returns to the feed station, no further feed is dispensed, the back gates remain unlocked and she has no incentive to stay there.

HOUSING THE BOAR

Good housing is essential because it prolongs the boar's life and use in the herd, and aids his fertility. Boars are very apt to 'go off their legs' and suffer from a number of 'mechanical' troubles with their limbs which may be less likely with good housing. Possibly the best way of keeping the boar is outside in a paddock with a simple protection of a hut and a run. Where more confined accommodation is required, a simple system of sty and run is all that is required, but the exercising area should be on generous lines. A covered area of around 3.7 m^2 and a yard of not less than 3.4 m^2 should be the aim. Part of the yarded area can form the service area or crate, which should be designed so that both the boar and the sow to be served can be easily moved around.

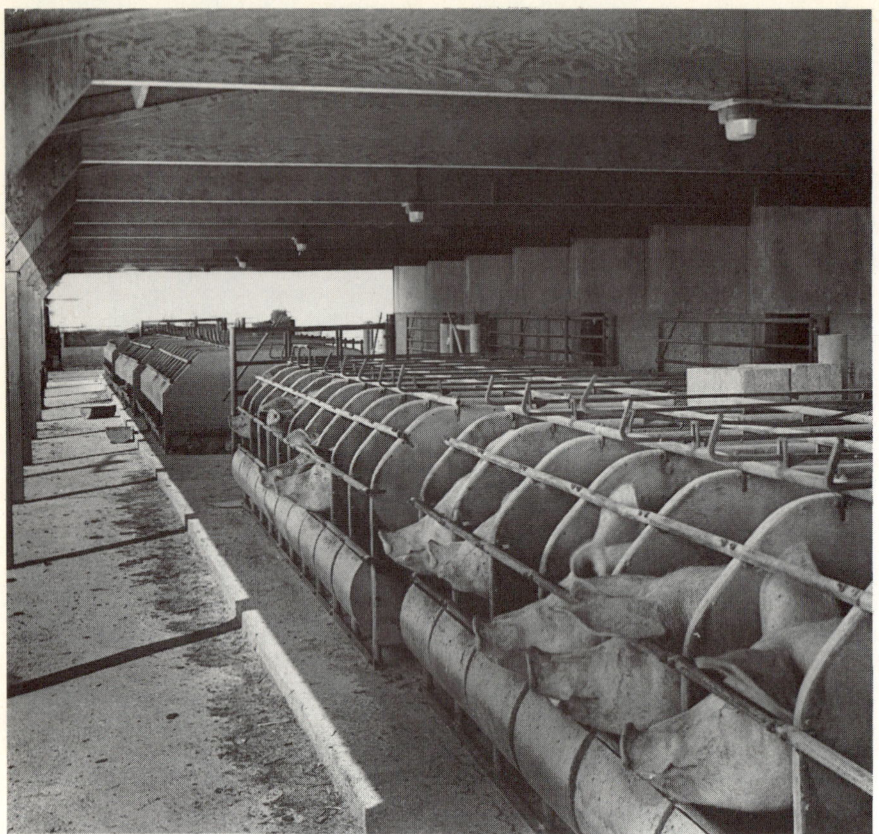

Fig. 13.26 A range of sow yards with individual feeders and kennels incorporating boar pens.

This type of unit is shown in Fig. 13.26 and can be installed in the middle or at the end of a range of sow yards. Another good way of keeping boars is to run them with a group of sows safely in-pig. No special accommodation is required in such cases – in fact, a boar can be run with a group of up to eight sows under any of the other systems shown. Whatever system is used, it is generally an advantage to have the boar within sight, sound and smell of the weaned sows awaiting service, as there is evidence that this can have a beneficial effect in stimulating the onset of heat in the sow. He should also be able to see plenty of people and the general farm activity which will tend to maintain his better temper and easier handling. It is certainly our experience that the most tractable boars are those who run with in-pig sows when not actually in use.

ACCOMMODATION FOR THE NEWLY WEANED SOW WITH BOARS

Because of the need to get sows served successfully as soon as possible after weaning and since it is most likely to be achieved if they are kept close to the boar, it is preferable to give special consideration to this period. Most of the accommodation considered in this chapter incorporates boar units close to the sows or gilts, and a design is illustrated in Fig. 13.27 which will help to make the process of detecting heat and serving the females an easier and less laborious job. Farmers often prefer to place sows in this type of accommodation for about four weeks after weaning before they enter cubicles, stalls or tethers, or any other systems, for the last three months of pregnancy.

EQUIPMENT FOR THE PIGGERY

Pen gates

Weak features in many piggeries are the gates. Pigs are strong and can easily damage equipment. Satisfactory gates can be made of a number of materials. Metal is only suitable if it is well galvanized. Timber gates are satisfactory if protected with sheet metal at any point at which the pig can make contact. Gates of 12 mm thick asbestos have been marketed for some years giving a corrosion-free material. The gate must also be well secured on its hinged side and is strongest if it hangs on a steel post or channel independent of the dividing wall. Likewise, the gate must be closed with a latch that is secure, pig-proof and still easy to operate, preferably with one hand.

The weighing room

As methods of feeding and dung cleaning become more efficient, weighing becomes one of the most labour-intensive activities in the fattening house and every effort should be made to make it efficient.

In most piggeries the preferred arrangement is to take a portable weighing machine round the pig fattening unit pen by pen. This does have certain unsatisfactory features. The machine is neither very acurate nor easily damped and the recorder cannot take the figures under ideal conditions.

In many respects a more satisfactory arrangement is to have a fixed weighing machine in a separate place with arrangements to ease the task of the recorder and the stockman and also to allow a quick circulation of the pigs. If pigs are weighed in the pen or passage attached to the pen, careful thought must be given to the direction in which the doors open or close, to ensure correct holding and movement of the pigs.

Loading pens

It is a most risky procedure to allow the lorries collecting the pigs for market to come into close proximity to the rest of the pig unit, owing to the great dangers of bringing in disease. To prevent this a passageway should be provided from the piggery to the loading bay holding the maximum number of pigs that are likely to be sent off at one time. A further help is to provide a raised loading

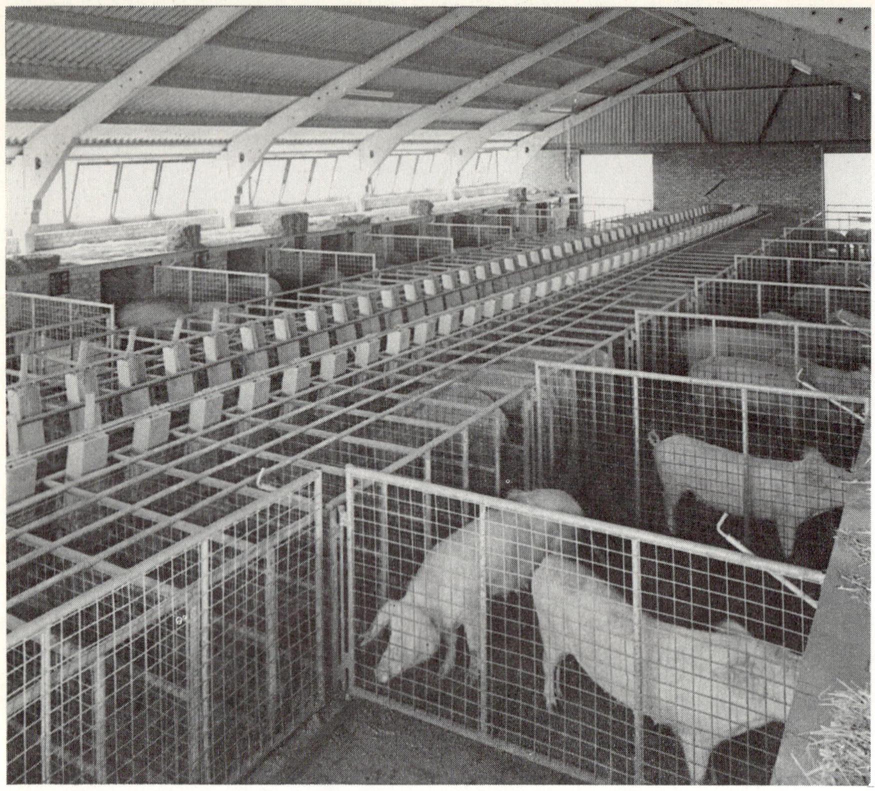

Fig. 13.27 Arrangement of pens for sows in the service period.

bay to allow the pigs to walk on level with the lorry. If this whole set-up is near the highway but at least 30 m from the fattening house, the danger of disease introduction is virtually eliminated and the job of loading itself becomes a straightforward, if not an easy one.

Self-feeders

With self-feeders it is wise to allow three pigs to 0.3 m of feeder space. Self-feeders of wood, metal or plastic are satisfactory and may be used as part of the pen divisions with economy. A useful procedure is to use the self-feeders as the pen fronts; these can slide forward or backwards to give the variable size to a pen which is a great help in ensuring clenliness in the stock.

Individual feeders

There are great advantages in providing individual feeders in sow yards to ensure fair shares and prevent bullying (Fig. 13.28). The usual type of feeder is

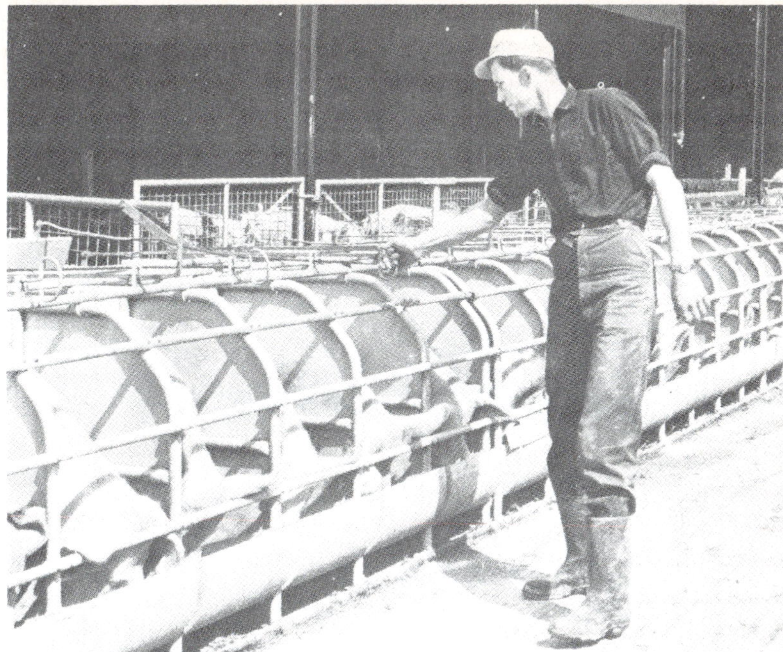

Fig. 13.28 Individual feeders for sows.

of metal construction measuring 550 mm across and being 2.05 m long. The gate at the back for the sow should be remotely controlled from the front which will also contain a built-in trough.

Water bowls and nozzle drinkers

A necessary permanent fitting in the piggery is the automatic water bowl. As self-filling bowls are generally used and there is always some spillage, it is most satisfactory to place them in the dunging area; where this is impossible, they should at least be situated at the lowest point in the pen adjoining the dunging area, so that spillage does not run back on to the bed.

The bowl is best placed well within the dunging area, so that the pig has its whole body out of the pen when drinking. It is also important that the bowl does not project into the passage when it has a solid floor to interfere with cleaning out operations. To satisfy this requirement the bowl may be either placed on the dunging passage door, connected with flexible piping, or recessed into the dividing wall between pen and passageway. The bowl lip should be 150 mm above floor level, but where young pigs before weaning are using it, it is good practice to place a step up to it. This keeps it cleaner and less likely to be fouled.

An important consideration is that the bowl should not be placed in a position where frost may affect it. Care must be taken when it is in an outside yard, therefore, to ensure that the bowl is as near the pen as possible and pipes are kept warm either by running them within the pen or by efficient lagging. It is obligatory to have a storage tank to serve the bowls rather than direct from the mains. If this tank is placed within the piggery it should be sealed as far as possible to keep the water clean and dust-free, and also by lagging it condensation will be prevented.

As an alternative to water bowls, nozzle drinkers have achieved a large measure of popularity in recent years, the water flowing when the pigs depress a valve on the end of a brass nozzle projecting from the wall, gate or pen division. The system is economical and hygienic, and should give little mechanical trouble, but cheap products have a short life and soon drip or run excessively. Pigs are also inclined to play with them and waste water.

There is some evidence that the pigs will benefit from the water being warmed in winter; a tank housed within a piggery will ensure that the water has the chill taken off it. Alternatively, bowls can be purchased which incorporate small heating units. Where restricted water is given rather than ad lib, to save physical handling of the water, the bottom rail over the trough can be a waterpipe. The pipe is individually controlled by a valve to each pen and is punctured on the base by a series of small apertures of 3 mm diameter at 230 mm centres.

Troughs

When fixed troughs are used in the piggery, great care should be given to the small details in their design and construction, particularly bearing in mind the importance of eliminating food wastage at all costs, food representing 80 per cent of the cost of rearing pigs. The general requirements are that they hold the necessary food and allow the pigs ready access at all ages within the group, yet provide as little wastage as posible. A trough must also be hygienic, easily cleaned and able to withstand acidic elements. The arrangement must enable the pigman to put the food in easily without wastage from his side, and also without undue interference from pigs. Trough space allowances should be:

150 mm at weaning
230 mm for small porkers
250 mm for heavy porkers
300 mm for baconers
350 mm for heavy hogs.

Undoubtedly the best trough is made of half-round salt-glazed pipe. Although this is expensive, it satisfies all the requirements for the trough itself that have been specified above and there seems to be no substitute that is as satisfactory. Pipes used are 250 or 300 mm in diameter, the latter being preferred. Fig. 13.29 shows the details of this with a tubular rail trough front. The trough is tilted towards the pig and should be 125 mm above the floor on the pen side, while the front should extend 375 mm above the feeding passage. The lip at the top of the trough nearest to the pigs should be a maximum of 50 mm wide. The

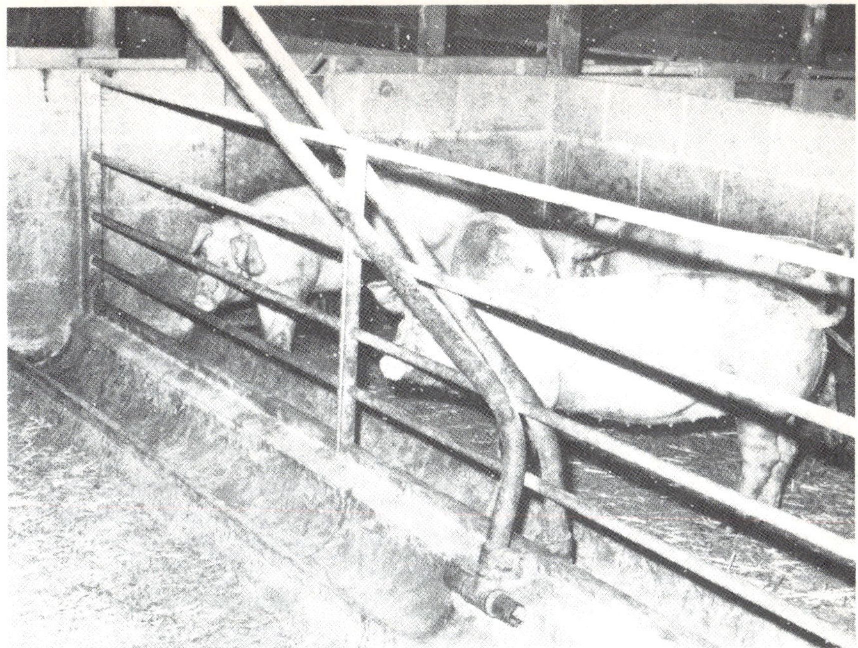

Fig. 13.29 Salt-glazed double troughs with tubular rail front for automatic liquid feeding.

rails over the trough front must be set accurately, in the way shown, to ensure first, that pigs cannot escape; and secondly, that food is easily put into the pen. A recess under the trough front, as shown in the diagram, should be 37–50 mm to help the pigs to stand right up to the front. A more elaborate front than the railed one is the swinging panel, which is pivoted above the trough and can be fixed for access either by the pigs or by the pigman only for filling the trough without interference from the pigs.

Dividing walls

Walls between pens for fatteners need not be more than 1.05 m high. For farrowing pens 1.2 m is advised. Walls between the dunging passage and the pens are normally the same, or in case of slatted floor arrangements, they are either omitted or a dwarf wall only is used. Wherever possible divisions between pens and between pens and dunging passage are taken to the ceiling. Ceiling high pen divisions taken at regular intervals across a large piggery, together with doorways between the individual compartments of the piggery so formed, do have the most favourable effect on health and the environment.

Service room

The pigman must have a place for washing, for protective clothing and to take and collate the records required in an efficient unit. An adequate, warmed, well-lit, well-insulated room, attached to the farrowing house and with lighting and heating points, is an ideal arrangement.

Isolation area

Every pig unit should be equipped with an adequate number of solid floored and bedded pens that may be used for the isolation of sick or injured pigs, or the quarantining of new arrivals.

Automatic feeding systems

There are two main choices of automatic feeding systems for pigs. The first is to feed dry in the form of meal or pellets and provide water separately. The second is to feed a fully balanced ration mixed with a liquid (usually water) but in some cases whey or skimmed milk. Evidence suggests that wet feeding systems can give better food conversion efficiencies than dry rations, and since control of intake is now technically possible, with automatic systems the method has much to commend it. It is also likely that wet feeding will give better liveweight gains than dry feeding which occurs with the latter because of dust. Pelleting feed offsets this to some extent, but involves an additional cost which must be compared with the extra cost of providing equipment for wet feeding.

Dry-feeding systems for pigs

Pigs may be dry fed on the floor, or in self-feed troughs (Fig. 13.30). If on-the-floor feeding is practised, pellets are better than meal as they create less dust. One system of feeding pellets is to convey them by auger from a bulk hopper outside the building into small hoppers above each pig pen. The quantity of pellets for each pen is varied by moving a slide within the hopper, and the underside outlet of the hopper is closed by means of a moving shutter. All the moving shutters are coupled by means of a long rod and controlled by a linear actuator or geared motor. In operation, after the augers have filled the hopper to the required amount for each pen, a time switch operates the linear actuator. One actuator can control up to 75 m of rod length and opens all the feed hoppers together, so that the dry feed is discharged simultaneously on to the floor of all the pens. Afterwards a microswitch reverses the actuator drive and closes the hopper flaps. Following this a further microswitch, operated by a timer, energizes the starters of the auger motors to bring in replacement feed automatically. When all the hoppers are full, a diaphragm switch in the last hopper switches off all the augers and the equipment is then ready for the next feed.

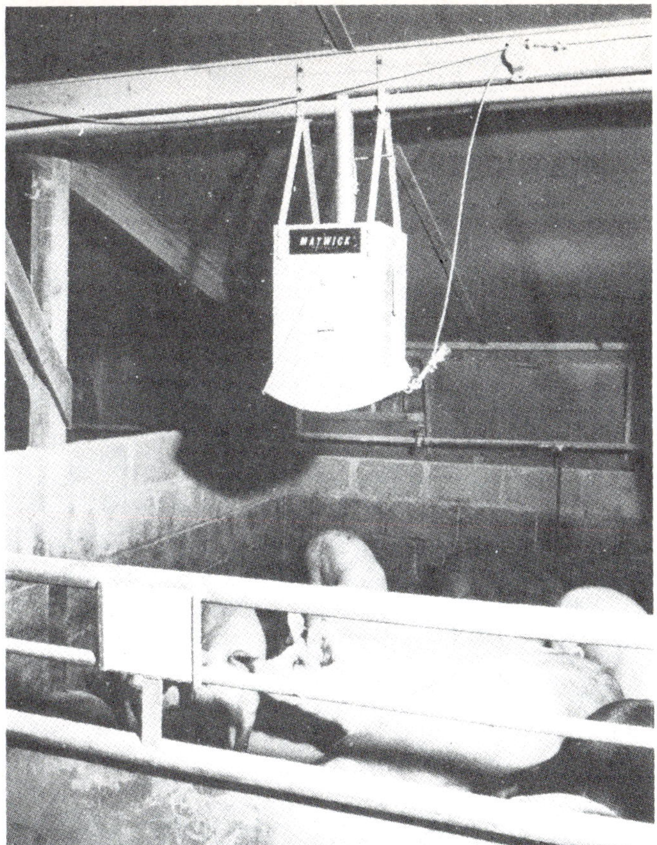

Fig. 13.30 Maywick floor feeder, one of several systems for bulk handling of pig feeds.

Feeding in troughs

Tubular conveyors are also used for trough feeding for pigs. Down-drop tubes at intervals along a trough can then be used to dispense feed. By telescoping the tube, adjustment according to age, weight and number of pigs is achieved, and calibrated slots are normally provided by the manufacturer to enable this to be done quickly by the pigman. The length of conveyor required for a particular size of herd can be worked out assuming that 0.25 m of trough length will be needed per pig on restricted feeding.

Self-feeders

Automatic conveying can be arranged as for trough feeding, using down-spouts to each feeder and stopping the flow in the last feeder by fitting a pressure flap switch near the top to switch off the auger motor.

Wet-feeding systems for pigs

Two main systems for wet-feeding pigs are available in batch and continuous flow. Both systems are available for hand operation and for automatic delivery of feed to the pig by means of main pipelines with branch feeds to the pig troughs controlled by valves (Fig. 13.31).

SLATTED FLOORS

Slatted floors for pigs may be constructed of several materials – concrete, metal, welded wire mesh or polypropylene and other plastics. Reinforced concrete is probably the most popular and generally successful material and wire mesh the cheapest. Common measurements for all types of pigs for concrete slats are a slat width of 50–75 mm at the top tapering to 38–50 mm at the base, a depth of 60–75 mm, and a gap of 21 mm between the slats. Welded mesh is best using 75 × 12 mm mesh at 10 gauge or 75 × 15 mm at 5 gauge. Also very popular are pre-perforated steel panels, 14 gauge. Panel sizes are usually about 1 × 0.2 m or 1.2 × 0.2 m and holes are punched to give about a 50 per cent void. They can be hot-dip galvanized to prolong the life greatly and are suited to all ages of pigs. Other metal arrangements are flattened expanded metal 17 mm 10 gauge or steel straps 30–37 mm wide and 5–7 mm thick with a space between of 9 mm for farrowing and 17 mm for nursery units. The pig farmer is warned that all types of slats, if not properly made or fitted, can cause a frightening degree of discomfort or damage to the pigs.

There have been important advances in the design of slats. In the early use of concrete slats it was usual to use one of about 50–75 mm in width. But

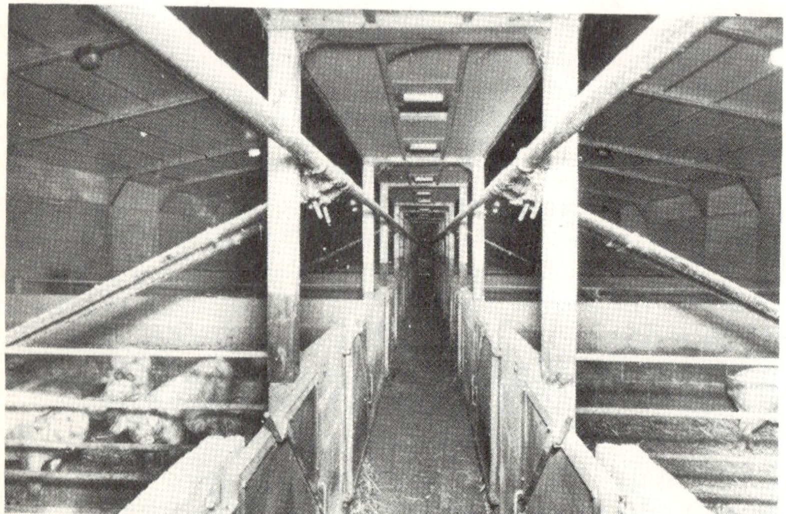

Fig. 13.31 Automatic wet feeding systems for pigs.

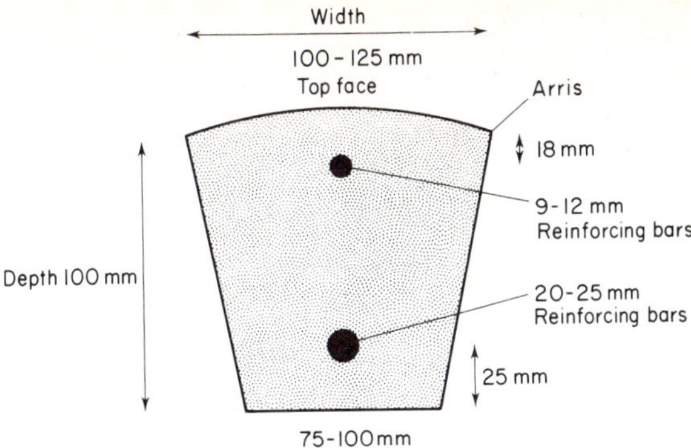

Fig. 13.32 Cambered slat.

narrow concrete slats of about 50 mm width are usually more prone to lodging of the faeces than slats of, say, 100 mm width, for in order to ensure a comfortable floor, narrower gaps also have to be used and the sides of the concrete slat must be perpendicular to the face in order to provide adequate cover to the steel reinforcement. Narrower slats bounded by parallel concrete faces 75 mm deep are subject to bridging of the manure. Where solid slats are used a bevel of at least 1 : 5 is advised and the width of slat should not be less than four times the width of the gap. Slats may be made up in panels with a fixed gap or in single units, so that spaces can be made to suit any class of stock.

Slats for fatteners

In general the larger the pig the wider the slat that can be used without sacrificing cleaning efficiency. Small pigs provide less effective traffic to work waste material through the spacings. Slats even as wide as 200 mm and 25 mm apart have performed satisfactorily for fatteners. And indeed extra wide slats have some of the advantages of both a solid floor and a slatted floor. We have used, with considerable success, a slat of 125 mm width with a 25 mm gap, with a slight camber on the surface and with pencil-smooth edges and bevelled sides. The form of this is shown in Fig. 13.32. Such a slat keeps very dry and appears to be extremely comfortable for the pigs.

14

The Housing of Sheep

There have been marked trends within the past two decades towards the more intensive management of sheep indoors. There have been three principal reasons for this. First, the in-wintering of sheep of all ages enables better conditions and management to be provided during the winter months, thereby also eliminating poaching of the land. Secondly, housing provides an ideal environment for the production of early fat lambs to satisfy the demands of the profitable spring and Easter markets, when especially high prices are paid. Finally, sheep may be housed permanently in environmentally controlled conditions to enable round-the-year production of lambs by the provision of artificial lighting patterns which enable a ewe to produce up to two crops of lambs per year.

It is only within fairly recent times that sheep have been housed to any great extent and in consequence there has been considerable uncertainty as to the best way of keeping them indoors. The position is summarized as follows.

THE CONTROLLED ENVIRONMENT SHEEP HOUSE

If light cycles and intensity are to be controlled to enable out-of-season breeding to take place, the ewes must be kept in windowless houses in which artificial light cycles are maintained. The onset of oestrus cycles in ewes is stimulated by subjecting them to decreasing periods of light, similar to the natural cycle in the autumn in the northern hemisphere.

The controlled environment house must be a thermally insulated structure dependent on mechanical fan-controlled ventilation, because the elimination of windows or ventilating flaps, which would permit the entry of light, prevents sufficient natural air flow taking place. It is thus a relatively expensive house both to construct and maintain and the only chance of its being economic is to house the sheep at a fairly high density. For example, a ewe would be provided with about 1.2 m^2 on a bedded area or approximately 1 m^2 if the ewe is housed on a form of perforated or slatted floor (see Table 14.1). Thermal insulation of the surfaces of the building is necessary in a controlled environment house to prevent condensation and dampness in the winter, which is anathema to housed sheep, or overheating in the summer, which may be equally harmful. A ewe with lambs requires an additional 0.3 m^2. Mechanical ventilation for sheep should be provided at the rate of a maximum of 3 m^3 per hour per kg body weight.

Table 14.1 *Some essential data for sheep*

Type of sheep	Requirements	
	Slat (m^2)	Straw (m^2)
Covered area		
Ewe: large	1.0	1.2
small	0.8	1.2
With lambs, add	0.3	
Hoggs up to 30 kg	0.6	0.7
Lamb creeps to 5 weeks		0.3
Ventilation		
Mechanical	Up to 3 m^3/h/kg body weight	
Natural	Open ridge up to 0.6 m	
	Side walls at least 1 m all round building	
Troughs and racks	Troughs (mm)	Hay rack (mm)
Ewe: large	450	200
small	400	150
Lambs: Up to 50 kg	350	150
Up to 40 kg	300	125

The slatted or slotted floor

There is little doubt that the best flooring for sheep is a soft bedded surface of straw or shavings, or a mixture of the two. However, this is an expensive floor to maintain: the bedding has to be purchased or harvested, stored and put into the house and then the dung plus straw removed. A much more attractive proposition is the slatted or slotted floor, which, if carefully designed, has been shown to be eminently satisfactory. Much investigation of slats and slots for sheep has been done at the National Agricultural Centre.[1,2]

Constructions have been tried using concrete, timber, welded mesh, woven mesh, expanded steel, punched steel and punched aluminium. Gap size has proved vital with a much smaller gap (not more than 16 mm wide) being needed for lambs. There is also a considerable danger with welded mesh or expanded metal that the small lamb's feet can divide over these materials and get trapped. The long slatted slats in timber and concrete allow spillage of hay from feed racks to get through, whereas the various meshes eventually block. For concentrate-fed lambs all meshes prove satisfactory, with the expanded steel being probably the cheapest and the best. The conclusions reached from the work at the National Agricultural Centre are that sheep should be stocked more intensively than on straw. Such flooring is not particularly good for ewes with very young lambs but is ideal for dry sheep or finishing lambs.

Feed racks must be a carefully designed to prevent spillage without restricting feed intake. Figs. 14.1 and 14.2 show suitable types of slatting which provide a clean and comfortable surface for sheep.

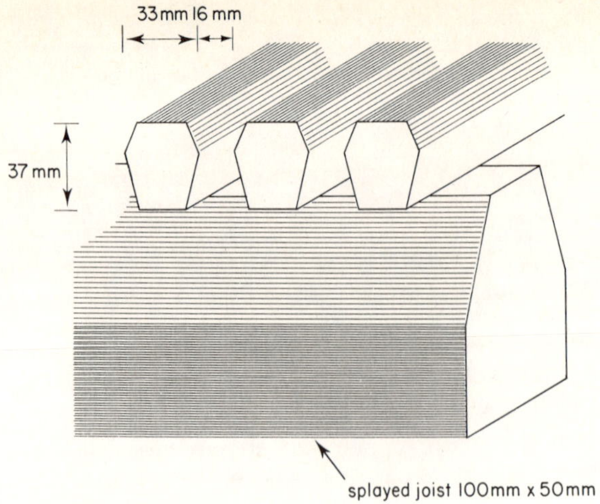

Fig. 14.1 Splayed slatted floor for sheep.

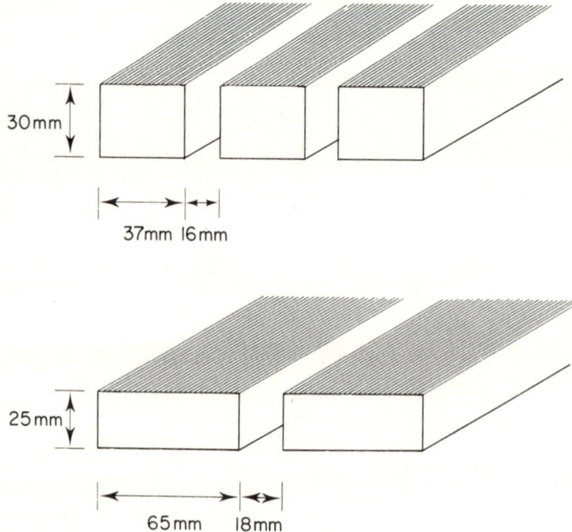

Fig. 14.2 Rectangular slats for sheep.

Troughs and hay racks

Designs based on the Scandinavian feed box have been found most suitable and can perform the dual function of trough and hay rack (hake).[3] They will also be useful in a dual function as pen divisions, and passageways are frequently constructed for feeding into the trough from one or both sides. The feed box is illustrated in Fig. 14.3.

Space allowances for troughs are given in Table 14.1. A plentiful supply of

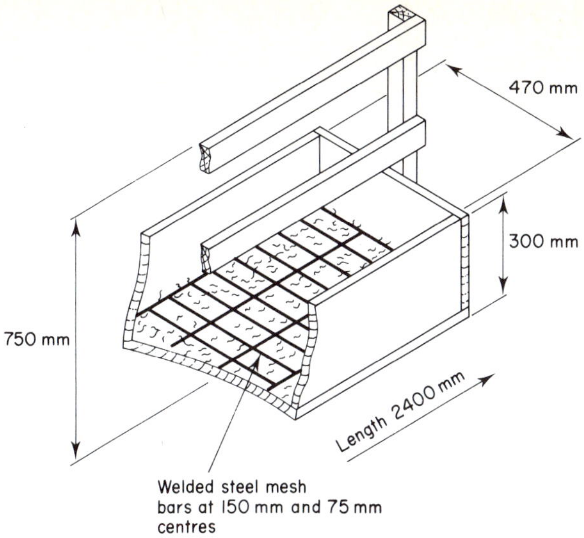

Fig. 14.3 Scandinavian feed box.

clean water must also be provided; to avoid fouling, troughs should be raised and a wood or concrete surround provided so that the sheep can put their forefeet on it to drink.

Low-cost sheep housing

For the in-wintering of sheep there is no necessity for elaboration and the basic requirements are simple – a roof and side cladding to give protection from the rain and wind, and copious ventilation without draughts. Fig. 14.4 shows the various forms of sheep housing and yarding in profile.

Pens

There is a strong case for the division of sheep into small pens in order to place the sheep into uniform groups that are evenly disposed throughout the building. Divisions should be made of posts and rails that ensure an unobstructed flow of air across the building. A satisfactory size of pen would accommodate about ten sheep.

The mono-pitch house

A popular basic shape for low-cost housing is the mono-pitch house (Fig. 14.4). The building is highest at the front, being high enough to allow mucking out with a tractor and fore-loader. There must also be adequate trough space and racking for hay or silage which can be taken ad lib. Straw bedding is usually

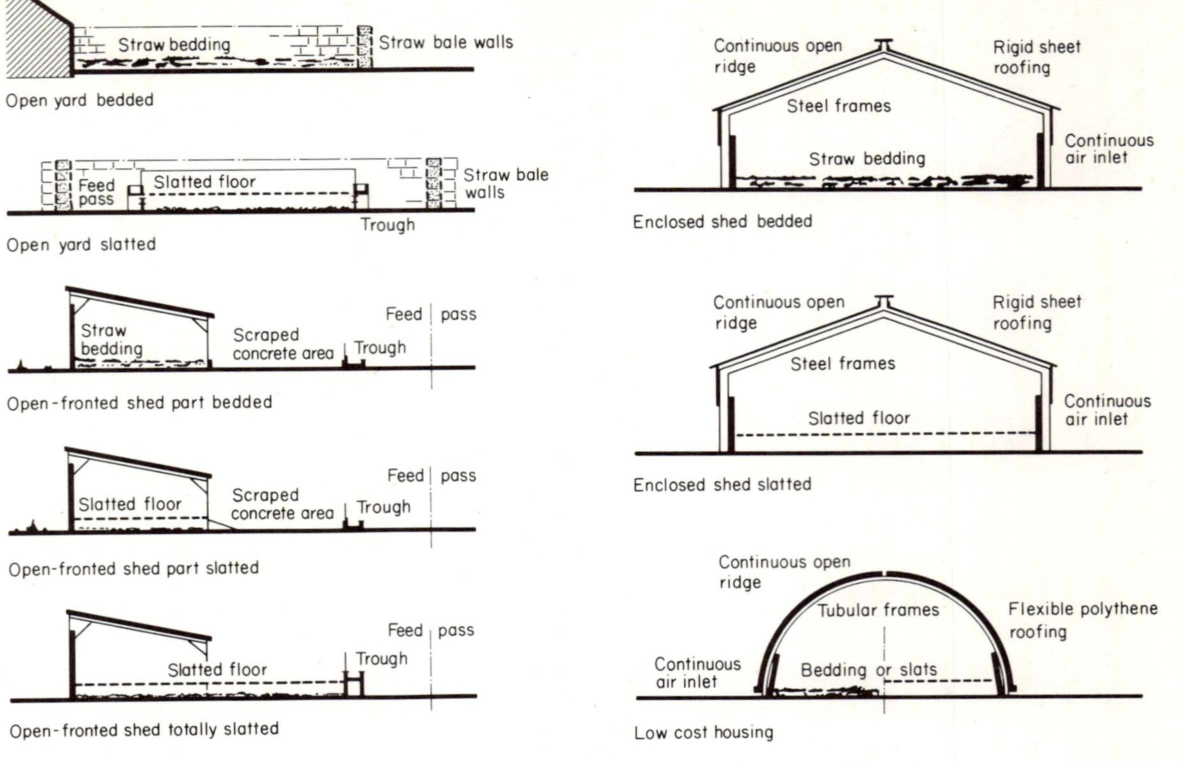

Fig. 14.4 Various forms of sheep housing.

placed on the floor, which is of earth, unless slats or slatted floors should be preferred. It is usual to build a mono-pitch (lean-to) design of timber. Second-hand timber and sheeting can be satisfactorily employed and the whole house erected by farm labour. The front of the building is approximately 4 m high, the rear 3 m and the depth is most satisfactory at about 6 m maximum. The rear and end walls are usually of corrugated galvanized steel sheeting. At the rear there is a substantial gap under the eaves of about 700 mm or more, and the front of the mono-pitch house should be open, apart from the gate. The roof is also usually of corrugated steel sheets. Feed troughs are commonly placed between the pens with a central walk which can also serve as a lambing area and the hay racks can be placed on the gates.

Whilst the mono-pitch house generally has a clear economic advantage over pitched roof buildings so far as costs are concerned, the latter are often used. In many cases existing buildings are available, or a more elaborate but multi-purpose building may be preferred. Cheap pitched roof buildings, such as the pole barn, can be made with rough-cut poles and second-hand steel sheeting to give good protection though at a low cost.

The plastic sheep house

Great interest has focused in recent years on low-cost polythene covered buildings for a whole range of livestock, but in particular for sheep. The construction is quite simple. There is a frame of tubular steel arches at about 2.5 m centres. In addition three lines of galvanized steel purlins and lines of coated wire support the polythene cladding. The first 1 m height down each side of the building is clad with a perforated polyethylene windbreak giving approximately half the area 'open'. The remainder of the 'tunnel' is clad with white polythene 125 μm (600 gauge) thick, supported on horizontal wires. The gables are usually clad entirely in perforated polythene.

Ventilation is usually highly effective with the air entering the sides and the ends quite freely, but without draughts. Gaps in the roof should be provided for the escape of stale air. Buildings of the polythene tunnel form are usually 9 m wide, about 3 m high, and can be to any convenient length. The polythene sheeting is supposed to last about three years and can be replaced quite cheaply but the main structure has a potentially long life. The environment in the building is light and airy and is suitable for all forms of sheep. It also provides first-class lambing accommodation. The width of buildings allows for pens on each side of a wide central passage to take a tractor and trailer.

'Topless' in-wintering shed

The ultimate in sheep housing is the 'topless' in-wintering yard, which can house ewes during the wettest months in the cheapest way possible. Typical construction consists of a layer of stone on top of soil but separated from the soil by a fibre mat. This is surrounded by a windbreak of fencing or straw bales. Straw is placed over the stones but its usage can be quite heavy, varying from some 4–6 bales per ewe. Whilst the sheep can certainly be better off than on grass, there can be difficulties with the drainage of topless accommodation and it is frankly difficult to achieve this satisfactorily. There is, therefore, no doubt of the merits of the roof over all housed sheep, even though it may be of a semi-permanent nature, as with the polythene-clad house.

Ventilation

It is of the utmost importance that the ventilation of all sheep housing is on the most generous lines. It is almost impossible to over-ventilate housed sheep. With a pitched roof there should be a wide open ridge and approximately one metre opening all round the house under the eaves. This area may be protected with some form of wind baffle on the colder side, spaced boards with 25 mm gaps are popular, or alternatively the whole open area may be temporarily covered with polythene netting when required. Sheep will greatly appreciate the ability to breathe in fresh air wherever they may be penned.

The lambing pen

This can be the simplest of all forms of housing on the farm. It usually consists of a series of pens about 0.5 m^2, arranged to form a hollow square. Each pen has a low roof and is walled behind with timber, thatched hurdles or sheep nets filled with straw. The unit may be permanent or preferably a temporary erection dismantled at the end of the lambing season. Normally the centre of the square is left open, but it is sometimes the practice with pedigree flocks to have the whole area covered for added protection. The unit is provided to protect the ewe and lambs during and around the lambing period and also to give adequate protection to the shepherd during this important period. The principal danger in the lambing pen is of a build-up of infection in the building, the flooring and its surrounds, and this can best be avoided by moving the site of the lambing each year. In fixed buildings this is not possible so that thorough disinfection and resting is absolutely essential.

Sheep handling unit

An essential requirement for all sheep farms is a thoroughly efficient sheep handling unit, including a race, dipping tank and footbath. A design must enable all operations to be done as quickly as possible with the minimum number of helpers and an absence of stress and strain on both men and sheep (Figs. 14.5 and 14.6).

Procedures that will be carried out in the handling unit will be dipping, spraying, care of the feet, drafting, dosing and inoculating and dagging. Essential features for all handling systems will be:

1 A *gathering pen* large enough to take all the sheep to be dealt with at one time.
2 A *forcing pen* which acts as a funnel to the race – the narrow passage which sheep are forced into in single file with gates in the side to enable the sheep to be sorted into separate pens. Circular pens which can be reduced in size as dipping proceeds are the most satisfactory arrangement.
3 A *dipping bath* with draining pens.
4 A *footbath.*
5 *Handling or treatment pens.*
6 *Holding or drafting pens* into which sheep pass after treatment and sorting.

The sheep handling unit should be sited centrally to the grazing areas, free draining, shaded and convenient for access and loading. All constructions must be free of sharp edges and posts must be on the outside of rails or sheeting. It is preferable if the main working area is roofed over to assist with the many operations that may need to be carried out under all kinds of weather conditions.

The sorting race will be the most frequently used part of the unit as its use normally precedes all other procedures. The purpose of the sorting race is to present the operator with a continuous stream of sheep one at a time. A narrow sorting race is the best to achieve this. It must be long enough to permit an unobstructed view to identify sheep well in advance. A race with sloping sides is best since, being narrower at the bottom, it gives less footroom for sheep to pass one enother. Races of this type are usually made 200–300 mm at the base, increasing to 430–600 mm at the top. The sides are best of solid construction with a gap at the bottom of 100 mm to allow the operator to get closer to the sheep and also to assist in the inspection of the sheep's feet.

Because sheep follow one another, provision should be made for sheep to see other sheep to draw them in the intended direction. Their preference to move uphill should be utilized by siting races and the working area so that sheep go through them up an incline. If a solid drafting gate blocks their view or apparent exit, a see-through gate should be used.

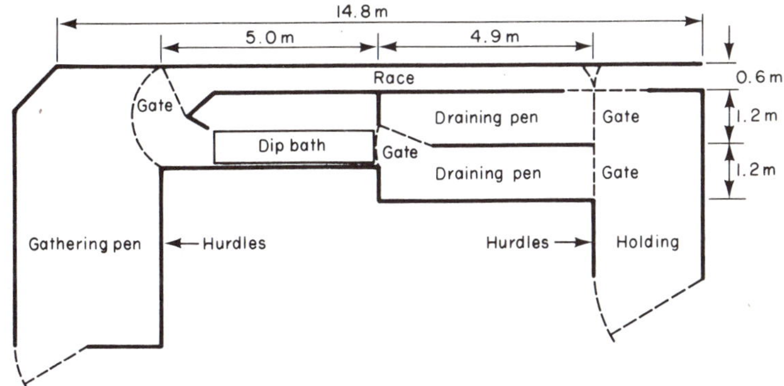

Fig. 14.5 Small sheep-handling unit for small flocks or batches.

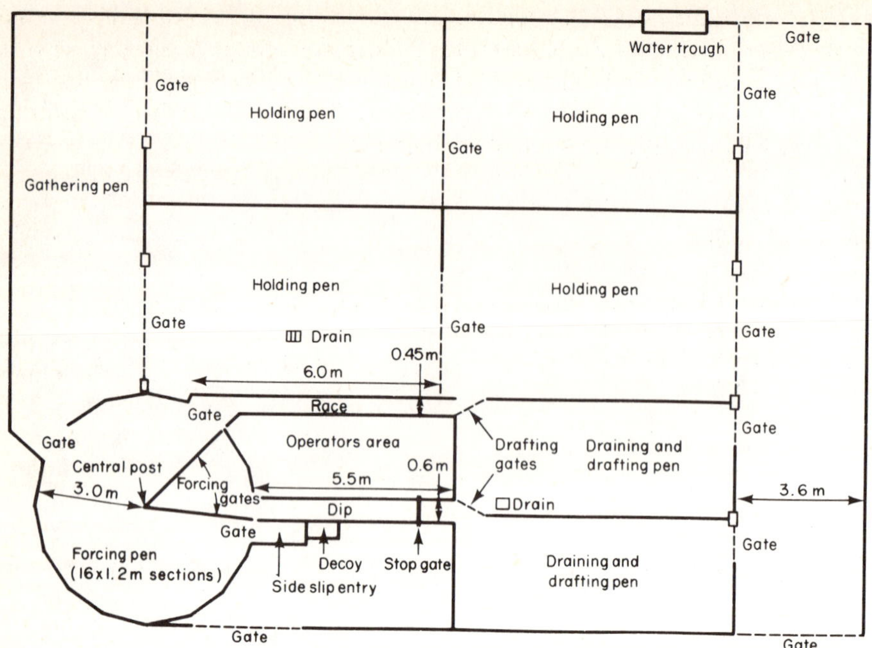

Fig. 14.6 Large unit incorporating a circular forcing pen and gates remotely controlled by cords.

Draining pens at the exit end of the bath are essential because of the amount of dip fluid which a sheep has in its fleece when it emerges from the bath. It is best to use two or three draining pens and diverting gates at the exit of the bath so that dipping is continuous. A two-way sump in the draining pens should be fitted to divert rain water away from the dip when not in use but to drain fluid back to the dip when dipping is in progress.

Sorting gates at the end of races can be two-way, or even three-way for the most experienced, and some excellent arrangements have been designed to assist.

Dipping baths exist in a very wide range of sizes from small dips of about 1000 litres, to hold one or two sheep at a time, to swim baths of from 2000 litres to nearly 6000 litres capacity. The capacity of tank selected will depend

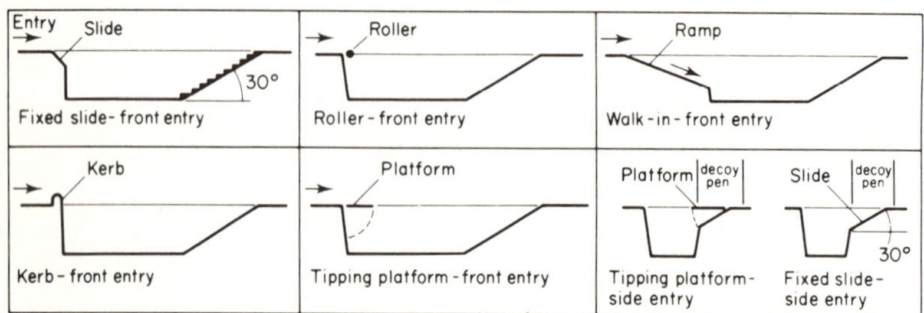

Fig. 14.7 Various dip entry arrangements.

on the size of the flock, the really big ones which dip about 500 sheep an hour only being suitable for the largest flocks. There are a range of different ways of getting the sheep into the dip, which is illustrated diagrammatically in Fig. 14.7.

Finally it should be emphasized that it is very convenient to have a shearing and wool shed at the end of the handling unit.

REFERENCES

1 Court, K. (1978) *Farm Buildings Digest* **13**, 19–20.
2 Dymond, A. (1979) *J.R. Agric. Soc.*, **140**, 175–181.
3 Cunningham, I. M. M. and Soutar, D. S. (1967–8) Sheep housing. *Scott. Agric.*, 5–10.

15

The Housing of Domestic Fowls, Turkeys and Ducks

This chapter deals with the main method of housing from a practical viewpoint. The underlying principles of environmental and health control have been dealt with in earlier chapters.

REARING CHICKENS

Methods of rearing chickens have become so standardized in the U.K. that many of the more traditional arrangements that will at least be briefly mentioned in this chapter have very nearly disappeared. However, they still have their place in a limited number of circumstances, even in the U.K., and elsewhere, especially in the countries with less intensively developed systems and where therefore they may be more appropriate.

The simplest methods of rearing chicks are those known as 'single-stage' systems, in which the chicks are taken from day-old to maturity in the same house. The simplest of all these systems are the single-stage systems in which chicks are reared on built-up (deep) litter from day-old until they are ready to enter the laying quarters. They are suited to certain types of layers and almost all breeders. There are no 'checks' in the growth created by changes in the housing, and immunity to parasitic diseases, such as coccidiosis, develop naturally without hindrance. From the husbandry and health aspects the systems are definitely the best. Another scheme in elaboration of this is to take breeding stock from day-old right through to the end of the laying period in the same quarters; some commercial layers are similarly housed. It is rather wasteful of space as the birds have to grow into the space provided which must be sufficient for the mature stock. However, poultrymen using single-stage housing for birds from 'day-old to death' are enthusiastic about the benefits and convinced of its merits. The extra space for the young birds undoubtedly assists in uniform growth, and the fact that there is no change in housing prevents the stress that is inevitable when they are moved, however much care is taken.

Floor space allowances for birds kept in this way vary from 0.12 m^2 per bird for the lighter breeds up to 0.24 m^2 for the heaviest birds, the maximum figure being required for broiler breeding stock. The floor area per bird can be reduced by about one-third by using partly deep litter and partly slats or wire. With this arrangement a proportion of the droppings falls into a pit under the slats or wire and the litter remains in better condition. Also, by placing the food and water points largely on the slats, not only are the birds encouraged to make more use of this area, but also water spillage goes safely into the droppings pit and keeps the litter drier, which is a major requirement of good management.

Where a combination of litter and slats is used, the birds may be brooded on the slats, which are covered first with paper bags and litter, and given access at a later stage to the littered area. More commonly the birds are brooded on the litter and at about 4–8 weeks are trained to use the slats by the provision of a sloping run-up and the addition of water and food troughs to the raised area. Rearing on slats and wire only is comparatively new and raises management problems, not the least being difficulties from excitability, cannibalism and feather pecking. Wire with a mesh of 75 × 25 mm is satisfactory for all birds from six weeks of age, but if used earlier than this, a cover of smaller mesh wire, approximately 12 × 50 mm, is required.

Single-stage rearing is also carried out widely and successfully in special pullet-rearing battery cages, in which the birds are taken from day-old through to placement in the laying cages. The usual method is to start by putting all the chicks in the top tiers where the temperature can be kept to the required level and where management and observation are most easily carried out. They can be spread through all the tiers within a few weeks of hatching and indeed this change should on no account be delayed or the high density in the one tier used will cause serious problems. Birds which are reared in cages should be housed subsequently in battery cages and not on deep litter, straw yard or free range, since they are likely to have a poor resistance to parasitic infection.

Single-stage intensive systems require careful hygiene, nutrition and management in order to minimize the risk of vices and disease, especially as they often contain thousands of birds. They do, however, have the enormous advantage we have mentioned and simplify the whole process of management.

Cages are now produced that are so flexible in design that the chicks can be brooded in them and yet they may also serve for the birds when they are laying. They have, as in the floor systems that parallel them, advantages in favour of labour economy; in addition, they tend to ensure that the chicks are in small groups, parasitic diseases are unlikely and the food and water are very accessible. Stress can be reduced to an absolute minimum, as changes that cause it are either absent altogether or at least very mild. Great care must be taken to choose good equipment that has all food and water points easily adjustable, and where nipple drinkers are provided it is desirable that founts should be used when the chicks first go into the cages. The floors may be of 20 mm wire netting or 25 × 12.5 mm 16 gauge welded mesh.

MULTI-STAGE SYSTEMS

Traditionally birds are brooded in one house and then moved on afterwards, when the period of artificial heating is over, to a variety of other forms of accommodation. Some of these methods remain because the equipment is still available or those who have experience of them are very convinced of their virtue. This is not to decry them, since anyone who had experience of livestock husbandry will be well aware that systems come and go but the older arrangements often make a come-back under a modified guise. For example, a rather out-dated arrangement is to rear chicks in a tier brooder, which is suitable for the first 3–5 weeks of life. Tier brooders have the advantage that they can be placed in many forms of adapted and non-specialist buildings, but as room for expansion is limited, the chicks soon have to be moved on. The tier brooder consists of two or three warmed brooder compartments largely enclosed and placed one on top of another, with runs in front with wire side and top. The base is all of wire and droppings trays are provided underneath. A typical size of tier brooder is 3 × 1 m, taking about 50 chicks to four weeks of age.

The tier brooder and the building within which it is housed are areas of great disease risk because of the quick succession of populations that can result. It is therefore essential that the building be depopulated after each batch and then cleaned, fumigated and disinfected. The risk is further exacerbated by the high density of birds the brooder house can contain. and slats, straw yard or free range. However, it is always best to reduce the different forms of flooring used to a miminum, otherwise there is an increased hazard from parasitic diseases, such as coccidiosis, and the danger of a more prolonged check in growth. If tier-brooders are used, a system which has much to commend it is to keep the chicks in tier-brooders for a maximum of six weeks and then put them straight into laying cages which are specially designed to cope with the feeding and modified flooring required for younger birds.

Outdoor rearing

A procedure that was once very common was to rear the chicks from hatching to about four weeks either in tier-brooders or on the floor below an ordinary radiant brooder. They were then transferred to a 'haybox' brooder. This consisted of a covered compartment 1 × 1 m with a run in front approximately twice as long. No artificial heating was required because the covered section was packed round with hay or straw to conserve the chicks' heat and prevent draughts. Whilst this latter part was constructed of solid wooden sides and roof, the run had wire mesh sides and roof. The units were designed to be moved over the ground (which had to be good pasture) but they were also sometimes used as fixed units mounted on straw bales.

The system is healthy and can produce hardy, vigorous stock at economic running costs as no heat is used, but it has unfortunately serious faults in other ways – it is labour-intensive and places high demands on capital, maintenance and, above all, on stockmanship.

After the haybox stage birds were normally reared in range shelters or, indeed, this system may be used for other systems of management, especially if the birds have been reared until then on the floor. Range shelters are a simple, easily made and light form of protection and consist of an ark approximately 3 × 2 m with a height of 1.7 m at the ridge and 0.85 m at the eaves. A unit of this size will take 60 growers from 8 weeks to about 18 weeks. The roof can be built of metal, plywood, hardboard or felt and wire for extreme economy; the sides are of wire, but a large overhang on the roof protects the stock from wind and rain.

Alternative housing systems for birds reared on range are the night ark and the apex hut. The former is a hut of 2 × 1 m with a slatted floor and solid walls and roof, whilst the apex hut is essentially similar to the other two, but is of triangular cross-section.

These systems discussed above for outdoor rearing are little used in Great Britain but they have considerable possibilities for use in warmer areas of the world where simpler systems are appropriate.

THE PRODUCTION OF MEAT-CHICK ('BROILERS')

The systems used for rearing broilers are probably more standardized than any other arrangement (Figs. 15.1 and 15.2). Invariably the birds are reared from day-old to about 40–63 days in a controlled environment house on built-up

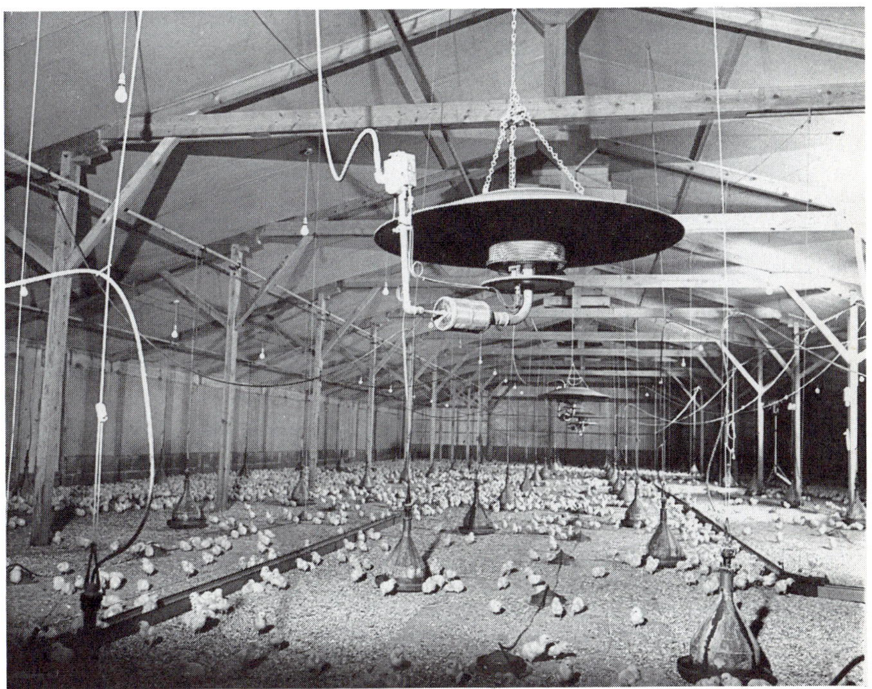

Fig. 15.1 A large broiler house showing the centrally placed brooder/space heaters, the numerous circular automatic drinkers and the automatic track feeders.

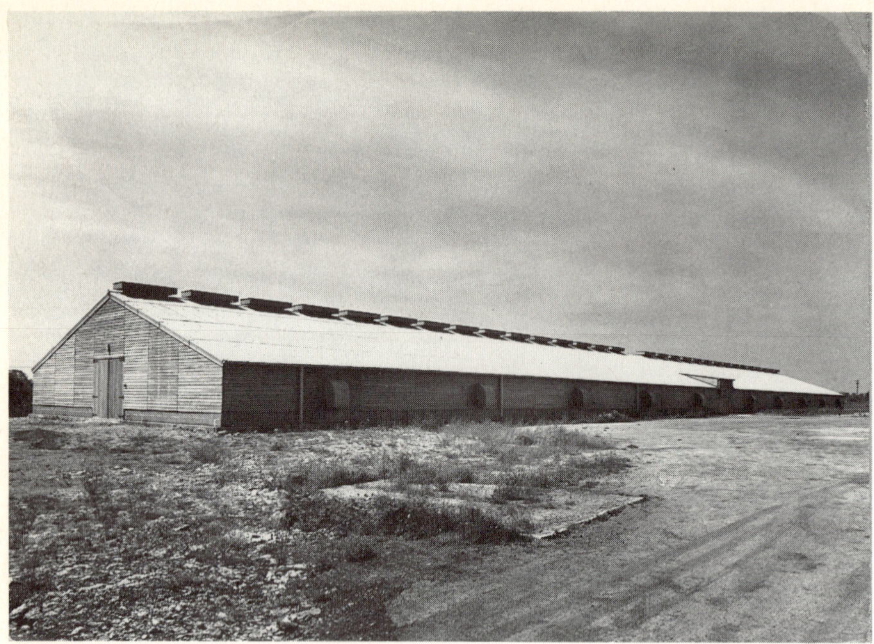

Fig. 15.2 A large controlled environment poultry house with ridge intake ventilation and wall mounted extract fans.

litter of wood shavings or straw, or a mixture of the two types. Because the birds grow so quickly any upset in the condition of the litter, which must be soft and friable, will be likely to lead to a damaged carcase due to bruising of the breast muscles which are the most valuable part of the meat.

A typical broiler house consists of a building of 10 000 to 20 000 capacity, reactangular in shape, and from 14 m to 28 m wide. Birds are reared commercially to give a maximum liveweight at the end of the growing period of 34 kg per m^2. The lightest weights of birds are marketed at about 1.4 kg liveweight, though the more typical weight now sought by the market is a 1.8–2 kg bird. Broiler management is probably the most intensive system in which poultry are kept on the floor and success depends on most diligent care in rearing the birds over their short 7–10-week existence. The maintenance of good environmental conditions and a perfect litter are the basis of good management and are explained in some detail in a later section.

LAYING SYSTEMS

Free range

Only relatively few layers are now kept on free range; nevertheless certain purchasers are still willing to pay a premium price for the 'genuine' free range egg so that it may still be profitable under some circumstances to keep birds in this way. With free range systems housing is simple and cheap but any real environmental control of heating and air movement is impossible. The birds may be housed in a movable colony house of 3.3 × 1.7 m on skids or wheels holding up to 50 birds. This type of hut has a solid wooden base and is fitted with perches, droppings board and a nest. An alternative is the slatted floor house which is similar but does allow a heavier concentration of stock, a hut of 2.7 × 2 m holds 60 birds comfortably. It has skids or wheels and is fitted with nests, broody coop, troughs and drinkers. A more recent development is the use of insulated, semi-circular, plastic-clad houses which may be moved at about yearly intervals. The houses are fitted with automatic drinkers, tube feeders, nests and lighting.

Free range systems can provide a healthy environment but it is wrong to believe that they are inherently healthier than indoor systems. They have disadvantages in that the birds and the stockmen are at the mercy of the elements, and winter egg production can be particularly poor. Some of these disadvantages may be overcome by keeping the birds in a fold unit, as the environmental control is somewhat better. The fold unit consists of a covered-in roost with slatted floor, measuring about 1.7 m^2 with a height of 1 m and with a totally wire-enclosed run in front of about 4 m long. The whole unit is built strongly of timber to withstand movement daily on to fresh ground.

The fold unit has a capacity for 25–35 birds, depending on the type of bird housed. Whilst the birds do benefit from the advantages inherent in keeping stock in small groups, and in the movement of them to fresh clean ground each day, the cost of the system is out of proportion to the economic return. Using either housing system, production can cease altogether under very severe wintry conditions and it is difficult to see how such costly methods can return to popularity.

The semi-intensive system

The fixed house or 'cabin', with either single or two or more alternative runs, is a system that is only used to any extent now by the domestic poultry keeper. A typical unit consists of 50 birds kept in a house 3 m^2 with two runs each 10 m^2, the birds alternating between them at six-monthly intervals. The cost of such a system is high both in capital and labour, while the climatic control over the birds is poor. Even when alternating between two runs a certain build up of disease organisms may ocur. Eggs are often dirty. It ranks as being perhaps the worst system of all in theory and in practice, but can function in the hands of the domestic poultry keeper where the normal economics of the market place do not operate.

Fully intensive housing systems

Deep litter systems

One of the first really successful methods of housing layers intensively was the built-up or deep litter system. After some 40 years of use it remains as a thoroughly satisfactory system though of rather high capital cost. Now, because of this, commercial egg layers are rarely kept on deep litter but breeders and broilers are. The litter is either wood shavings about 350 mm deep, or increasingly popular is the use of chopper straw and shredded paper.

In some designs of deep litter housing movable perches, drinkers and feeders are used so that, as far as possible, the control of the distribution of droppings and water splashings is maintained. However, under this system, birds require about 0.27 to 0.36 m^2 of floor space per bird if the litter is to work properly. It is preferable to have part of the floor as a slatted area over a droppings pit with perches and food and water troughs situated there as well. In this way the litter receives proportionally less droppings so the density of stocking can be increased. If the nest boxes are suitably disposed, with feeding and egg collection by hand, the two operations can be combined in a single movement round the house. Automatic feeding is more usual and there are now several systems for automatic egg collection, greatly reducing the labour costs.

With an area of deep litter combined with a droppings pit of roughly equal proportion, 0.18 m^2 per bird is sufficient for 'heavies' and 0.14 m^2 is enough for the 'lights'. In more recent years it has become quite popular to keep breeding stock on deep litter without a droppings pit, but in some houses, in order to assist heat conservation, heat-exchangers are installed. This keeps the litter in good condition even in winter but even without such equipment, provided there is very good insulation, the absence of a droppings-pit can be tolerated. By eliminating the droppings-pit the capital cost is lowered and management, particularly cleaning, is made easier. It also helps to make ventilation better without the obstruction of the pit and it promotes the better distribution of the birds on the floor since there is a general uniformity of the conditions and there is no reason for certain areas to be favoured.

The covered straw yard (Fig. 15.3)

The covered straw yard is a much cheaper version of the deep litter house, using a thick bedding of straw only as the litter and a different approach to environmental control. It was introduced in its orginal form about 30 years ago as a cheaper system suitable for the arable farmer who had abundant straw and a selection of old and otherwise redundant buildings. Because it often included a large uncovered yard area in its original form it failed to compete with fully intensive systems since it gave lower yields and often dirty eggs. The disadvantages had to be balanced against the very low capital cost of the system, assuming some cover was already available.

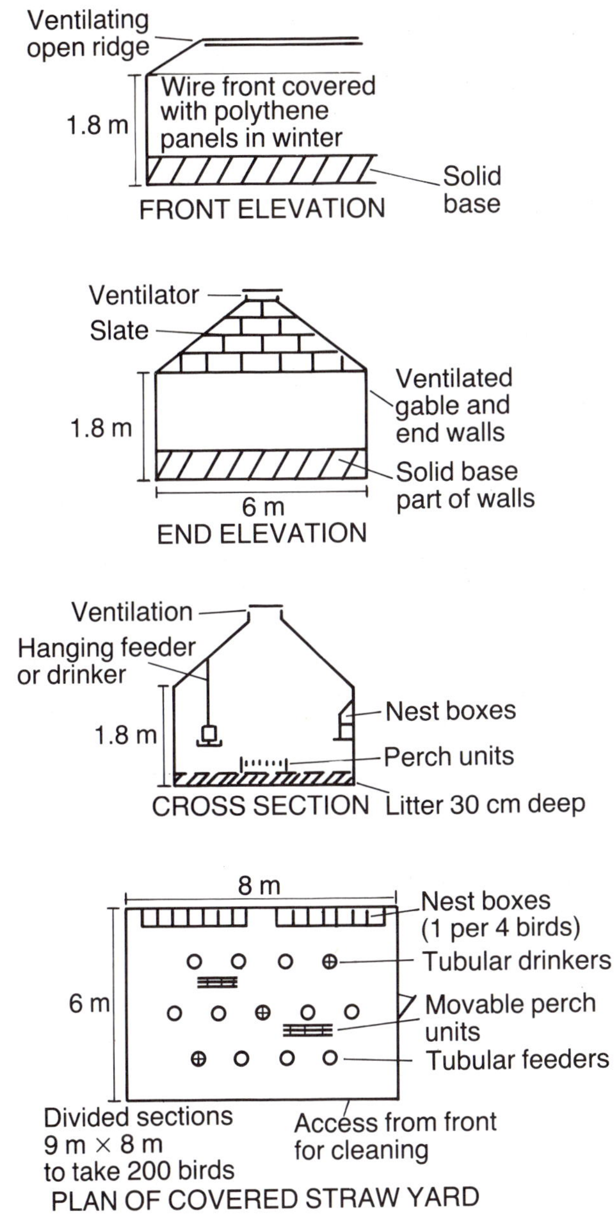

Fig. 15.3 Diagram of covered straw-yard.

One of the worst disease problems that occurred was an infestation with intestinal worms, the viability of the worm eggs being favoured by the damp conditions. If plenty of straw was used and good drainage arranged, the danger could be somewhat reduced. Data have been produced that show that as good a profit may be obtained per bird from this system as from some of the more popular ones but the arrangement requires a high degree of skill in management and has no widespread application at present.

The totally covered straw yard is of uninsulated construction and depends on natural ventilation. The roof and walls are clad only with a single layer of sheeting and the whole structure is usually placed on a dwarf brick wall and a concrete base. For ventilation there may be an open ridge. The birds can roost on movable perch units.

The wall height may be of 2 m so there is plenty of air flow well above the birds. The front of the yard may be of wire mesh and can be closed off in the colder weather with frames clad in polythene. Tubular feeders and automatic drinkers complete the equipment required.

In a comparison of the results with those from birds kept in multi-bird cages in a fully controlled environment house, it has been found that those kept in a straw yard performed as well.

The straw yard has certain other advantages. Running costs are low, there are no fans and a minimum of lighting; there is nothing mechanical to go wrong: it converts straw into valuable manure; the quality of the eggs is good, and is comparable to eggs in a cage system, but the straw yard eggs are richer in colour and much richer in vitamin B_{12}. Also there appear to be no welfare problems.

It is interesting to speculate on the reasons for a reasonable food conversion by chickens in a straw yard. The birds are well-feathered, probably improving their heat retention, and it is also found that they produce much firmer droppings and spend less time in eating. It may well be that caged birds eat and drink more than they want, due to the boredom of their existence, whilst straw yard birds spend time in activity on and in the litter and derive certain beneficial by-products from it.

The slatted floor system

Some years ago an arrangement was developed for keeping layers on totally slatted or totally wire floored housing. It is the most concentrated method of housing layers on the floor at a stocking rate of $0.09\ m^2$ per bird. Labour requirements are low, housing costs can be competitive, but apart from the continuing enthusiasm of the few poultry farmers who make it work, and still do, in general it has been a failure with an excessive number of floor eggs, which are lost. Extreme behavioural problems can also be created, probably by the boredom inherent in a system such as this, allied to the very close proximity of a large number of birds. Nevertheless in some areas of the world it is still a very popular form of housing, especially in the northeast of the USA which is an area climatically not dissimilar to Western Europe where it has lost its popularity.

Layout of floor-laying houses

Equipment in a floor-laying house must be arranged to ease the work associated with such management jobs as feeding and egg collection. In a small building holding up to 500 layers, a service room may be placed at one end of the house and the nests arranged so that collection is from this room. The nests form the upper part of the dividing wall between the house and the service room. In larger buildings, with automatic feeding, the more usual arrangement is to have a central service passage and nests on each side so that a quick collection is easily made. If the birds are manually fed it is preferable to have the nests against the wall and an overhead monorail and conveyor adjoining the nests. The conveyor can then be used both to collect the eggs and to take the food to the tubular or trough feeders which are placed on the opposite side towards the centre of the house. When this design is used in a deep litter house, a central droppings-pit is installed and the majority of the waterers are placed over this to minimize the harmful effects of splashing. It is preferable if the birds can walk across the slats before they enter the nest box, for the same reason as in the straw yard, that it tends to keep the feet cleaner and the egg is less likely to be soiled. With such an arrangement in a wide-span building, a centre passage would be used with nest boxes on each side and droppings-pit immediately adjoining.

There are, however, those who prefer to site the droppings-pit at the side of the house for ease of construction, the usual pattern being to have it on one side and a central deep-litter area and nests adjoining a passage on the other side. This passageway will also take the food trolley where hand feeding is practised. The house will usually be cleaned out annually and to assist this the slats, perches and divisions should be easily demountable and the doors should be sufficiently large to allow tractor entry.

Laying cages

The system of keeping birds in cages, often three or four tiers high, exceeds all other housing systems in popularity. The most popular cage systems house 3–5 birds in a cage. With a multi-bird cage system the *total* floor area per bird can be no more than 0.06 m^2. Cages vary in width as follows:

225–300 mm for a single light hybrid
300–325 mm for a single heavy hybrid or two light hybrids
350–375 mm for two heavier hybrids or three light hybrids
525 mm for four heavy hybrids or five light hybrids.

Cages are usually 450 mm deep and 450 mm high at the front, sloping to 350 mm high at the back. The floor extends at least 150 mm in front to form an egg cradle and the droppings-tray or belt, if there is one, has a minimum clearance of 100 mm below the floor of the cage. Each bird should have 100 mm of trough space.

THE VARIOUS CAGE SYSTEMS (Fig. 15.4)

There are several different types of cages that can be used. The three major groups are as follows: *stacked cages*, one on top of another are three or four tiers high and are mostly mechanically cleaned by a scraper, a plastic belt or occasionally using disposable paper belts. Some are still hand-cleaned. Occasionally more than four tiers are used, up to six or seven. An intermediate catwalk is required to service the top tiers.

The next group of cages are the *Californian* or *stair-step* often called the *deep pit system* because of the way it is installed. These cages are staggered, as in the diagram, so the droppings go into a large pit under the cages and can build-up right through the laying cycle when they are cleaned out by a tractor and foreloader. These also may be two or more tiers high, three being usual and four now becoming popular. A recent form of stair-step is the 'semi' form in which the upper cages are set partly over the lower ones, thus economizing on space.

Stacked cages used to be the most popular; probably the main difficulty with these units is the cleaning system, whether it be by belt or scraper, since the 'runs' should not be much longer than about 30 m or the mechanical equipment can be troublesome. Travelling food hoppers and belt egg collection should not be on long runs otherwise mechanical problems occur. Manufacturers tend to be too optimistic about the robustness of their equipment under the extremely exacting conditions of the poultry house. When equipment breaks down it may be extremely difficult to get it repaired, and even then the attention needed to repair the equipment may cause considerable disturbance to the birds and so affect production. In the period between breakdown and repair attention to the birds may also be very difficult.

Adequate passageways between rows of tiered or stacked cages are very important for ease of all procedures. If a unit is a hand-cleaning one, then 1 m is advisable, but if it is not possible 850 mm will suffice. Passageways 600 mm wide are general with systems where there is automatic egg collection. Whilst this is in theory adequate, and in practice sufficient with flat-deck cages, it is unwise to have birds so close if it can be avoided. In any system of cage disposition the passageways serve to some extent as the means of distributing the air to the birds and wider passageways contribute to the maintenance of a uniform, draught-free environment.

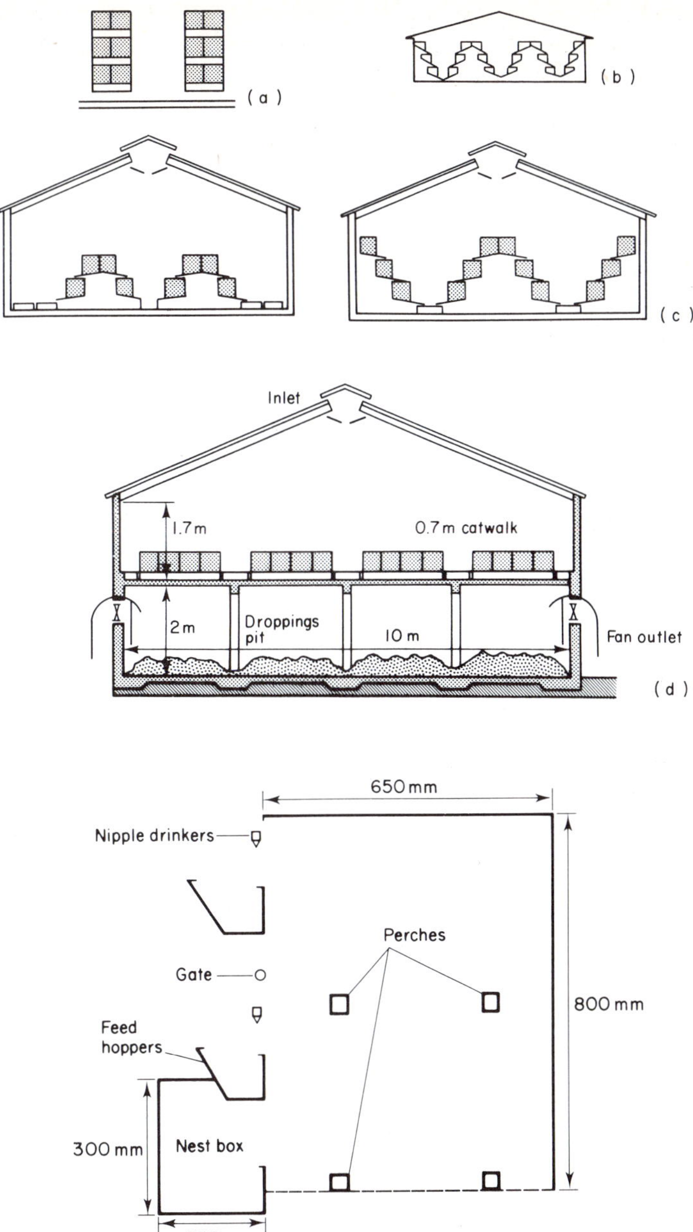

Fig. 15.4 Top: (a) vertical cages; (b) semi-stepped cages; (c) fully stepped cages; (d) flat-deck cages over deep pit for droppings. Bottom: Get-away cage.

'ALTERNATIVE SYSTEMS'

In view of public objections to cage systems for laying birds there has been considerable interest in the adoption of alternative arrangements that give the birds a more natural environment and can still be economic. Several systems have been examined for this purpose. Of the existing systems there are the various deep litter arrangements and the straw yard. In addition there has been the development of the 'aviary' and 'modified free range system'.

Aviary system for layers

An aviary is essentially similar to a conventional deep litter or slatted floor system but has the addition of extra floors of wire or slats (Fig. 15.5). The feeders, drinkers and nest boxes are provided on each of the floors and the various levels are interconnected with ladders which are able to take both the birds and the attendants.

The great advantage of this system is that it allows the stocking density within the house to be much increased above that possible in an ordinary deep litter or slatted floor house. This reduces the capital cost per bird, enables a warmer house temperature to be maintained more akin to that in a cage laying house, and reduces feed consumption. Also, because of this extra warmth, ventilation may be increased, thereby improving the litter conditions and generally eliminating condensation.

Modified free range system

Traditional free range systems allowed birds to roam freely over farm land at concentrations of up to 200 birds to an acre; the night roosting and egg nesting accommodation is simple and usually placed on sleds or wheels for regular

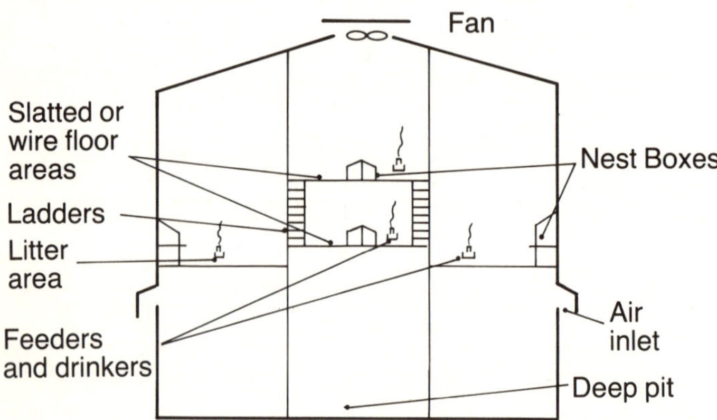

Fig. 15.5 Diagrammatic cross section of Gleadthorpe aviary.

movement. The problems of this system, already touched on earlier, are so considerable leading to such high costs of production that modified systems are now practised in the following way.

The housing is usually fully insulated and is capable of containing the birds entirely during poor weather, for example, deep snow, very hard frosts or in very wet conditions, all of which can be most harmful to the laying chicken (Fig. 15.6). This housing may be permanent on a concrete base, or of a semi-permanent type such as a semi-circular polythene 'poly-pen' which can be moved from time to time. Electricity must be provided to give lighting to keep up winter egg production. Thus this part of the house is essentially a deep litter or covered straw yard.

An essential of the free range is that the birds must be able to go outside at all times during good weather and there should be palatable greenstuff for the birds to eat. Runs must be capable of being used in rotation and should be surrounded by fencing that is predator (fox)-proof. Birds must be shut up at night for safety and also to keep them warm.

It is highly dangerous to allow runs to become fowl-sick and once the pasture has been denuded it should be vacated, ploughed up and re-seeded. If pasture is used carefully for birds, in a rotational programme, there will be several benefits. The good health of the birds will be assisted and the stocking density can be increased far above 200 birds per acre in a particular run at any time; a factor of four times this will be acceptable and also of great benefit to the pasture before it is ploughed up.

It is probable that the use of modified free range systems will have less application in temperate climates than in the warmer parts of the world, though in all areas there appears to be a definite place for it on well-drained and dry

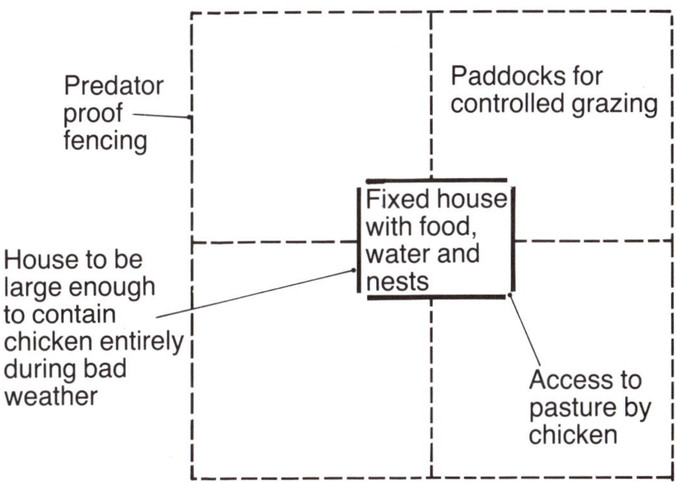

Fig. 15.6 A plan of a modified free range chicken unit.

land such as chalk downs, or sandy soil such as the Brecklands of Norfolk. Great credit is due to the pioneering farmers who are developing this arrangement by ingenious cost saving methods. One farmer has recently built sheds with straw bales using internally an aviary layout of multi-tiers of birds. With care this sort of housing may last as long as ten years with a very low capital input.

CONCLUSIONS

It is not easy to see clearly ahead where the welfare controversy is going to lead. Research and investigation may eventually provide some sort of a scientific answer but in many ways the moral issue has tended to make the running. Our legislators, moved by public demand, may consider the keeping of layers in multi-bird cages is unacceptable, in which case it is good to know that there are a number of alternative arrangements that can be used and which will provide eggs of good quality at very little extra cost than those laid by the battery bird.

Index